AMERICAN
SEXUAL BEHAVIOR

Demographics of Sexual Activity, Fertility, and Childbearing

AMERICAN SEXUAL BEHAVIOR

Demographics of Sexual Activity, Fertility, and Childbearing

BY THE EDITORS OF NEW STRATEGIST PUBLICATIONS

New Strategist Publications, Inc.
Ithaca, New York

New Strategist Publications, Inc.
P.O. Box 242, Ithaca, New York 14851
800/848-0842; 607/273-0913
www.newstrategist.com

ISBN 978-1-933588-09-4

Printed in the United States of America

Table of Contents

Tables

Illustrations

Introduction

Perhaps no issue is more important to a society than the reproductive health of its population. Family formation is central to the wellbeing of individuals. Individual success in coping with sexuality, fertility, marriage, and childbirth determines the quality of life in society as a whole.

To assess the status of Americans' reproductive health, the federal government periodically collects data on the factors affecting the formation, growth, and dissolution of families, including sexual activity, contraception, cohabitation, marriage, divorce, sterilization, infertility, pregnancy outcomes, and births. It does this through the National Survey of Family Growth (NSFG), first fielded in 1973 and conducted periodically since then. In publishing the NSFG data, the National Center for Health Statistics produces a variety of reports focused on particular topics such as teenage sexual activity, women's reproductive health, and men's fertility and fatherhood. *American Sexual Behavior: Demographics of Sexual Activity, Fertility, and Childbearing,* a new addition to New Strategist's demographic reference book offerings, presents in one volume the latest results from this important government effort.

American Sexual Behavior includes more than the NSFG results, allowing researchers easy access to the facts about the sexual activity and reproductive behavior of teenagers, men, and women. In these pages you will find birth data from the National Vital Statistics System, fertility and marital history data from the Census Bureau, the latest estimates from the HIV/AIDS and STD surveillance programs of the Centers for Disease Control and Prevention, and profiles of adopted children from the 2000 Census. *American Sexual Behavior* is a compendium of facts about reproductive health and family formation practices in the United States.

How to use this book

American Sexual Behavior is divided into 11 chapters, each exploring a different facet of reproductive health. The topics are Sexual Initiation, Teenage Sexual Activity, Adult Sexual Activity, Sexual Orientation, AIDS and STDs, Cohabitation and Marriage, Fertility and Infertility, Contraception, Pregnancy, Births, and Caring for Children. Each chapter includes a variety of tables showing the behavior—and the attitudes—of a nationally representative sample of Americans. The book also includes explanatory text and charts revealing the most important trends. Most of the tables in the book show how reproductive and family formation behaviors vary by demographic characteristics such as age, marital status, number of children, race, education, region, metropolitan status, and even religion.

The tables in *American Sexual Behavior* are based on data collected by the federal government, primarily the National Center for Health Statistics. The federal government continues to be the best source of up-to-date, reliable information on the activities and characteristics of Americans. In the area of sexual and reproductive behavior, the federal government is often the only source of reliable information.

While the federal government collected the data appearing in *American Sexual Behavior*, most of the tables published here are not just reprints of the government's tabulations. Instead, New Strategist's editors individually compiled and created the tables to reveal the trends—the story behind the statistics. If you need more information, you can explore the data source cited at the bottom of each table.

American Sexual Behavior includes a list of tables to help you locate the information you need. For a more detailed search, use the index at the back of the book. Also at the back of the book are a bibliography of data sources, more information about the National Survey of Family Growth, and a comprehensive glossary defining the terms used in the tables and text.

American Sexual Behavior is the reference book on the American family. With this book in hand, you will be armed with the facts about some of the most important issues of the day.

Sexual Initiation

■ For most Americans, sexual activity begins during the teenage years. Although many have mixed feelings about their first sexual experience, the majority uses birth control the first time they have sex—condoms being most popular.

■ Most men and women lose their virginity before age 18. Among women aged 15 to 44, average age at first sexual intercourse was 17.3 years. Their male counterparts lost their virginity at 17.0 years on average.

■ Most women lose their virginity to someone with whom they are "going steady." Among women aged 15 to 44 who have ever had sex, 61 percent say they first had sex with a steady boyfriend.

■ Most women had mixed feelings about first sexual intercourse. Only 34 percent "really wanted it to happen at the time." In contrast, 62 percent of men say they really wanted it to happen.

■ Birth control is used by most teens the first time. Seventy-five percent of teen girls and 82 percent of teen boys who have had sex say they used some form of birth control the first time. Most commonly, they report using a condom.

■ Regardless of religious background, few Americans wait for marriage before they have sex. Among men, fundamentalist Protestants are more likely to wait than those from other religious backgrounds, but only 23 percent do.

■ Morals is the number-one reason teens have not yet had sex. Among teenagers aged 15 to 19 who are virgins, a 31 to 38 percent plurality say they have avoided sex for moral or religious reasons.

Seventeen Is the Average Age at First Sexual Intercourse

Average age at sexual initiation is about the same for men and women.

Among women aged 15 to 44, average age at first sexual intercourse was 17.3 years. Their male counterparts lost their virginity at 17.0 years on average. Several demographic characteristics are associated with the loss of virginity at a younger or older age. Black men and women lost their virginity at a younger age than non-Hispanic whites and Hispanics, for example. People who lived with both parents at age 14 waited longer to engage in sex for the first time than did those in other family situations.

For most women, sexual initiation occurs with a slightly older man, while most men first have intercourse with a woman their own age or younger. Among teen girls, the younger the woman at first intercourse, the more likely it was that her partner was considerably older. Eleven percent of girls who were age 15 at first sexual intercourse, and 10 percent of those under age 15, lost their virginity to men who were aged 20 or older.

■ Most men and women have their first sexual experience with someone relatively close in age.

Religion has some impact on the age of sexual initiation

(average age at first sexual intercourse among women aged 15 to 44, by religion raised, 2002)

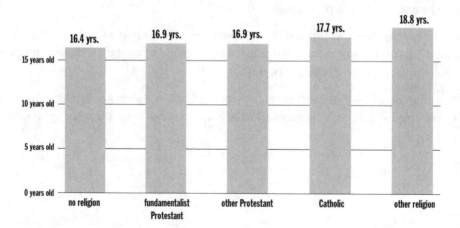

16.4 yrs.	16.9 yrs.	16.9 yrs.	17.7 yrs.	18.8 yrs.
no religion	fundamentalist Protestant	other Protestant	Catholic	other religion

Table 1.1 Average Age at First Sexual Intercourse among Women, 2002

(average age of women aged 15 to 44 at first sexual intercourse, by selected characteristics, 2002)

	average age at first sexual intercourse
Total women aged 15 to 44	**17.3 years**
Race and Hispanic origin	
Black, non-Hispanic	16.3
Hispanic	18.0
White, non-Hispanic	17.2
Family structure at age 14	
Living with both parents	17.8
Other	16.1
Religion raised	
None	16.4
Fundamentalist Protestant	16.9
Other Protestant	16.9
Catholic	17.7
Other religion	18.8

Source: National Center for Health Statistics, Fertility, Family Planning, and Reproductive Health of U.S. Women: Data from the 2002 National Survey of Family Growth, Vital and Health Statistics, Series 23, No. 25, 2005; Internet site http://www.cdc.gov/nchs/nsfg.htm

Table 1.2 Average Age at First Sexual Intercourse among Men, 2002

(average age of men aged 15 to 44 at first sexual intercourse, by selected characteristics, 2002)

	average age at first sexual intercourse
Total men aged 15 to 44	**17.0 years**
Race and Hispanic origin	
Black, non-Hispanic	15.5
Hispanic	16.5
White, non-Hispanic	17.1
Family structure at age 14	
Living with both parents	17.0
Other	15.8
Religion raised	
None	15.8
Fundamentalist Protestant	16.4
Other Protestant	16.3
Catholic	16.8
Other religion	18.1

Source: National Center for Health Statistics, Fertility, Contraception, and Fatherhood: Data on Men and Women from Cycle 6 of the 2002 National Survey of Family Growth, Vital and Health Statistics, Series 23, No. 26, 2006; Internet site http://www.cdc.gov/nchs/nsfg.htm

Table 1.3 Age Difference between First Male Sexual Partner and Women Aged 15 to 19 at First Sexual Intercourse, 2002

(number of women aged 15 to 19 who have ever had sexual intercourse and percent distribution by age difference between female and first male sexual intercourse partner, by selected characteristics, 2002; numbers in thousands)

| | total | | | | first male partner's age | | |
	number	percent	younger	same age	one to three years older	four to five years older	six or more years older
Women aged 15 to 19 who have ever had sexual intercourse	**4,598**	**100.0%**	**4.1%**	**14.9%**	**58.7%**	**14.7%**	**7.7%**
Age at first sexual intercourse							
Aged 14 or younger	1,289	100.0	–	4.2	58.3	26.7	9.8
Aged 15	1,200	100.0	–	9.8	65.6	12.8	10.8
Aged 16	1,035	100.0	6.5	23.5	59.6	5.8	4.6
Aged 17 to 19	1,074	100.0	8.8	25.0	50.6	10.8	4.9
Race and Hispanic origin							
Black, non-Hispanic	854	100.0	2.9	18.3	59.8	11.9	7.1
Hispanic	615	100.0	4.1	22.1	38.6	24.3	11.0
White, non-Hispanic	2,905	100.0	4.7	13.4	62.4	13.6	6.0
Family structure at age 14							
Living with both parents	2,507	100.0	5.1	16.4	58.1	14.5	5.9
Other	2,092	100.0	2.8	13.1	59.4	14.8	9.9

Note: "–" means sample is too small to make a reliable estimate.
Source: National Center for Health Statistics, Teenagers in the United States: Sexual Activity, Contraceptive Use, and Childbearing, 2002, Vital and Health Statistics, Series 23, No. 24, 2004; Internet site http://www.cdc.gov/nchs/nsfg.htm

Table 1.4 Age Difference between First Male Sexual Partner and Women Aged 15 to 44 at First Sexual Intercourse, 2002

(number of women aged 15 to 44 who have ever had sexual intercourse and percent distribution by age difference between female and first male sexual intercourse partner, by selected characteristics, 2002; numbers in thousands)

| | total | | first male partner's age | | | | |
	number	percent	younger	same age	one to three years older	four to five years older	six or more years older
Women aged 15 to 44 who have ever had sexual intercourse	**54,190**	**100.0%**	**7.2%**	**17.8%**	**49.1%**	**15.5%**	**10.5%**
Age at first sexual intercourse							
Under age 16	15,549	100.0	1.2	10.1	54.2	21.6	12.8
Aged 16	9,348	100.0	4.6	18.6	57.9	11.4	7.4
Aged 17	8,210	100.0	6.7	24.0	50.4	12.3	6.6
Aged 18	7,025	100.0	7.0	23.5	46.7	11.5	11.4
Aged 19	4,111	100.0	10.8	21.4	41.1	17.2	9.6
Aged 20	2,477	100.0	8.3	18.7	49.3	15.1	8.5
Aged 21 to 22	3,692	100.0	12.5	22.8	38.0	12.8	13.9
Aged 23 or older	3,777	100.0	29.5	13.4	27.0	15.3	14.9
Race and Hispanic origin							
Black, non-Hispanic	7,403	100.0	6.3	16.0	50.9	18.0	8.9
Hispanic	7,887	100.0	9.6	14.9	39.9	19.9	15.7
White, non-Hispanic	34,999	100.0	6.9	19.1	50.9	14.0	9.1

Source: National Center for Health Statistics, Fertility, Family Planning, and Reproductive Health of U.S. Women: Data from the 2002 National Survey of Family Growth, Vital and Health Statistics, Series 23, No. 25, 2005; Internet site http://www.cdc.gov/nchs/nsfg.htm

Table 1.5 Age Difference between First Female Sexual Partner and Men Aged 15 to 44 at First Sexual Intercourse, 2002

(number of men aged 15 to 44 who have ever had sexual intercourse and percent distribution by age difference between male and first female sexual intercourse partner, by selected characteristics, 2002; numbers in thousands)

| | total | | first female partner's age | | | | |
	number	percent	more than one year younger	one year younger	same age	one to two years older	more than two years older
Men aged 15 to 44 who have ever had sexual intercourse	**53,257**	**100.0%**	**11.9%**	**16.0%**	**36.1%**	**22.2%**	**14.0%**
Age							
Aged 15 to 24	13,332	100.0	8.7	13.2	36.4	29.9	11.8
Aged 25 to 29	8,836	100.0	11.2	19.2	28.5	25.4	15.8
Aged 30 to 34	9,823	100.0	15.1	11.8	37.4	20.6	15.1
Aged 35 to 39	10,328	100.0	13.3	14.3	36.9	18.6	16.9
Aged 40 to 44	10,938	100.0	11.9	22.1	39.8	14.9	11.3
Age at first sexual intercourse							
Under age 16	17,600	100.0	1.8	6.8	39.8	30.7	20.9
Aged 16	9,359	100.0	5.0	18.0	43.0	24.7	9.3
Aged 17	8,348	100.0	7.2	25.2	38.9	20.2	8.6
Aged 18	5,890	100.0	12.7	23.3	43.1	13.3	7.6
Aged 19	2,938	100.0	19.4	32.8	20.3	15.0	12.6
Aged 20 or older	9,121	100.0	39.7	13.1	19.7	12.9	14.6
Race and Hispanic origin							
Black, non-Hispanic	6,258	100.0	6.9	11.3	39.3	22.8	19.7
Hispanic	9,173	100.0	14.0	13.7	26.8	21.1	24.4
White, non-Hispanic	33,362	100.0	11.5	18.3	38.2	21.6	10.4

Source: National Center for Health Statistics, Fertility, Contraception, and Fatherhood: Data on Men and Women from Cycle 6 of the 2002 National Survey of Family Growth, Vital and Health Statistics, Series 23, No. 26, 2006; Internet site http://www.cdc .gov/nchs/nsfg.htm

Most Are "Going Steady" with First Sexual Partner

The younger the age at first sexual intercourse, the less serious the relationship.

Few men and women wait for marriage before they have sex. The husband was the first sexual partner for only 10 percent of women aged 15 to 44 who have ever had sex. A much large 61 percent lost their virginity to men with whom they were "going steady." The younger the woman at first intercourse, the more likely the relationship with her partner was not serious. Fourteen percent of women who were under age 16 at first intercourse had a partner who was "just a friend," but the share was only 5 percent among women who waited until they were at least 20 to have sex for the first time.

Hispanic women are most likely to wait for marriage. Eighteen percent of Hispanic women aged 15 to 44 had their first sexual experience with their husband. This compares with only 2 percent of black women and 8 percent of non-Hispanic white women. Non-Hispanic black women were most likely to first have sex with a man who was just a friend. Women who were living with both parents at age 14 are more likely to wait until marriage to have sex for the first time, although the share is still a low 12 percent.

■ Efforts to convince young people to remain abstinent until marriage face a steep uphill battle, especially as the age of marriage rises.

Three out of four teenage girls were "going steady" with their first sexual partner

(percent distribution of women aged 15 to 19 who have ever had sexual intercourse, by relationship with first sexual partner, 2002)

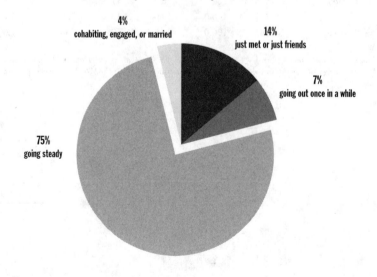

4%
cohabiting, engaged, or married

14%
just met or just friends

7%
going out once in a while

75%
going steady

Table 1.6 Relationship with First Male Sexual Partner among Women Aged 15 to 19, 2002

(number of women aged 15 to 19 who have ever had sexual intercourse and percent distribution by type of relationship with first male sexual intercourse partner, by selected characteristics, 2002; numbers in thousands)

	total		just met or just friends	going out once in a while	going steady	cohabiting, engaged, or married
	number	percent				
Women aged 15 to 19 who have ever had sexual intercourse	**4,598**	**100.0%**	**14.0%**	**6.6%**	**74.6%**	**3.7%**
Age at first sexual intercourse						
Aged 14 or younger	1,289	100.0	24.0	9.0	63.5	–
Aged 15 to 16	2,235	100.0	11.5	6.7	78.9	2.0
Aged 17 to 19	1,074	100.0	7.1	–	78.8	10.1
Race and Hispanic origin						
Black, non-Hispanic	854	100.0	18.6	6.6	74.4	–
Hispanic	615	100.0	12.4	–	69.3	13.0
White, non-Hispanic	2,905	100.0	13.2	6.7	75.9	2.9
Family structure at age 14						
Living with both parents	2,507	100.0	13.5	5.0	76.7	3.6
Other	2,092	100.0	14.5	8.5	72.0	3.8
Importance of religion						
Very important	1,551	100.0	10.2	5.4	77.2	5.3
Somewhat important	1,882	100.0	10.8	8.6	77.0	3.0
Not important	1,152	100.0	24.4	5.0	66.8	–

Note: Numbers may not sum to 100 because "other" types of relationships are not shown. "–" means sample is too small to make a reliable estimate.
Source: National Center for Health Statistics, Teenagers in the United States: Sexual Activity, Contraceptive Use, and Childbearing, 2002, Vital and Health Statistics, Series 23, No. 24, 2004; Internet site http://www.cdc.gov/nchs/nsfg.htm

Table 1.7 Relationship with First Male Sexual Partner among Women Aged 15 to 44, 2002

(number of women aged 15 to 44 who have ever had sexual intercourse and percent distribution by relationship with first male sexual intercourse partner, by selected characteristics, 2002; numbers in thousands)

	total number	total percent	just met	just friends	going out once in a while	going steady	cohabiting	engaged	married	other
Women aged 15 to 44 who have ever had sexual intercourse	54,190	100.0%	2.2%	8.9%	7.2%	61.2%	2.2%	4.5%	9.6%	3.8%
Age										
Aged 15 to 19	4,598	100.0	3.3	10.6	6.6	74.3	1.4	1.2	1.1	1.2
Aged 20 to 24	8,530	100.0	2.3	8.8	8.4	64.5	2.5	3.3	6.8	3.5
Aged 25 to 29	8,939	100.0	1.3	8.6	5.5	63.7	2.6	4.0	9.8	4.5
Aged 30 to 34	10,077	100.0	1.8	9.2	7.1	61.6	1.7	4.8	9.1	4.2
Aged 35 to 39	10,686	100.0	3.2	10.0	7.0	56.5	2.9	5.1	11.6	3.4
Aged 40 to 44	11,360	100.0	1.8	7.5	8.0	55.8	1.8	6.2	13.7	4.4
Age at first sexual intercourse										
Under age 16	15,549	100.0	4.0	14.1	8.2	59.6	1.8	1.7	1.2	8.7
Aged 16	9,348	100.0	1.5	7.9	7.6	75.9	1.4	1.9	1.5	2.1
Aged 17	8,210	100.0	1.1	8.5	6.4	71.8	1.5	6.1	2.9	1.6
Aged 18	7,025	100.0	2.1	5.3	9.1	65.9	2.5	5.8	6.7	2.6
Aged 19	4,111	100.0	2.1	7.9	7.4	56.7	3.9	7.4	13.1	1.3
Aged 20 or older	9,646	100.0	1.2	5.2	4.4	39.9	3.3	7.8	36.6	1.3
Race and Hispanic origin										
Black, non-Hispanic	7,403	100.0	1.6	14.1	7.3	68.5	1.7	1.3	1.9	3.2
Hispanic	7,887	100.0	1.7	6.8	5.9	47.6	7.2	9.5	18.4	2.8
White, non-Hispanic	34,999	100.0	2.5	8.3	7.4	64.2	1.2	4.2	8.1	4.0
Family structure at age 14										
Living with both parents	38,480	100.0	2.0	8.1	7.4	60.1	1.9	5.2	11.8	3.2
Other	15,710	100.0	2.8	10.9	6.6	64.1	2.9	2.8	4.3	5.3
Religion raised										
None	4,255	100.0	6.2	12.0	8.6	56.9	2.7	3.0	5.8	4.7
Fundamentalist Protestant	3,062	100.0	0.8	11.9	4.7	56.9	3.4	5.0	11.9	5.4
Other Protestant	24,898	100.0	1.9	10.1	7.2	63.6	1.0	4.0	7.9	4.1
Catholic	19,119	100.0	1.8	6.1	7.4	62.4	3.5	5.6	9.9	2.8
Other religion	2,664	100.0	2.8	10.1	6.6	44.7	1.5	3.5	26.6	4.3

Source: National Center for Health Statistics, Fertility, Family Planning, and Reproductive Health of U.S. Women: Data from the 2002 National Survey of Family Growth, Vital and Health Statistics, Series 23, No. 25, 2005; Internet site Internet site http://www .cdc.gov/nchs/nsfg.htm

Most Women Had Mixed Feelings about First Sexual Intercourse

Most men really wanted it to happen.

More than half (53 percent) of women aged 18 to 24 who have ever had intercourse say they had mixed feelings about the first time: "Part of me wanted it to happen at the time and part of me didn't." Thirty-four percent "really wanted it to happen at the time." In contrast, only one-third of men were conflicted about having sex the first time, while 62 percent say they really wanted it to happen.

One out of ten women aged 18 to 24 who first had intercourse before age 20 say the encounter was involuntary. The younger the women at sexual initiation, the more likely first intercourse was coerced. Eighteen percent of women aged 14 or younger at first intercourse say it was involuntary compared with 5 percent of those aged 18 to 19 the first time. The older the male partner, the more likely the sex was involuntary on the part of the female.

Among all women aged 18 to 44 who have ever had sex, 20 percent of those who had sex before age 15 say their first intercourse was coerced. Nineteen percent of women say they were pressured into having sex the first time, while 9 percent say they were given alcohol or drugs.

■ Among men aged 18 to 24 who had sex before age 20, the older they were at first intercourse, the more likely they felt conflicted about it. This suggests that at least some men who wait until they are older may end up losing their virginity for reasons such as peer pressure rather than a genuine desire to have sex.

Women become less conflicted, men more when they wait to have sex

(percent of men and women aged 18 to 24 who had mixed feelings about their first sexual intercourse, by age at first sexual intercourse, 2002)

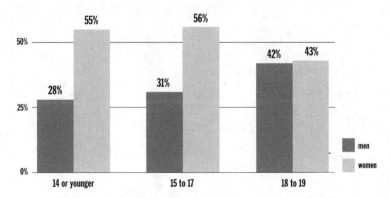

Table 1.8 How Much First Sexual Intercourse Was Wanted among Women Aged 18 to 24, 2002

(number of women aged 18 to 24 who had sex before age 20 and percent distribution by how much first sexual intercourse was wanted, by selected characteristics, 2002; numbers in thousands)

	total number	total percent	I didn't really want it to happen at the time	I had mixed feelings; part of me wanted it to happen at the time and part of me didn't	I really wanted it to happen at the time
Women aged 18 to 24 who had sexual intercourse before age 20	**10,234**	**100.0%**	**13.4%**	**52.7%**	**33.9%**
Age at first sexual intercourse					
Aged 14 or younger	1,980	100.0	26.8	55.0	18.2
Aged 15 to 17	5,948	100.0	12.0	55.7	32.3
Aged 18 to 19	2,306	100.0	5.2	42.9	51.9
Age of male partner					
Younger	506	100.0	1.8	62.2	36.1
Same age or one year older	1,857	100.0	12.8	44.9	42.4
One to two years older	4,075	100.0	10.3	55.4	34.4
Three or more years older	3,796	100.0	18.6	52.4	29.0
Race and Hispanic origin					
Black, non-Hispanic	1,666	100.0	10.2	63.0	26.8
Hispanic	1,681	100.0	13.5	60.0	26.4
White, non-Hispanic	6,332	100.0	13.8	47.9	38.3

Source: National Center for Health Statistics, Teenagers in the United States: Sexual Activity, Contraceptive Use, and Childbearing, 2002, Vital and Health Statistics, Series 23, No. 24, 2004; Internet site http://www.cdc.gov/nchs/nsfg.htm

Table 1.9 How Much First Sexual Intercourse Was Wanted among Men Aged 18 to 24, 2002

(number of men aged 18 to 24 who had sex before age 20 and percent distribution by how much first sexual inter-course was wanted, by selected characteristics, 2002; numbers in thousands)

	total		I didn't really want it to happen at the time	I had mixed feelings; part of me wanted it to happen at the time and part of me didn't	I really wanted it to happen at the time
	number	percent			
Men aged 18 to 24 who had sexual intercourse before age 20	**10,389**	**100.0%**	**5.8%**	**32.7%**	**61.6%**
Age at first sexual intercourse					
Aged 14 or younger	2,171	100.0	4.7	28.1	67.2
Aged 15 to 17	6,175	100.0	6.6	31.2	62.3
Aged 18 to 19	2,044	100.0	4.6	41.7	53.7
Age of female partner					
Three or more years younger	1,358	100.0	5.4	33.4	61.2
One to two years younger	3,027	100.0	4.7	32.8	62.5
Same age	3,858	100.0	7.3	32.6	60.0
Older	2,146	100.0	4.6	32.1	63.3
Race and Hispanic origin					
Black, non-Hispanic	1,502	100.0	9.4	34.9	55.7
Hispanic	2,282	100.0	3.7	33.3	63.0
White, non-Hispanic	6,145	100.0	5.0	31.0	64.0

Source: National Center for Health Statistics, Teenagers in the United States: Sexual Activity, Contraceptive Use, and Childbearing, 2002, Vital and Health Statistics, Series 23, No. 24, 2004; Internet site http://www.cdc.gov/nchs/nsfg.htm

Table 1.10 How Much First Sexual Intercourse Was Wanted among Men Aged 18 to 44, 2002

(number of men aged 18 to 44 who have ever had sexual intercourse and percent distribution by how much first sexual intercourse was wanted, by selected characteristics, 2002; numbers in thousands)

	total		I didn't really want it to happen at the time	I had mixed feelings; part of me wanted it to happen at the time and part of me didn't	I really wanted it to happen at the time
	number	percent			
Men aged 18 to 44 who have ever had sexual intercourse	**51,442**	**100.0%**	**4.7%**	**27.3%**	**68.1%**
Age at first sexual intercourse					
Under age 15	9,378	100.0	6.8	30.1	63.1
Aged 15	6,952	100.0	4.7	25.6	69.7
Aged 16	9,002	100.0	4.3	23.0	72.7
Aged 17	8,161	100.0	2.7	25.6	71.8
Aged 18	5,890	100.0	4.8	25.7	69.5
Aged 19	2,938	100.0	1.9	36.9	61.2
Aged 20 or older	9,121	100.0	5.3	29.5	65.2
Race and Hispanic origin					
Black, non-Hispanic	5,839	100.0	8.7	31.9	59.4
Hispanic	8,811	100.0	6.3	28.4	65.3
White, non-Hispanic	32,465	100.0	3.3	25.0	71.7
Family structure at age 14					
Living with both parents	37,990	100.0	4.9	25.9	69.2
Other	13,452	100.0	4.0	31.0	65.0

Source: National Center for Health Statistics, Fertility, Contraception, and Fatherhood: Data on Men and Women from Cycle 6 of the 2002 National Survey of Family Growth, Vital and Health Statistics, Series 23, No. 26, 2006; Internet site http://www.cdc.gov/nchs/nsfg.htm

Table 1.11 Women Aged 18 to 24 Whose First Sexual Intercourse Was Involuntary, 2002

(number of women aged 18 to 24 who had sex before age 20 and percent whose first intercourse was involuntary, by selected characteristics, 2002; numbers in thousands)

	total	percent whose first intercourse was involuntary
Women aged 18 to 24 who had sexual intercourse before age 20	**10,234**	**9.6%**
Age at first sexual intercourse		
Aged 14 or younger	1,980	18.1
Aged 15 to 17	5,948	10.3
Aged 18 to 19	2,306	4.7
Age of male partner		
Younger	506	–
Same age or one year older	1,857	8.1
One to two years older	4,075	7.9
Three or more years older	3,796	13.4
Race and Hispanic origin		
Black, non-Hispanic	1,666	10.3
Hispanic	1,681	10.5
White, non-Hispanic	6,332	8.8
Family structure at age 14		
Living with both parents	6,595	8.2
Other	3,639	12.2

Note: "–" means sample is too small to make a reliable estimate.
Source: National Center for Health Statistics, Teenagers in the United States: Sexual Activity, Contraceptive Use, and Childbearing, 2002, Vital and Health Statistics, Series 23, No. 24, 2004; Internet site http://www.cdc.gov/nchs/nsfg.htm

Table 1.12 Women Aged 18 to 44 Whose First Sexual Intercourse Was Involuntary, 2002

(number of women aged 18 to 44 who have ever had sexual intercourse and percent whose first intercourse was involuntary, by selected characteristics, 2002; numbers in thousands)

	total	percent whose first intercourse was involuntary
Women aged 18 to 44 who have ever had sexual intercourse	**52,425**	**8.3%**
Age at first sexual intercourse		
Under age 15	7,404	20.0
Aged 15	6,823	10.2
Aged 16	9,002	8.5
Aged 17	8,113	5.3
Aged 18	7,025	6.1
Aged 19	4,111	3.1
Aged 20 or older	9,946	4.3
Year of first sexual intercourse		
1995 or later	12,311	7.1
1990 to 1994	9,391	6.7
1980 to 1989	20,675	7.9
Before 1980	10,048	12.3
Race and Hispanic origin		
Black, non-Hispanic	7,048	7.0
Hispanic	7,658	8.8
White, non-Hispanic	33,915	8.2
Family structure at age 14		
Living with both parents	37,666	7.3
Other	14,759	11.0

Source: National Center for Health Statistics, Fertility, Family Planning, and Reproductive Health of U.S. Women: Data from the 2002 National Survey of Family Growth, Vital and Health Statistics, Series 23, No. 25, 2005; Internet site http://www.cdc.gov/nchs/nsfg.htm

Table 1.13   Women Forced to Have First Sexual Intercourse, 2002

(number of women aged 18 to 44 who have ever had sexual intercourse and percent distribution by whether force was used at first intercourse, by type of force, 2002; numbers in thousands)

Women aged 18 to 44 who have ever had sexual intercourse, number	**52,425**
Women aged 18 to 44 who have ever had sexual intercourse, percent	**100.0%**
No type of force reported	74.0
One or more types of force reported	26.0
Pressured into it by his words or actions, but without threats of harm	18.6
Given alcohol or drugs	8.7
Did what he said because he was bigger or grown-up, and you were young	7.8
Physically held down	5.2
Told that the relationship would end if you didn't have sex	3.9
Physically hurt or injured	3.0
Threatened with physical harm or injury	2.9

Note: Numbers will not sum to 100 because more than one type of force may have been used.
Source: National Center for Health Statistics, Fertility, Family Planning, and Reproductive Health of U.S. Women: Data from the 2002 National Survey of Family Growth, Vital and Health Statistics, Series 23, No. 25, 2005; Internet site http://www.cdc .gov/nchs/nsfg.htm

Most Use Birth Control during First Sexual Intercourse

Fundamentalist Protestants are among those least likely to use birth control the first time they have sex.

Among teenagers aged 15 to 19 who have ever had sex, the great majority (75 to 82 percent) say they used some form of birth control the first time. Most commonly, they report having used a condom. Younger teens are less likely than older teens to use some type of birth control. Teen boys and girls who first have sex with a significantly older (four or more years) partner are less likely to use protection than those with partners closer to their own age.

The advent of HIV infection and AIDS has clearly had an impact on the use of some type of protection, particularly condoms, during first intercourse. Men and women aged 15 to 44 who had sex the first time prior to 1980 were unlikely to have used any form of birth control, and only about one in five said they used a condom. By the early 1990s, most were using condoms. Those least likely to have used a condom at first sexual intercourse were Hispanics, fundamentalist Protestants, and Catholics.

■ In recent years, more than 60 percent of men and women aged 15 to 44 report having used a condom at first sexual intercourse.

Most Hispanics do not use birth control at first sexual intercourse

(percentage of women aged 15 to 44 who have ever had sexual intercourse who used birth control at first sexual intercourse, by race and Hispanic origin, 2002)

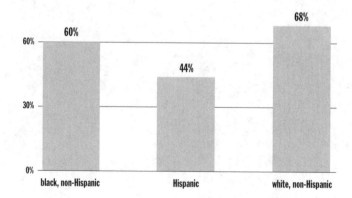

Table 1.14 Teenage Girls Who Report Birth Control Use at First Sexual Intercourse, 2002

(number of women aged 15 to 19 who have ever had sexual intercourse and percent having used birth control at first sexual intercourse, by selected characteristics, 2002; numbers in thousands)

		percent having used birth control at first sexual intercourse	
	number	any method	condom
Total women aged 15 to 19 ever having had sexual intercourse	**4,598**	**74.5%**	**66.4%**
Age			
Age 14 or younger	1,290	65.2	58.5
Age 15 to 16	2,235	75.9	68.6
Age 17 to 18	1,074	82.6	71.3
Race and Hispanic origin			
Black, non-Hispanic	854	71.2	61.2
Hispanic	615	71.4	55.5
White, non-Hispanic	2,905	78.0	71.8
Age difference between female and first male partner			
Male partner same age or younger	871	79.8	71.6
Male partner one year older	1,107	77.1	67.9
Male partner two to three years older	1,590	77.8	69.5
Male partner four or more years older	1,030	62.0	55.6

Source: National Center for Health Statistics, Teenagers in the United States: Sexual Activity, Contraceptive Use, and Childbearing, 2002, Vital and Health Statistics, Series 23, No. 24, 2004; Internet site http://www.cdc.gov/nchs/nsfg.htm

Table 1.15 Teenage Boys Who Report Birth Control Use at First Sexual Intercourse, 2002

(number of men aged 15 to 19 who have ever had sexual intercourse and percent having used birth control at first sexual intercourse, by selected characteristics, 2002; numbers in thousands)

	number	percent having used birth control at first sexual intercourse	
		any method	condom
Total men aged 15 to 19 ever having had sexual intercourse	**4,697**	**82.0%**	**70.9%**
Age			
Age 14 or younger	1,513	75.9	72
Age 15 to 16	1,977	88.1	77.3
Age 17 to 18	1,207	79.6	59.1
Race and Hispanic origin			
Black, non-Hispanic	934	85.6	84.9
Hispanic	903	73.4	67.4
White, non-Hispanic	2,672	84.8	68.2
Age difference between male and first female partner			
Female partner younger	773	84.1	71.5
Female partner same age	1,727	82.8	72.3
Female partner one year older	1,101	82.8	75.1
Female partner two or more years older	1,096	78.3	64.2

Source: National Center for Health Statistics, Teenagers in the United States: Sexual Activity, Contraceptive Use, and Childbearing, 2002, Vital and Health Statistics, Series 23, No. 24, 2004; Internet site http://www.cdc.gov/nchs/nsfg.htm

Table 1.16   Women Who Report Birth Control Use at First Sexual Intercourse, 2002

(number of women aged 15 to 44 who have ever had sexual intercourse and percent having used birth control at first sexual intercourse, by selected characteristics, 2002; numbers in thousands)

	number	percent having used birth control at first sexual intercourse		
		any method	condom	pill
Total women aged 15 to 44 ever having had sexual intercourse	**54,190**	**62.9%**	**42.2%**	**20.2%**
Year of first sexual intercourse				
1999–2002	6,953	78.1	60.3	24.7
1995–1998	7,254	71.7	57.1	21.3
1990–1994	9,363	68.6	53.3	18.0
1980–1989	20,683	61.7	36.0	22.4
Before 1980	9,882	43.1	21.1	13.5
Race and Hispanic origin				
Black, non-Hispanic	7,403	60.2	43.6	22.9
Hispanic	7,887	44.1	28.7	11.0
White, non-Hispanic	34,999	68.3	45.3	21.9
Religion raised				
None	4,255	64.7	49.9	17.7
Fundamentalist Protestant	3,062	53.2	35.5	16.5
Other Protestant	24,898	67.0	43.7	24.9
Catholic	19,119	58.7	38.9	15.7
Other religion	2,664	65.9	50.0	17.7

Source: National Center for Health Statistics, Fertility, Family Planning, and Reproductive Health of U.S. Women: Data from the 2002 National Survey of Family Growth, Vital and Health Statistics, Series 23, No. 25, 2005; Internet site http://www.cdc .gov/nchs/nsfg.htm

Table 1.17 Men Who Report Birth Control Use at First Sexual Intercourse, 2002

(number of men aged 15 to 44 who have ever had sexual intercourse and percent having used birth control at first sexual intercourse, by selected characteristics, 2002; numbers in thousands)

| | number | percent having used birth control at first sexual intercourse | | |
		any method	condom	pill
Total men aged 15 to 44 ever having had sexual intercourse	**53,257**	**63.1%**	**47.7%**	**13.6%**
Age at first sexual intercourse				
Under age 16	17,600	52.9	43.3	6.6
Age 16	9,359	65.9	52.9	9.7
Age 17	8,348	69.8	51.3	14.9
Age 18	5,890	63.6	52.6	16.3
Age 19	2,938	72.6	51.4	16.7
Age 20 or older	9,121	70.3	42.8	27.0
Year of first sexual intercourse				
1995–2002	14,469	81.8	67.8	17.2
1990–1994	8,203	68.8	55.5	13.7
1980–1989	19,705	60.5	43.9	13.3
Before 1980	10,880	38.5	21.8	9.1
Race and Hispanic origin				
Black, non-Hispanic	6,258	56.6	51.8	8.0
Hispanic	9,173	48.8	40.2	7.2
White, non-Hispanic	33,362	68.7	48.9	17.1
Religion raised				
None	4,303	70.4	59.2	12.9
Fundamentalist Protestant	2,413	58.6	45.0	13.1
Other Protestant	23,556	65.7	48.4	16.5
Catholic	19,206	58.6	43.9	10.8
Other religion	3,626	65.4	51.5	10.5

Source: National Center for Health Statistics, Fertility, Contraception, and Fatherhood: Data on Men and Women from Cycle 6 of the 2002 National Survey of Family Growth, Vital and Health Statistics, Series 23, No. 26, 2006; Internet site http://www.cdc .gov/nchs/nsfg.htm

Few Wait until Marriage before Having Sex

Only 15 percent of ever-married women waited until marriage.

American men and women have been waiting longer to marry—the median age at first marriage was 27.1 years for men and 25.8 years for women in 2005. This may be one reason why so few remain virgins until they marry. Only 9 percent of ever-married men aged 20 to 44 and 15 percent of their female counterparts aged 15 to 44 had sex for the first time either within a month of their wedding or after the nuptials. The largest share of men (65 percent) had intercourse for the first time five or more years before they married. Among women, 46 percent had sex for the first time at least five years before marriage.

Some demographic segments are more likely to wait for marriage than others. Hispanics are more likely than blacks or non-Hispanic whites to wait, as are people who were living with both parents at age 14. Among men, fundamentalist Protestants are more likely to wait than those from other religious backgrounds, but among women those with a religion other than Protestant or Catholic are most likely to wait.

■ Regardless of religious background, most men and women do not wait for marriage before having sex.

Women are more likely than men to wait for marriage

(percent of ever-married men aged 20 to 44 and ever-married women aged 15 to 44 who first had sexual intercourse in the same month of or after marriage, 2002)

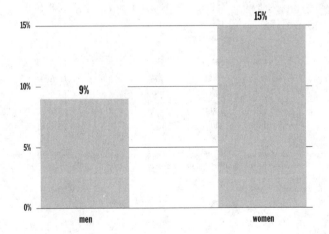

Table 1.18 Time between First Sexual Intercourse and Marriage among Women, 2002

(number of ever-married women aged 15 to 44 and percent distribution by timing of first sexual intercourse in relation to first marriage, by selected characteristics, 2002; numbers in thousands)

| | total | | time from first sexual intercourse to marriage | | | | |
	number	percent	same month or after	less than 12 months	one to three years	three to five years	five years or more
Ever-married women aged 15 to 44	**35,849**	**100.0%**	**15.1%**	**7.1%**	**16.4%**	**15.9%**	**45.6%**
Age							
Aged 15 to 24	2,926	100.0	19.6	9.1	23.8	23.1	24.4
Aged 25 to 29	5,566	100.0	15.9	6.4	14.2	14.6	48.9
Aged 30 to 34	7,971	100.0	12.2	6.1	12.3	13.8	55.7
Aged 35 to 39	9,041	100.0	13.4	6.9	16.8	15.8	47.1
Aged 40 to 44	10,345	100.0	17.2	7.9	18.1	16.2	40.6
Year of first marriage							
1995–2002	12,453	100.0	13.3	3.7	9.9	12.1	61.0
1990–1994	7,507	100.0	12.2	4.8	12.1	13.1	57.7
1980–1989	13,065	100.0	17.3	9.1	21.1	20.3	32.1
Before 1980	2,823	100.0	20.4	19.6	33.8	18.9	7.3
Race and Hispanic origin							
Black, non-Hispanic	3,242	100.0	4.1	3.5	12.9	16.1	63.5
Hispanic	5,269	100.0	28.5	12.1	15.9	13.3	30.2
White, non-Hispanic	24,817	100.0	12.0	6.5	17.2	17.2	47.1
Family structure at age 14							
Living with both parents	26,839	100.0	17.2	7.7	16.8	15.5	42.9
Other	9,009	100.0	8.8	5.6	15.1	16.9	53.6
Religion raised							
None	2,196	100.0	11.8	4.3	17.5	13.9	52.5
Fundamentalist Protestant	2,169	100.0	17.2	13.6	18.6	21.3	29.3
Other Protestant	16,290	100.0	12.9	6.6	14.9	17.4	48.1
Catholic	13,113	100.0	14.6	8.0	18.1	14.3	45.0
Other religion	1,933	100.0	38.1	2.1	12.4	9.1	38.3

Source: National Center for Health Statistics, Fertility, Family Planning, and Reproductive Health of U.S. Women: Data from the 2002 National Survey of Family Growth, Vital and Health Statistics, Series 23, No. 25, 2005; Internet site http://www.cdc.gov/nchs/nsfg.htm

Table 1.19 Time between First Sexual Intercourse and Marriage among Men, 2002

(number of ever-married men aged 20 to 44 and percent distribution by timing of first sexual intercourse in relation to first marriage, by selected characteristics, 2002; numbers in thousands)

	total		time from first sexual intercourse to marriage				
	number	percent	same month or after	less than 12 months	one to three years	three to five years	five years or more
Ever-married men aged 20 to 44	**30,903**	**100.0%**	**8.7%**	**3.9%**	**10.4%**	**12.2%**	**64.9%**
Age							
Aged 20 to 24	1,658	100.0	28.8	4.0	12.2	20.8	34.2
Aged 25 to 29	4,590	100.0	9.9	2.8	12.5	11.3	63.5
Aged 30 to 34	7,105	100.0	7.1	5.3	7.2	13.1	67.4
Aged 35 to 39	8,260	100.0	8.7	2.6	6.0	11.3	71.5
Aged 40 to 44	9,290	100.0	5.6	4.5	15.5	11.2	63.2
Year of first marriage							
1995–2002	12,750	100.0	10.3	3.0	6.1	6.9	73.7
1990–1994	6,559	100.0	5.8	2.8	6.3	14.4	70.8
1980–1989	10,003	100.0	8.2	3.7	13.0	17.1	57.9
Before 1980	1,592	100.0	9.7	16.6	45.2	15.3	13.2
Race and Hispanic origin							
Black, non-Hispanic	2,889	100.0	2.6	1.9	3.4	10.5	81.7
Hispanic	5,039	100.0	12.1	5.1	10.3	10.1	62.3
White, non-Hispanic	20,572	100.0	8.2	3.4	11.4	11.8	65.2
Family structure at age 14							
Living with both parents	23,227	100.0	9.4	3.5	9.6	12.9	64.6
Other	7,676	100.0	6.4	5.0	12.9	10.0	65.8
Religion raised							
None	1,986	100.0	1.9	0.5	11.3	9.2	77.2
Fundamentalist Protestant	1,401	100.0	23.0	1.6	4.1	19.1	52.2
Other Protestant	14,657	100.0	8.1	4.5	12.5	15.2	59.7
Catholic	10,758	100.0	7.1	4.1	8.0	8.8	72.1
Other religion	2,047	100.0	18.3	3.7	12.1	6.6	59.4

Source: National Center for Health Statistics, Fertility, Contraception, and Fatherhood: Data on Men and Women from Cycle 6 of the 2002 National Survey of Family Growth, Vital and Health Statistics, Series 23, No. 26, 2006; Internet site http://www.cdc .gov/nchs/nsfg.htm

Among Teens Who Have Not Had Sex, Morals Is the Number-One Reason

Fear of pregnancy is reason number two.

Most teens have had some form of sexual education at school. More than 80 percent say they received instruction on how to say no to sex; two-thirds were taught birth control methods. Relatively few teens aged 15 to 19 say they have taken a pledge to remain a virgin until marriage—13 percent of girls and 11 percent of boys.

Among teenagers aged 15 to 19 who have not yet had sex, a plurality say they have avoided it because of moral or religious reasons. Fear of pregnancy is the second most commonly cited reason, mentioned by 19 percent of girls and 25 percent of boys. There are sharp differences among boys by race and Hispanic origin, however. Hispanic boys are most likely to say they are still virgins because they fear getting a girl pregnant (42 percent). Blacks are more likely than others to abstain because of concerns about sexually transmitted diseases.

■ The average girl is 12.6 years old at first menstruation, with little variation by race or Hispanic origin.

Girls are slightly more likely than boys to cite moral or religious reasons for not having sex

(percent of teenagers aged 15 to 19 who have never had sexual intercourse primarily because it is against their religion or morals, by sex, 2002)

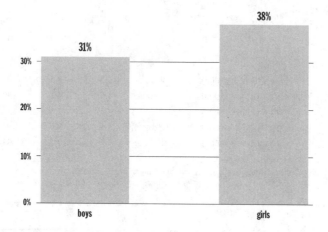

Table 1.20 Average Age at First Menstrual Period by Age, Race, and Hispanic Origin, 2002

(average age at first menstrual period among women aged 15 to 44, by age, race, and Hispanic origin, 2002)

	average age
Total women aged 15 to 44	**12.6 years**
Aged 15 to 19	12.4
Aged 20 to 24	12.5
Aged 25 to 29	12.5
Aged 30 to 34	12.6
Aged 35 to 39	12.7
Aged 40 to 44	12.7
Black, non-Hispanic	12.4
Hispanic	12.5
White, non-Hispanic	12.6

Source: National Center for Health Statistics, Fertility, Family Planning, and Reproductive Health of U.S. Women: Data from the 2002 National Survey of Family Growth, Vital and Health Statistics, Series 23, No. 25, 2005; Internet site http://www.cdc .gov/nchs/nsfg.htm

Table 1.21 Sex Education Experience among Teenagers, 2002

(percentage of people aged 15 to 19 who received school instruction or talked with a parent about sex before age 18, by sex, 2002)

	boys	girls
School instruction on how to say no to sex	82.6%	85.5%
School instruction on methods of birth control	66.2	69.9
Talked with a parent about how to say no to sex	45.2	57.5
Talked with a parent about methods of birth control	33.2	51.0
Talked with a parent about where to get birth control	23.0	38.0
Talked with a parent about sexually transmitted diseases	51.8	51.3
Talked with a parent about how to use a condom	33.9	29.3
Took a pledge to remain a virgin until marriage	10.7	13.0

Source: National Center for Health Statistics, Teenagers in the United States: Sexual Activity, Contraceptive Use, and Childbearing, 2002, Vital and Health Statistics, Series 23, No. 24, 2004; Internet site http://www.cdc.gov/nchs/nsfg.htm

Table 1.22 Reason for Not Having Sexual Intercourse among Teenage Girls by Age, 2002

(number of women aged 15 to 19 who have never had sexual intercourse and percent distribution by main reason for not having intercourse, by age, 2002; numbers in thousands)

	total	15 to 17	18 to 19
Women aged 15 to 19 who have never had sexual intercourse, number	**5,236**	**4,054**	**1,182**
Women aged 15 to 19 who have never had sexual intercourse, percent	**100.0%**	**100.0%**	**100.0%**
Against religion or morals	37.8	37.5	38.7
Don't want to get pregnant	18.7	19.1	17.3
Haven't found the right person yet	17.2	15.9	21.8
Don't want to get a sexually transmitted disease	7.4	9.1	–
In a relationship, but waiting for the right time	6.6	6.1	8.0
Other reason	12.4	12.3	12.7

Note: "–" means sample is too small to make a reliable estimate.
Source: National Center for Health Statistics, Teenagers in the United States: Sexual Activity, Contraceptive Use, and Childbearing, 2002, Vital and Health Statistics, Series 23, No. 24, 2004; Internet site http://www.cdc.gov/nchs/nsfg.htm

Table 1.23 Reason for Not Having Sexual Intercourse among Teenage Boys by Age, 2002

(number of men aged 15 to 19 who have never had sexual intercourse and percent distribution by main reason for not having intercourse, by age, 2002; numbers in thousands)

	total	15 to 17	18 to 19
Men aged 15 to 19 who have never had sexual intercourse, number	**5,511**	**3,934**	**1,577**
Men aged 15 to 19 who have never had sexual intercourse, percent	**100.0%**	**100.0%**	**100.0%**
Against religion or morals	31.4	29.3	36.9
Don't want to get a female pregnant	25.2	27.4	19.5
Haven't found the right person yet	20.8	17.9	28.2
Don't want to get a sexually transmitted disease	9.9	12.0	–
In a relationship, but waiting for the right time	4.8	4.3	5.9
Other reason	7.9	9.2	4.7

Note: "–" means sample is too small to make a reliable estimate.
Source: National Center for Health Statistics, Teenagers in the United States: Sexual Activity, Contraceptive Use, and Childbearing, 2002, Vital and Health Statistics, Series 23, No. 24, 2004; Internet site http://www.cdc.gov/nchs/nsfg.htm

Table 1.24   **Reason for Not Having Sexual Intercourse among Teenage Girls by Race and Hispanic Origin, 2002**

(number of women aged 15 to 19 who have never had sexual intercourse and percent distribution by main reason for not having intercourse, by race and Hispanic origin, 2002; numbers in thousands)

	total	black non-Hispanic	Hispanic	white non-Hispanic
Women aged 15 to 19 who have never had sexual intercourse, number	5,236	645	906	3,351
Women aged 15 to 19 who have never had sexual intercourse, percent	100.0%	100.0%	100.0%	100.0%
Against religion or morals	37.8	19.2	29.8	42.1
Don't want to get pregnant	18.7	14.0	24.2	18.3
Haven't found the right person yet	17.2	18.6	13.5	19.3
Don't want to get a sexually transmitted disease	7.4	25.9	8.6	3.7
In a relationship, but waiting for the right time	6.6	5.1	11.4	4.9
Other reason	12.4	17.2	12.4	11.6

Source: National Center for Health Statistics, Teenagers in the United States: Sexual Activity, Contraceptive Use, and Childbearing, 2002, Vital and Health Statistics, Series 23, No. 24, 2004; Internet site http://www.cdc.gov/nchs/nsfg.htm

Table 1.25   **Reason for Not Having Sexual Intercourse among Teenage Boys by Race and Hispanic Origin, 2002**

(number of men aged 15 to 19 who have never had sexual intercourse and percent distribution by main reason for not having intercourse, by race and Hispanic origin, 2002; numbers in thousands)

	total	black non-Hispanic	Hispanic	white non-Hispanic
Men aged 15 to 19 who have never had sexual intercourse, number	5,511	540	725	3,829
Men aged 15 to 19 who have never had sexual intercourse, percent	100.0%	100.0%	100.0%	100.0%
Against religion or morals	31.4	21.4	18.9	35.9
Don't want to get a female pregnant	25.2	28.1	42.1	23.1
Haven't found the right person yet	20.8	13.6	19.0	19.4
Don't want to get a sexually transmitted disease	9.9	20.2	11.7	9.0
In a relationship, but waiting for the right time	4.8	–	–	4.5
Other reason	7.9	9.9	5.6	8.2

Note: "–" means sample is too small to make a reliable estimate.
Source: National Center for Health Statistics, Teenagers in the United States: Sexual Activity, Contraceptive Use, and Childbearing, 2002, Vital and Health Statistics, Series 23, No. 24, 2004; Internet site http://www.cdc.gov/nchs/nsfg.htm

Teenage Sexual Activity

■ The nation's teenagers are sexually active, but less so than they used to be. They have surprisingly conservative views toward sexual activity between 16-year-olds, but are more tolerant of premarital sex between 18-year-olds.

■ Teenagers today are less sexually experienced than in the past. The percentage of never-married boys aged 15 to 19 who have ever had sexual intercourse fell from 60 to 46 percent between 1988 and 2002. Among girls, the percentage fell from 51 to 46 percent.

■ Many teens have had more than one sexual partner. Sexually experienced teens aged 15 to 19 are more likely to have had multiple partners than to have engaged in sex with only one person.

■ Most teens have experienced oral sex, but few stop there. Among boys aged 15 to 19, only 12 percent have had oral sex but no intercourse, while among girls the share is 10 percent.

■ Teens are surprisingly conservative about sex. Most do not think it is all right for unmarried 16-year-olds to have sexual relations. Among 15-to-19-year-olds, 68 percent of girls and 63 percent of boys disapprove of sex between 16-year-olds.

Most Teenagers Have Sex before Age 18

Boys and girls are equally likely to have had sexual intercourse.

Teenage sexual activity has declined significantly over the past 12 years, according to the National Survey of Family Growth. In 2002, 46 percent of never-married boys aged 15 to 19 had had sexual intercourse, down from 60 percent in 1988. The percentage of girls in the age group who have had sexual intercourse fell from 51 to 46 percent. Despite the decline, 54 percent of boys and 58 percent of girls have had sex by age 18.

Teens aged 15 to 19 who live in two-parent families are much less likely to have sexual intercourse than those in other family situations. Only 30 to 34 percent of those in two-parent families have had sex compared with 52 to 54 percent of those in other types of families. Among 15-to-19-year-olds, Hispanic girls and non-Hispanic white boys are least likely to have had sexual intercourse (37 and 41 percent, respectively).

■ The decline in teen sexual activity may be due to concerns about sexually transmitted diseases.

The decline in sexual experience has been greater for teenage boys than teenage girls

(percent of people aged 15 to 19 who have ever had sexual intercourse, by sex, 1988 and 2002)

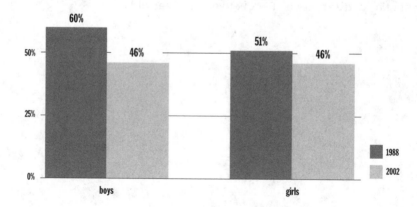

Table 2.1 Sexual Intercourse among Teenagers, 1988 and 2002

(percent of never-married people aged 15 to 19 who have ever had sexual intercourse, by selected characteristics and sex, 1988 and 2002; percentage point change, 1988–2002)

	percent who have ever had sexual intercourse		percentage point change, 1988–2002
	2002	1988	
BOYS			
Total aged 15 to 19	**45.7%**	**60.4%**	**–14.7**
Aged 15 to 17	31.3	50.0	–18.7
Aged 18 to 19	64.3	77.3	–13.0
Race and Hispanic origin			
Black, non-Hispanic	63.3	80.6	–17.3
Hispanic	54.8	59.7	–4.9
White, non-Hispanic	40.8	56.8	–16.0
Family structure at age 14			
Living with both parents	40.4	57.0	–16.6
Other	57.1	68.3	–11.2
GIRLS			
Total aged 15 to 19	**45.5**	**51.1**	**–5.6**
Aged 15 to 17	30.3	37.2	–6.9
Aged 18 to 19	68.8	72.6	–3.8
Race and Hispanic origin			
Black, non-Hispanic	56.9	60.4	–3.5
Hispanic	37.4	45.8	–8.4
White, non-Hispanic	45.1	50.4	–5.3
Family structure at age 14			
Living with both parents	38.7	44.9	–6.2
Other	57.2	62.2	–5.0

Source: National Center for Health Statistics, Teenagers in the United States: Sexual Activity, Contraceptive Use, and Childbearing, 2002; Vital and Health Statistics Series 23, No. 24, 2004; Internet site http://www.cdc.gov/nchs/nsfg.htm

Table 2.2 Cumulative Percentage of Teenagers Aged 15 to 19 Who Have Ever Had Sexual Intercourse, 2002

(cumulative percentage of never-married people aged 15 to 19 who had sexual intercourse before reaching specified age, by sex, 2002)

	percent having sexual intercourse before reaching specified age	
	boys	girls
Total aged 15 to 19	**45.7%**	**45.5%**
By age 14	7.9	5.7
By age 15	14.6	13.0
By age 16	25.3	26.8
By age 17	39.4	43.1
By age 18	54.3	58.0
By age 19	65.2	70.1

Source: National Center for Health Statistics, Teenagers in the United States: Sexual Activity, Contraceptive Use, and Childbearing, 2002; Vital and Health Statistics Series 23, No. 24, 2004; Internet site http://www.cdc.gov/nchs/nsfg.htm

Table 2.3 Teenage Girls' Experience with Sexual Intercourse in Lifetime and Past Year, 2002

(number of total and never-married women aged 15 to 19, and percent who have ever had sexual intercourse in lifetime, in past 12 months, and in past three months, by selected characteristics, 2002; numbers in thousands)

		percent having had sexual intercourse			
	number	in lifetime	in past 12 months	in past three months	once
Total women aged 15 to 19	**9,834**	**46.8%**	**42.5%**	**35.7%**	**4.1%**
Never-married women aged 15 to 19	**9,598**	**45.5**	**41.3**	**34.4**	**4.2**
Age					
Aged 15 to 17	5,815	30.3	26.1	21.7	4.3
Aged 18 to 19	3,783	68.8	64.6	54.0	4.1
Race and Hispanic origin					
Black, non-Hispanic	1,496	56.9	46.2	34.8	3.7
Hispanic	1,447	37.4	33.0	28.7	3.4
White, non-Hispanic	6,099	45.1	42.6	36.2	6.4
Family structure					
Living with both parents	4,406	30.3	27.1	21.8	5.1
Other	4,233	52.4	46.9	37.5	4.2

Source: National Center for Health Statistics, Teenagers in the United States: Sexual Activity, Contraceptive Use, and Childbearing, 2002; Vital and Health Statistics Series 23, No. 24, 2004; Internet site http://www.cdc.gov/nchs/nsfg.htm

Table 2.4 Teenage Boys' Experience with Sexual Intercourse in Lifetime and Past Year, 2002

(number of total and never-married men aged 15 to 19, and percent who have ever had sexual intercourse in lifetime, in past 12 months, and in past three months, by selected characteristics, 2002; numbers in thousands)

| | | percent having had sexual intercourse | | | |
	number	in lifetime	in past 12 months	in past three months	once
Total men aged 15 to 19	**10,208**	**46.0%**	**39.8%**	**31.7%**	**4.1%**
Never-married men aged 15 to 19	**10,139**	**45.7**	**39.4**	**31.2**	**4.1**
Age					
Aged 15 to 17	5,726	31.3	25.6	18.1	5.0
Aged 18 to 19	4,413	64.3	57.2	48.2	3.0
Race and Hispanic origin					
Black, non-Hispanic	1,468	63.3	51.6	40.4	6.2
Hispanic	1,603	54.8	47.0	38.1	4.9
White, non-Hispanic	6,462	40.8	36.4	28.9	2.6
Family structure					
Living with both parents	5,181	33.5	30.1	23.6	3.1
Other	4,277	54.0	43.6	34.1	5.7

Source: National Center for Health Statistics, Teenagers in the United States: Sexual Activity, Contraceptive Use, and Childbearing, 2002; Vital and Health Statistics Series 23, No. 24, 2004; Internet site http://www.cdc.gov/nchs/nsfg.htm

Many Teens Have Had More than One Sexual Partner

Eighteen percent of teen boys have had two or more partners in the past year.

When teenagers lose their virginity, many no doubt believe they are "giving themselves" to the person they will ultimately marry. But it rarely ends up that way. Teen romance usually has a short life span. But having already had sex once can make it easier to have sex again without assuming the relationship is destined to last.

Sexually experienced teens aged 15 to 19 are more likely to have had multiple partners than to have engaged in sex with only one person. Among girls, 55 percent say they have never had sex, 28 percent report having had more than one sexual partner, and 18 percent have had just one partner. Their male counterparts show a similar distribution, with 54 percent still virgins, 30 percent having had multiple partners, and 16 percent having had only one sex partner.

The largest share of sexually experienced teens have had only one sex partner in the prior year. Among never-married girls aged 15 to 19, 29 percent had only one partner in the past year compared with 14 percent with two or more partners. Among their male counterparts, 22 percent had one partner and 18 percent had two or more.

■ A younger age at first sexual intercourse is associated with a larger number of sex partners.

Boys are more likely to have had multiple sex partners in the past year

(percent of never-married people aged 15 to 19 who have had more than one sexual partner in the past 12 months, by sex, 2002)

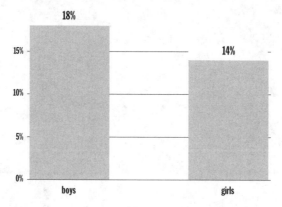

Table 2.5 Number of Sexual Intercourse Partners Teenage Girls Had in Lifetime, 2002

(number of total and never-married women aged 15 to 19, and percent distribution by number of partners with whom they have had sexual intercourse in lifetime, by selected characteristics, 2002; numbers in thousands)

	total		number of sexual intercourse partners in lifetime				
	number	percent	none	one	two to three	four to six	seven or more
Total women aged 15 to 19	9,834	100.0%	53.2%	18.2%	14.3%	8.0%	6.2%
Never-married women aged 15 to 19	9,598	100.0	54.6	17.7	13.6	7.9	6.3
Age							
Aged 15 to 17	5,815	100.0	69.7	13.7	10.0	4.5	2.2
Aged 18 to 19	3,783	100.0	31.2	23.9	19.3	13.0	12.6
Age at first sexual intercourse							
Never had sex	5,236	100.0	100.0	–	–	–	–
Under age 15	1,248	100.0	–	13.5	29.5	31.7	25.4
Aged 15 to 16	2,095	100.0	–	40.8	37.7	11.1	10.4
Aged 17 to 19	1,019	100.0	–	66.4	14.7	12.5	6.5
Race and Hispanic origin							
Black, non-Hispanic	1,496	100.0	43.1	20.6	21.0	10.8	4.5
Hispanic	1,447	100.0	62.6	17.5	13.1	5.4	1.5
White, non-Hispanic	6,099	100.0	54.9	17.3	12.0	7.8	7.9

Note: "–" means not applicable.
Source: National Center for Health Statistics, Teenagers in the United States: Sexual Activity, Contraceptive Use, and Childbearing, 2002; Vital and Health Statistics Series 23, No. 24, 2004; Internet site http://www.cdc.gov/nchs/nsfg.htm

Table 2.6 Number of Sexual Intercourse Partners Teenage Boys Had in Lifetime, 2002

(number of total and never-married men aged 15 to 19, and percent distribution by number of partners with whom they have had sexual intercourse in lifetime, by selected characteristics, 2002; numbers in thousands)

	total		number of sexual intercourse partners in lifetime				
	number	percent	none	one	two to three	four to six	seven or more
Total men aged 15 to 19	10,208	100.0%	54.0%	15.5%	13.6%	9.6%	7.3%
Never-married men aged 15 to 19	10,139	100.0	54.4	15.5	13.5	9.4	7.2
Age							
Aged 15 to 17	5,726	100.0	68.7	13.3	9.2	4.8	4.0
Aged 18 to 19	4,413	100.0	35.7	18.5	19.1	15.4	11.3
Age at first sexual intercourse							
Never had sex	5,511	100.0	100.0	–	–	–	–
Under age 15	1,483	100.0	–	12.2	26.9	29.7	31.2
Aged 15 to 16	1,947	100.0	–	33.1	33.9	21.9	11.2
Aged 17 to 19	1,199	100.0	–	62.7	26.2	7.3	3.8
Race and Hispanic origin							
Black, non-Hispanic	1,468	100.0	36.8	18.9	15.1	16.5	12.8
Hispanic	1,603	100.0	45.2	17.4	12.7	15.1	9.6
White, non-Hispanic	6,462	100.0	59.3	15.3	13.7	6.8	5.0

Note: "–" means not applicable.
Source: National Center for Health Statistics, Teenagers in the United States: Sexual Activity, Contraceptive Use, and Childbearing, 2002; Vital and Health Statistics Series 23, No. 24, 2004; Internet site http://www.cdc.gov/nchs/nsfg.htm

Table 2.7 Number of Sexual Intercourse Partners Teenage Girls Had in Past Year, 2002

(number of total and never-married women aged 15 to 19, and percent distribution by number of partners with whom they have had sexual intercourse in past 12 months, by selected characteristics, 2002; numbers in thousands)

| | total | | no partners | | | | |
| | | | number of sexual intercourse partners in past 12 months | | | | |
	number	percent	never had sexual intercourse	had sex, but not in past 12 months	one partner	two to three partners	four or more partners
Total women aged 15 to 19	9,834	100.0%	53.2%	4.2%	28.6%	10.3%	3.6%
Never-married women aged 15 to 19	9,598	100.0	54.6	4.2	27.5	10.2	3.7
Age							
Aged 15 to 17	5,815	100.0	69.7	4.2	18.6	6.5	1.0
Aged 18 to 19	3,783	100.0	31.2	4.1	41.0	15.9	7.7
Race and Hispanic origin							
Black, non-Hispanic	1,496	100.0	43.1	10.7	27.5	14.6	4.1
Hispanic	1,447	100.0	62.6	4.4	26.2	5.6	1.2
White, non-Hispanic	6,099	100.0	54.9	2.4	27.9	10.6	4.2
Family structure							
Living with both parents	4,406	100.0	69.7	3.2	19.9	5.7	1.5
Other	4,233	100.0	47.7	5.4	28.9	12.3	5.7

Source: National Center for Health Statistics, Teenagers in the United States: Sexual Activity, Contraceptive Use, and Childbearing, 2002; Vital and Health Statistics Series 23, No. 24, 2004; Internet site http://www.cdc.gov/nchs/nsfg.htm

Table 2.8 Number of Sexual Intercourse Partners among Teenage Boys in Past Year, 2002

(number of total and never-married men aged 15 to 19, and percent distribution by number of partners with whom they have had sexual intercourse in past 12 months, by selected characteristics, 2002; numbers in thousands)

| | total | | number of sexual intercourse partners in past 12 months | | | | |
| | | | no partners | | | | |
	number	percent	never had sexual intercourse	had sex, but not in past 12 months	one partner	two to three partners	four or more partners
Total men aged 15 to 19	10,208	100.0%	54.0%	6.3%	21.6%	14.6%	3.5%
Never-married men aged 15 to 19	10,139	100.0	54.4	6.3	21.4	14.5	3.5
Age							
Aged 15 to 17	5,726	100.0	68.7	5.7	15.5	7.2	2.9
Aged 18 to 19	4,413	100.0	35.7	7.0	28.9	23.9	4.4
Race and Hispanic origin							
Black, non-Hispanic	1,468	100.0	36.8	11.6	23.9	20.6	7.1
Hispanic	1,603	100.0	45.2	7.8	25.8	15.7	5.5
White, non-Hispanic	6,462	100.0	59.3	4.3	20.7	13.5	2.2
Family structure							
Living with both parents	5,181	100.0	66.5	3.4	18.2	10.5	1.4
Other	4,277	100.0	46.0	10.4	21.3	16.5	5.8

Source: National Center for Health Statistics, Teenagers in the United States: Sexual Activity, Contraceptive Use, and Childbearing, 2002; Vital and Health Statistics Series 23, No. 24, 2004; Internet site http://www.cdc.gov/nchs/nsfg.htm

Few Teens Limit Themselves to Oral Sex

But most of those aged 18 or older have taken part in oral sex.

For many young people sexual experimentation begins with touching and oral sex. But few stop there; most teens have either had no opposite-sex sexual contact or have "gone all the way"—engaging in sexual intercourse.

Among boys aged 15 to 19, only 12 percent have had oral sex but no intercourse, while among girls the share is 10 percent. By age, the percentage of teens having had no sexual contact declines from 57 to 66 percent among 15-year-olds to just 12 to 19 percent among 19-year-olds. The percentage of those who have had sexual intercourse rises in tandem.

There are differences in sexual experience by race and Hispanic origin. Non-Hispanic whites are most likely to limit themselves to oral sex, while non-Hispanic blacks are most likely to have had sexual intercourse. Hispanic girls are most likely to say they have had no type of sexual contact, while among boys, non-Hispanic whites are most likely to say this.

■ Although sexual activities that stop short of intercourse are virtually guaranteed to prevent pregnancy, it is uncommon for teenagers to say no for long.

The percentage of teen boys who have experienced oral sex rises with age

(percent of men aged 15 to 19 who have ever had oral sex, by age, 2002)

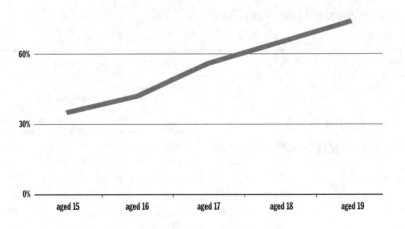

Table 2.9 Opposite-Sex Sexual Experience of Teenage Girls, 2002

(total number of women aged 15 to 19, and percent distribution by type of sexual contact ever experienced with a male, by selected characteristics, 2002; numbers in thousands)

	total		sexual intercourse	oral sex but no intercourse	no intercourse or oral sex, but other sexual contact	no opposite-sex sexual contact
	number	percent				
Total women aged 15 to 19	**9,834**	**100.0%**	**53.0%**	**10.3%**	**–**	**36.7%**
Aged 15	1,819	100.0	26.0	7.9	–	66.2
Aged 16	1,927	100.0	39.6	10.0	–	50.4
Aged 17	2,073	100.0	49.0	14.6	–	36.0
Aged 18	2,035	100.0	70.1	8.1	–	21.8
Aged 19	1,980	100.0	77.4	10.4	–	12.2
Race and Hispanic origin						
Black, non-Hispanic	1,409	100.0	61.7	5.8	–	32.5
Hispanic	1,521	100.0	48.8	9.9	–	41.3
White, non-Hispanic	6,069	100.0	51.7	12.0	–	36.3

Note: "–" means sample is too small to make a reliable estimate.
Source: National Center for Health Statistics, Sexual Behavior and Selected Health Measures: Men and Women 15–44 Years of Age, United States, 2002, Advance Data, No. 362, 2005; Internet site http://www.cdc.gov/nchs/nsfg.htm

Table 2.10 Opposite-Sex Sexual Experience of Teenage Boys, 2002

(total number of men aged 15 to 19, and percent distribution by type of sexual contact ever experienced with a female, by selected characteristics, 2002; numbers in thousands)

	total		sexual intercourse	oral sex but no intercourse	no intercourse or oral sex, but other sexual contact	no opposite-sex sexual contact
	number	percent				
Total men aged 15 to 19	**10,208**	**100.0%**	**48.9%**	**12.0%**	**3.1%**	**36.1%**
Aged 15	1,930	100.0	24.9	13.3	5.0	56.8
Aged 16	1,998	100.0	37.3	11.7	4.3	47.0
Aged 17	1,820	100.0	46.4	14.2	2.9	36.5
Aged 18	2,392	100.0	62.3	10.1	2.0	25.6
Aged 19	2,067	100.0	68.9	11.2	–	18.5
Race and Hispanic origin						
Black, non-Hispanic	1,352	100.0	65.6	7.6	–	25.3
Hispanic	1,628	100.0	56.0	7.3	3.2	33.5
White, non-Hispanic	6,324	100.0	44.5	14.7	3.7	37.2

Note: "–" means sample is too small to make a reliable estimate.
Source: National Center for Health Statistics, Sexual Behavior and Selected Health Measures: Men and Women 15–44 Years of Age, United States, 2002, Advance Data, No. 362, 2005; Internet site http://www.cdc.gov/nchs/nsfg.htm

Table 2.11 Sexual Experience of Teenage Girls, 2002

(total number of women aged 15 to 19, and percent distribution by type of sexual contact ever experienced, by selected characteristics, 2002; numbers in thousands)

| | total | | opposite-sex sexual contact | | | | | | any sexual experience with female | no sexual contact with another person |
| | | | any | sexual intercourse | oral | | | anal | | |
	number	percent			any oral	gave	received			
Total women aged 15 to 19	**9,834**	**100.0%**	**63.3%**	**53.0%**	**54.3%**	**43.6%**	**49.6%**	**10.9%**	**10.6%**	**35.5%**
Aged 15	1,819	100.0	33.8	26.0	26.0	18.3	23.9	2.4	7.2	63.7
Aged 16	1,927	100.0	49.6	39.6	42.4	30.4	39.3	6.9	13.1	48.8
Aged 17	2,073	100.0	64.0	49.0	55.5	41.1	49.1	7.3	5.1	35.2
Aged 18	2,035	100.0	78.2	70.3	70.2	61.3	62.4	18.8	13.7	21.2
Aged 19	1,980	100.0	87.8	77.4	74.4	64.2	71.1	18.6	13.9	11.7
Race and Hispanic origin										
Black, non-Hispanic	1,409	100.0	67.5	62.3	53.2	25.0	52.4	10.3	9.9	30.3
Hispanic	1,521	100.0	58.7	48.8	46.9	33.7	41.1	9.5	5.5	40.2
White, non-Hispanic	6,069	100.0	63.7	51.7	58.3	51.4	53.1	11.7	12.7	35.3

Note: The questions about same-sex sexual contact in the National Survey of Family Growth were worded differently for men and women. Women were asked whether they had ever had a sexual experience of any kind with another female. Men were asked whether they had performed any of four specific sexual acts with another male. The question asked of women may have elicited more "yes" answers than the questions asked of men.
Source: National Center for Health Statistics, Sexual Behavior and Selected Health Measures: Men and Women 15–44 Years of Age, United States, 2002, Advance Data, No. 362, 2005; Internet site http://www.cdc.gov/nchs/nsfg.htm

Table 2.12 Sexual Experience of Teenage Boys, 2002

(total number of men aged 15 to 19, and percent distribution by type of sexual contact ever experienced, by selected characteristics, 2002; numbers in thousands)

| | | total | | | opposite-sex sexual contact | | oral | | | | any oral or | no sexual |
	number	percent	any	sexual intercourse	any oral		gave	received	anal	female touched penis	anal sex with male	contact with another person
Total men aged 15 to 19	10,208	100.0%	63.9%	49.1%	55.2%		38.8%	51.5%	11.2%	52.4%	4.5%	35.4%
Aged 15	1,930	100.0	43.2	25.1	35.1		15.5	30.3	4.6	35.4	2.2	55.9
Aged 16	1,998	100.0	53.3	37.5	42.0		27.0	39.4	7.3	43.2	3.1	46.3
Aged 17	1,820	100.0	63.5	46.9	55.7		43.2	51.9	12.9	50.1	6.6	35.6
Aged 18	2,392	100.0	74.4	62.4	65.4		50.5	61.7	15.1	59.2	4.3	24.6
Aged 19	2,067	100.0	81.6	68.9	74.2		54.6	70.9	15.3	71.6	6.0	18.0
Race and Hispanic origin												
Black, non-Hispanic	1,352	100.0	74.7	66.0	58.6		20.2	57.4	11.2	55.7	5.2	24.1
Hispanic	1,628	100.0	66.5	56.6	52.7		36.5	48.1	16.1	54.4	7.0	32.2
White, non-Hispanic	6,324	100.0	62.8	44.6	57.0		44.5	53.5	10.1	54.0	3.5	36.7

Note: The questions about same-sex sexual contact in the National Survey of Family Growth were worded differently for men and women. Women were asked whether they had ever had a sexual experience of any kind with another female. Men were asked whether they had performed any of four specific sexual acts with another male. The question asked of women may have elicited more "yes" answers than the questions asked of men.
Source: National Center for Health Statistics, Sexual Behavior and Selected Health Measures: Men and Women 15–44 Years of Age, United States, 2002, Advance Data, No. 362, 2005; Internet site http://www.cdc.gov/nchs/nsfg.htm

Most Teenagers Have Not Had Sexual Intercourse in the Past Month

Although most older teens are sexually experienced, many are not sexually active.

Many teens may be sexually experienced, but the average 15-to-19-year-old has not had sexual intercourse in the past month. Seventy-two percent of never-married girls in the age group have not had sexual intercourse in the past four weeks. Among their male counterparts, an even larger 75 percent have not had sex in the past month.

Men and women aged 18 to 19 are more likely than those aged 15 to 17 to be sexually active. This is not surprising since the older group has reached the age of adulthood and has more freedom and opportunity to have sex. Many are undoubtedly in relationships they consider serious and committed. They may also simply be more ready to have sexual relations on a regular basis than younger—and less emotionally mature—teenagers.

■ Since it is unlikely that teenage marriage will become common again, sex between unmarried teenagers will remain a reality in spite of abstinence programs and pledges.

Younger teens are far less likely to be sexually active

(percent of never-married people aged 15 to 19 who have not had sexual intercourse in the past four weeks, by age and sex, 2002)

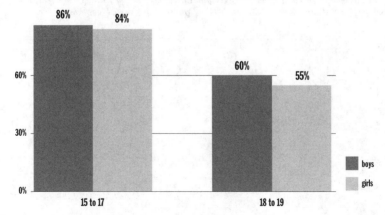

Table 2.13 Frequency of Sexual Intercourse among Teenage Girls in Past Four Weeks, 2002

(number of total and never-married women aged 15 to 19, and percent distribution by frequency of sexual intercourse in the past four weeks, by selected characteristics, 2002; numbers in thousands)

| | total | | frequency of sexual intercourse in past four weeks | | | | |
	number	percent	none	one time	two to three times	four to seven times	eight or more times
Total women aged 15 to 19	**9,834**	**100.0%**	**70.7%**	**4.2%**	**7.7%**	**6.7%**	**10.7%**
Never-married women aged 15 to 19	**9,598**	**100.0**	**72.2**	**4.3**	**7.3**	**6.8**	**9.4**
Age							
Aged 15 to 17	5,815	100.0	83.5	3.2	5.2	4.1	4.0
Aged 18 to 19	3,783	100.0	54.7	6.0	10.6	10.9	17.8
Race and Hispanic origin							
Black, non-Hispanic	1,496	100.0	70.6	5.1	11.2	7.0	6.2
Hispanic	1,447	100.0	75.3	4.7	7.5	2.5	10.1
White, non-Hispanic	6,099	100.0	71.2	3.8	6.4	8.0	10.6
Family structure							
Living with both parents	4,406	100.0	83.7	2.9	4.1	4.9	4.4
Other	4,233	100.0	67.7	5.4	10.4	6.6	9.9

Source: National Center for Health Statistics, Teenagers in the United States: Sexual Activity, Contraceptive Use, and Childbearing, 2002; Vital and Health Statistics Series 23, No. 24, 2004; Internet site http://www.cdc.gov/nchs/nsfg.htm

Table 2.14   Frequency of Sexual Intercourse among Teenage Boys in Past Four Weeks, 2002

(number of total and never-married men aged 15 to 19, and percent distribution by frequency of sexual intercourse in the past four weeks, by selected characteristics, 2002; numbers in thousands)

| | total | | frequency of sexual intercourse in past four weeks | | | | |
	number	percent	none	one time	two to three times	four to seven times	eight or more times
Total men aged 15 to 19	**10,208**	**100.0%**	**74.6%**	**6.7%**	**6.7%**	**6.2%**	**5.8%**
Never-married men aged 15 to 19	**10,139**	**100.0**	**75.0**	**6.7**	**6.5**	**6.0**	**5.8**
Age							
Aged 15 to 17	5,726	100.0	86.4	5.3	4.1	2.9	1.3
Aged 18 to 19	4,413	100.0	60.2	8.5	9.7	10.0	11.6
Race and Hispanic origin							
Black, non-Hispanic	1,468	100.0	67.7	10.2	10.9	9.0	2.2
Hispanic	1,603	100.0	70.5	6.9	10.7	8.9	3.0
White, non-Hispanic	6,462	100.0	76.8	6.0	4.9	4.9	7.4
Family structure							
Living with both parents	5,181	100.0	82.1	4.6	5.7	3.6	4.0
Other	4,277	100.0	72.7	8.9	7.3	6.6	4.6

Source: National Center for Health Statistics, Teenagers in the United States: Sexual Activity, Contraceptive Use, and Childbearing, 2002; Vital and Health Statistics Series 23, No. 24, 2004; Internet site http://www.cdc.gov/nchs/nsfg.htm

Teens Have Mixed Feelings about Sexual Activity

Most do not approve of unmarried 16-year-olds having sex.

Teens are surprisingly conservative about sex. Most do not think it is all right for unmarried 16-year-olds to have sexual relations. Among 15-to-19-year-olds, 68 percent of girls and 63 percent of boys disapprove of sex between 16-year-olds.

The majority of teens think it is OK for unmarried 18-year-olds to have sexual relations. Sixty-five percent of boys and 61 percent of girls think it is OK. And on the more general question about whether any sexual act between consenting adults is OK, nearly three out of four teens agree.

■ One-third of teenagers say it is not OK for unmarried 18-year-olds to have sexual relations.

Teens think age 18 is OK for sex

(percent of 15-to-19-year-olds who agree that it's all right for unmarried 18-year-olds to have sexual relations, by sex, 2002)

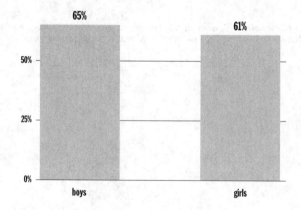

Table 2.15 Attitudes of Teenagers toward Sexual Activity by Sex, 2002

(percent distribution of people aged 15 to 19 by response to statements, by sex, 2002)

	boys	girls
"Any sexual act between two consenting adults is all right."		
Agree	73.7%	73.0%
Disagree	24.1	25.4
"It is all right for unmarried 18-year-olds to have sexual relations if they have strong affection for one another."		
Agree	65.0	60.9
Disagree	34.1	37.2
"It is all right for unmarried 16-year-olds to have sexual relations if they have strong affection for one another."		
Agree	35.7	30.5
Disagree	62.6	67.5

Note: Figues will not sum to 100 because "no opinion" is not shown.
Source: National Center for Health Statistics, Teenagers in the United States: Sexual Activity, Contraceptive Use, and Childbearing, 2002; Vital and Health Statistics Series 23, No. 24, 2004; Internet site http://www.cdc.gov/nchs/nsfg.htm

Adult Sexual Activity

■ If ever there was any doubt that sexual activity is a universal human drive, findings from the federal government's National Survey of Family Growth will put those doubts to rest. By age 18, most men and women have had sexual intercourse. By age 23, more than 90 percent are sexually experienced.

■ Marriage does not matter when it comes to sexual activity. Among never-married men and women aged 15 to 44, more than half have had sexual intercourse in the past year. Nearly half have had sex in the past three months.

■ Most Americans have had more than one sex partner. The majority of women aged 15 to 44 have had three or more opposite-sex partners in their lifetime.

■ Most men are in a committed relationship with their sexual partner. Among men aged 15 to 44 who have had sexual intercourse in the past three months, the 57 percent majority is married to their partner. Another 32 percent are living with or going steady with their partner.

■ Women are not the only gender vulnerable to sexual predation. Among men aged 18 to 44, a substantial 8 percent say they were forced to have sexual intercourse at some point in their life.

■ Americans think premarital sex is OK, within limits. Among 15-to-44-year-olds, 60 percent of men and 51 percent of women agree that premarital sex between unmarried 18-year-olds is all right.

Nearly Everyone Has Had Sex by Their Early Twenties

Most people aged 15 to 44 have had sex within the past three months.

If ever there was any doubt that sexual activity is a universal human drive, a look at the following tables would put those doubts to rest. By age 18, most men and women have had sexual intercourse. By age 23, more than 90 percent are sexually experienced.

The numbers barely change when the analysis is limited to the never-married. Among never-married men and women aged 15 to 44, fully 64 to 65 percent have had sexual intercourse in the past year. More than half have had sex in the past three months.

Interestingly, education dampens sexual activity. College graduates are less likely than those with less education to have had sex in the past three months—53 to 54 percent of college graduates have done so versus 67 to 70 percent of high school graduates.

■ With sexual activity universal, public health must focus on pregnancy and disease prevention.

Most single women have had sex in the past three months

(percent of never-married women aged 15 to 44 who have had sexual intercourse in the past three months, by age, 2002)

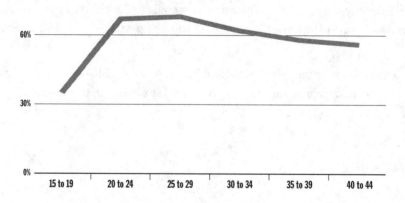

Table 3.1 Women Who Ever Had Sexual Intercourse by Age and Marital Status, 2002

(number of total and never-married women aged 15 to 44 and percent who have ever had sexual intercourse, by age at interview, 2002; numbers in thousands)

	total		never-married	
	number	percent ever having had sexual intercourse	number	percent ever having had sexual intercourse
Total women aged 15 to 44	**61,561**	**88.0%**	**25,712**	**71.3%**
Aged 15	1,819	14.0	1,819	14.0
Aged 16	1,927	29.5	1,927	29.5
Aged 17	2,073	45.5	2,069	45.4
Aged 18	2,035	66.6	1,887	64.0
Aged 19	1,980	74.7	1,896	73.5
Aged 20	1,958	77.6	1,646	73.3
Aged 21	2,047	79.2	1,709	75.1
Aged 22	2,147	90.3	1,695	87.7
Aged 23	1,895	95.0	1,141	91.7
Aged 24	1,793	92.1	959	85.2
Aged 25 to 29	9,249	96.6	3,684	91.6
Aged 30 to 44	32,638	98.4	5,280	90.3

Source: National Center for Health Statistics, Fertility, Family Planning, and Reproductive Health of U.S. Women: Data from the 2002 National Survey of Family Growth, Vital and Health Statistics, Series 23, No. 25, 2005; Internet site http://www.cdc.gov/nchs/nsfg.htm

Table 3.2 Men Who Ever Had Sexual Intercourse by Age and Marital Status, 2002

(number of total and never-married men aged 15 to 44 and percent who have ever had sexual intercourse, by age at interview, 2002; numbers in thousands)

	total		never-married	
	number	percent ever having had sexual intercourse	number	percent ever having had sexual intercourse
Total men aged 15 to 44	**61,147**	**87.1%**	**30,175**	**73.9%**
Aged 15	1,930	15.7	1,930	15.7
Aged 16	1,998	33.9	1,998	33.9
Aged 17	1,820	45.8	1,798	45.1
Aged 18	2,392	60.2	2,369	59.8
Aged 19	2,067	69.8	2,044	69.4
Aged 20	1,942	78.0	1,870	77.1
Aged 21	1,978	91.0	1,803	90.1
Aged 22	2,289	85.1	1,830	81.3
Aged 23	1,747	90.9	1,262	87.4
Aged 24	1,926	92.7	1,460	90.4
Aged 25 to 29	9,226	95.8	4,636	91.6
Aged 30 to 44	31,830	97.7	7,175	89.7

Source: National Center for Health Statistics, Fertility, Contraception, and Fatherhood: Data on Men and Women from Cycle 6 of the 2002 National Survey of Family Growth, Vital and Health Statistics, Series 23, No. 26, 2006; Internet site http://www.cdc .gov/nchs/nsfg.htm

Table 3.3 Sexual Intercourse Experience of Women Aged 15 to 44 in Lifetime and Past Year, 2002

(number of total and never-married women aged 15 to 44, and percent who have ever had sexual intercourse in lifetime, in past 12 months, and in past three months, by selected characteristics, 2002; numbers in thousands)

	number	percent having had sexual intercourse		
		in lifetime	in past 12 months	in past three months
Total women aged 15 to 44	**61,561**	**88.0%**	**79.2%**	**72.2%**
Never-married women aged 15 to 44	**33,234**	**77.8**	**64.3**	**54.8**
Age				
Aged 15 to 19	9,636	45.7	41.5	34.5
Aged 20 to 24	7,566	82.7	75.6	66.6
Aged 25 to 29	4,474	93.1	79.6	67.6
Aged 30 to 34	3,921	95.0	75.8	62.4
Aged 35 to 39	3,864	95.7	69.1	58.2
Aged 40 to 44	3,772	96.0	64.9	56.4
Marital status				
Currently cohabiting	5,570	100.0	95.7	93.0
Never married, not cohabiting	6,096	65.8	53.9	43.7
Formerly married, not cohabiting	21,568	100.0	72.5	59.4
Race and Hispanic origin				
Black, non-Hispanic	2,710	86.2	70.3	59.7
Hispanic	4,969	75.5	63.9	52.9
White, non-Hispanic	6,117	76.9	63.4	54.7
Education				
Not a high school graduate	2,863	96.4	78.9	68.3
High school graduate or GED	6,172	97.4	80.7	69.7
Some college, no degree	6,081	93.8	72.4	61.6
Bachelor's degree or more	5,030	87.6	65.1	54.1

Note: Education categories include only people aged 22 to 44.

Source: National Center for Health Statistics, Fertility, Family Planning, and Reproductive Health of U.S. Women: Data from the 2002 National Survey of Family Growth, Vital and Health Statistics, Series 23, No. 25, 2005; Internet site http://www.cdc .gov/nchs/nsfg.htm

Table 3.4 Sexual Intercourse Experience of Men Aged 15 to 44 in Lifetime and Past Year, 2002

(number of total and never-married men aged 15 to 44, and percent who have ever had sexual intercourse in lifetime, in past 12 months, and in past three months, by selected characteristics, 2002; numbers in thousands)

	number	percent having had sexual intercourse		
		in lifetime	in past 12 months	in past three months
Total men aged 15 to 44	**61,147**	**87.1%**	**78.9%**	**71.3%**
Never-married men aged 15 to 44	**35,340**	77.7	64.8	53.9
Age				
Aged 15 to 19	10,166	45.8	39.5	31.4
Aged 20 to 24	836	85.1	76.8	63.6
Aged 25 to 29	5,048	92.3	77.0	65.2
Aged 30 to 34	3,991	92.1	76.8	67.2
Aged 35 to 39	3,636	93.7	69.8	58.9
Aged 40 to 44	4,133	95.2	72.2	58.6
Marital status				
Currently cohabiting	5,653	100.0	98.3	97.4
Never married, not cohabiting	25,412	69.0	54.9	42.9
Formerly married, not cohabiting	4,274	100.0	79.5	61.9
Race and Hispanic origin				
Black, non-Hispanic	4,753	85.7	76.0	65.9
Hispanic	5,839	82.6	71.5	60.2
White, non-Hispanic	21,555	75.1	62.5	51.4
Education				
Not a high school graduate	2,976	93.7	77.5	66.1
High school graduate or GED	7,225	92.3	77.8	66.6
Some college, no degree	6,717	93.1	77.0	65.8
Bachelor's degree or more	4,562	87.6	64.0	53.0

Note: Education categories include only people aged 22 to 44.
Source: National Center for Health Statistics, Fertility, Contraception, and Fatherhood: Data on Men and Women from Cycle 6 of the 2002 National Survey of Family Growth, Vital and Health Statistics, Series 23, No. 26, 2006; Internet site http://www.cdc .gov/nchs/nsfg.htm

Most Women Have Had More than One Sex Partner

The 55 percent majority has had three or more partners.

Among women aged 15 to 44, only 12 percent have never had sexual intercourse. The proportion of women who are virgins ranges from a high of 53 percent among women aged 15 to 19 to fewer than 4 percent of women aged 25 to 44. The percentage of women with only one sexual partner in her lifetime does not vary much by age, ranging from 18 to 23 percent.

Most women in the 15-to-44 age group have had three or more opposite-sex partners. Only 15 percent have had ten or more. The younger the age at first sexual intercourse, the more sexual partners a woman is likely to have. Among women who first had sex when they were younger than age 16, nearly 30 percent have had ten or more partners.

■ Among married women aged 15 to 44, only one-third have had only one sexual partner in their lifetime. Sixty-seven percent have had two or more.

Hispanic women are most likely to have had only one sexual partner

(percent of women aged 15 to 44 with one opposite-sex sexual partner in lifetime, by race and Hispanic origin, 2002)

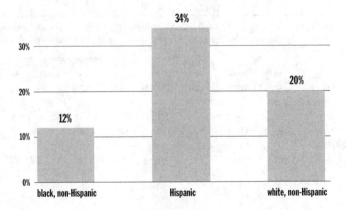

Table 3.5 Lifetime Sexual Experience of Women Aged 15 to 44 by Age, 2002

(total number of women aged 15 to 44 and percent distribution by number of opposite-sex partners with whom they have had sexual intercourse during their lifetime, by age, 2002; numbers in thousands)

	total		number of opposite-sex partners in lifetime							
	number	percent	none	one	two	three	four	five	six to nine	10 or more
Total women aged 15 to 44	**61,561**	**100.0%**	**12.0%**	**21.7%**	**11.1%**	**9.7%**	**8.8%**	**8.2%**	**13.5%**	**15.0%**
Aged 15 to 19	9,834	100.0	53.2	18.2	6.9	7.4	4.1	2.4	5.2	2.6
Aged 20 to 24	9,840	100.0	13.3	23.3	13.4	11.0	7.3	7.5	13.1	11.0
Aged 25 to 29	9,249	100.0	3.4	23.0	13.1	10.4	7.9	8.2	15.0	19.1
Aged 30 to 34	10,272	100.0	1.9	21.0	10.4	11.2	10.5	9.8	15.5	19.6
Aged 35 to 39	10,853	100.0	1.5	21.5	11.8	9.3	9.3	10.8	15.4	20.3
Aged 40 to 44	11,512	100.0	1.3	23.2	10.8	9.3	13.0	10.0	15.8	16.7

Source: National Center for Health Statistics, Fertility, Family Planning, and Reproductive Health of U.S. Women: Data from the 2002 National Survey of Family Growth, Vital and Health Statistics, Series 23, No. 25, 2005; Internet site http://www.cdc.gov/nchs/nsfg.htm

Table 3.6 Lifetime Sexual Experience of Women Aged 15 to 44 by Age at First Intercourse, 2002

(total number of women aged 15 to 44 and percent distribution by number of opposite-sex partners with whom they have had sexual intercourse during their lifetime, by age at first intercourse, 2002; numbers in thousands)

	total		number of opposite-sex partners in lifetime							
	number	percent	none	one	two	three	four	five	six to nine	10 or more
Total women aged 15 to 44	**61,561**	**100.0%**	**12.0%**	**21.7%**	**11.1%**	**9.7%**	**8.8%**	**8.2%**	**13.5%**	**15.0%**
Under age 16 at first intercourse	9,834	100.0	–	9.7	9.1	11.0	9.9	11.1	19.7	29.5
Aged 16 at first intercourse	9,840	100.0	–	14.1	12.0	11.1	12.8	11.9	18.6	19.5
Aged 17 at first intercourse	9,249	100.0	–	18.1	14.1	13.6	13.1	8.7	16.8	15.6
Aged 18 at first intercourse	10,272	100.0	–	25.0	14.9	13.1	9.4	10.1	15.7	11.7
Aged 19 at first intercourse	10,853	100.0	–	31.9	15.7	12.6	10.3	9.4	10.0	10.3
Aged 20 or older at first intercourse	11,512	100.0	–	60.3	14.3	6.9	5.4	4.2	5.8	3.2

Note: "–" means not applicable.
Source: National Center for Health Statistics, Fertility, Family Planning, and Reproductive Health of U.S. Women: Data from the 2002 National Survey of Family Growth, Vital and Health Statistics, Series 23, No. 25, 2005; Internet site http://www.cdc.gov/nchs/nsfg.htm

Table 3.7 Lifetime Sexual Experience of Women Aged 15 to 44 by Marital Status, 2002

(total number of women aged 15 to 44 and percent distribution by number of opposite-sex partners with whom they have had sexual intercourse during their lifetime, by marital status, 2002; numbers in thousands)

	total		number of opposite-sex partners in lifetime							
	number	percent	none	one	two	three	four	five	six to nine	10 or more
Total women aged 15 to 44	**61,561**	**100.0%**	**12.0%**	**21.7%**	**11.1%**	**9.7%**	**8.8%**	**8.2%**	**13.5%**	**15.0%**
Currently married	28,327	100.0	0.0	32.7	12.6	10.3	10.1	7.9	13.6	12.9
Currently cohabiting	5,570	100.0	0.0	15.1	13.8	11.0	10.7	12.1	15.3	22.0
Never married, not cohabiting	21,568	100.0	34.2	13.0	8.9	8.6	5.9	6.9	11.0	11.5
Formerly married, not cohabiting	6,096	100.0	0.0	7.7	8.9	10.3	11.3	11.3	19.4	31.0

Source: National Center for Health Statistics, Fertility, Family Planning, and Reproductive Health of U.S. Women: Data from the 2002 National Survey of Family Growth, Vital and Health Statistics, Series 23, No. 25, 2005; Internet site http://www.cdc.gov/nchs/nsfg.htm

Table 3.8 Lifetime Sexual Experience of Women Aged 15 to 44 by Race and Hispanic Origin, 2002

(total number of women aged 15 to 44 and percent distribution by number of opposite-sex partners with whom they have had sexual intercourse during their lifetime, by race and Hispanic origin, 2002; numbers in thousands)

	total		number of opposite-sex partners in lifetime							
	number	percent	none	one	two	three	four	five	six to nine	10 or more
Total women aged 15 to 44	**61,561**	**100.0%**	**12.0%**	**21.7%**	**11.1%**	**9.7%**	**8.8%**	**8.2%**	**13.5%**	**15.0%**
Black, non-Hispanic	8,250	100.0	10.3	11.6	9.0	12.1	11.6	13.1	17.3	15.1
Hispanic	9,107	100.0	13.4	34.1	15.8	9.9	8.1	4.7	7.3	6.7
White, non-Hispanic	39,498	100.0	11.4	19.9	10.9	9.3	8.6	8.3	14.4	17.2

Source: National Center for Health Statistics, Fertility, Family Planning, and Reproductive Health of U.S. Women: Data from the 2002 National Survey of Family Growth, Vital and Health Statistics, Series 23, No. 25, 2005; Internet site http://www.cdc.gov/nchs/nsfg.htm

Table 3.9 Lifetime Sexual Experience of Women Aged 15 to 44 by Education, 2002

(total number of women aged 15 to 44 and percent distribution by number of opposite-sex partners with whom they have had sexual intercourse during their lifetime, by education, 2002; numbers in thousands)

	total		number of opposite-sex partners in lifetime							
	number	percent	none	one	two	three	four	five	six to nine	10 or more
Total women aged 15 to 44	**61,561**	**100.0%**	**12.0%**	**21.7%**	**11.1%**	**9.7%**	**8.8%**	**8.2%**	**13.5%**	**15.0%**
Not a high school graduate	5,627	100.0	1.8	28.2	13.6	11.0	8.8	9.6	13.1	13.9
High school graduate or GED	14,264	100.0	1.1	18.6	11.6	9.6	10.1	10.3	17.5	21.3
Some college, no degree	14,279	100.0	2.7	20.6	10.4	11.4	10.6	9.6	14.8	19.9
Bachelor's degree or more	13,551	100.0	4.6	26.3	12.0	8.7	9.8	8.6	15.0	15.0

Note: Education categories include only people aged 22 to 44.
Source: National Center for Health Statistics, Fertility, Family Planning, and Reproductive Health of U.S. Women: Data from the 2002 National Survey of Family Growth, Vital and Health Statistics, Series 23, No. 25, 2005; Internet site http://www.cdc.gov/nchs/nsfg.htm

The Largest Share of Men Has Had Only One Sex Partner in the Past Year

Men aged 20 to 24 are most likely to have had two or more.

The average never-married man aged 15 to 44 has had 1.3 opposite-sex partners in the past year. The figure does not vary much by age among men aged 20 or older. Overall 22 percent of never-married men in the 15-to-44 age group are virgins, the figure ranging from 54 percent of those aged 15 to 19 to a low of 5 percent in the 40-to-44 age group.

Thirteen percent of never-married men in the 15-to-44 age group have had sexual intercourse in their lifetime, but not in the past year. Forty percent have had one sexual partner in the past year, and 25 percent have had two or more. The proportion of men with two or more partners peaks at 33 percent among 20-to-24-year-olds. By race, non-Hispanic white men had the greatest number of sexual partners in the past year, an average of 1.8. Hispanic men had the fewest, at 1.2.

■ Among never-married men, college graduates have less sexual experience than men with less education. Thirty-six percent of college graduates are virgins or have not had sex in the past year compared with a smaller 22 percent of high school graduates.

One in four never-married men has had more than one sex partner in the past year

(percent distribution of never-married men aged 15 to 44 by number of opposite-sex partners in past year, 2002)

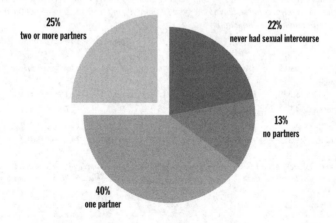

25%
two or more partners

22%
never had sexual intercourse

13%
no partners

40%
one partner

Table 3.10 Past Year Sexual Experience of Never-Married Men Aged 15 to 44 by Age, 2002

(number of never-married men aged 15 to 44 and percent distribution by number of opposite-sex partners with whom they have had sexual intercourse during the past 12 months, and average number of partners, by age, 2002; numbers in thousands)

	total		never had sexual intercourse	number of partners in past 12 months					average number
	number	total		none	one	two	three	four or more	
Never-married men aged 15 to 44	**35,340**	**100.0%**	**22.3%**	**12.8%**	**39.6%**	**12.1%**	**6.2%**	**7.0%**	**1.3**
Aged 15 to 19	10,166	100.0	54.2	6.3	21.5	10.6	3.9	3.5	0.7
Aged 20 to 24	8,366	100.0	14.9	8.3	43.6	15.2	8.7	9.3	1.6
Aged 25 to 29	5,048	100.0	7.7	15.3	50.7	12.0	6.3	8.1	1.4
Aged 30 to 34	3,991	100.0	7.9	15.3	49.9	11.5	4.5	11.0	1.6
Aged 35 to 39	3,636	100.0	6.3	23.9	44.4	12.0	7.0	6.3	1.5
Aged 40 to 44	4,133	100.0	4.8	23.1	48.3	9.9	7.4	6.6	1.3

Source: National Center for Health Statistics, Fertility, Contraception, and Fatherhood: Data on Men and Women from Cycle 6 of the 2002 National Survey of Family Growth, Vital and Health Statistics, Series 23, No. 26, 2006; Internet site http://www.cdc .gov/nchs/nsfg.htm

Table 3.11 Past Year Sexual Experience of Never-Married Men Aged 15 to 44 by Race and Hispanic Origin, 2002

(number of never-married men aged 15 to 44 and percent distribution by number of opposite-sex partners with whom they have had sexual intercourse during the past 12 months, and average number of partners, by race and Hispanic origin, 2002; numbers in thousands)

	total		never had sexual intercourse	number of partners in past 12 months					average number
	number	total		none	one	two	three	four or more	
Never-married men aged 15 to 44	**35,340**	**100.0%**	**22.3%**	**12.8%**	**39.6%**	**12.1%**	**6.2%**	**7.0%**	**1.3**
Black, non-Hispanic	4,753	100.0	17.4	11.1	44.3	12.0	8.1	7.2	1.4
Hispanic	5,839	100.0	24.9	12.5	39.6	12.1	5.0	5.9	1.2
White, non-Hispanic	21,555	100.0	14.3	9.7	38.8	14.2	10.2	12.8	1.8

Source: National Center for Health Statistics, Fertility, Contraception, and Fatherhood: Data on Men and Women from Cycle 6 of the 2002 National Survey of Family Growth, Vital and Health Statistics, Series 23, No. 26, 2006; Internet site http://www.cdc .gov/nchs/nsfg.htm

Table 3.12 Past Year Sexual Experience of Never-Married Men Aged 15 to 44 by Education, 2002

(number of never-married men aged 15 to 44 and percent distribution by number of opposite-sex partners with whom they have had sexual intercourse during the past 12 months, and average number of partners, by education, 2002; numbers in thousands)

| | total | | never had sexual intercourse | number of partners in past 12 months | | | | | average number |
	number	total		none	one	two	three three	four or more	
Never-married men aged 15 to 44	**35,340**	**100.0%**	**22.3%**	**12.8%**	**39.6%**	**12.1%**	**6.2%**	**7.0%**	**1.3**
Not a high school graduate	2,976	100.0	6.3	16.3	53.5	8.4	7.7	7.9	1.5
High school graduate or GED	7,225	100.0	7.7	14.5	53.0	11.4	5.1	8.4	1.5
Some college, no degree	6,717	100.0	6.9	16.1	44.2	14.1	10.1	8.6	1.5
Bachelor's degree or more	4,562	100.0	12.4	23.6	38.1	11.2	5.5	9.2	1.5

Note: Education categories include only people aged 22 to 44.
Source: National Center for Health Statistics, Fertility, Contraception, and Fatherhood: Data on Men and Women from Cycle 6 of the 2002 National Survey of Family Growth, Vital and Health Statistics, Series 23, No. 26, 2006; Internet site http://www.cdc .gov/nchs/nsfg.htm

Oral Sex Is Common

Few have had same-sex experiences.

Sexual activity is nearly universal among young and middle-aged adults. The percentage of people aged 15 to 44 who have had opposite-sex sexual contact in their lifetime ranges from about half of 15-to-17-year-olds to more than 90 percent of people aged 20 or older. More than 80 percent of 15-to-44-year-olds have had oral sex, and one-third have had anal sex. Six percent of men and 11 percent of women have had same-sex sexual contact. (The figure may be greater for women than men because the questions about same-sex contact were worded differently depending on the sex of the respondent.)

Among young adults, Hispanic women and non-Hispanic white men are the least sexually experienced. In the 15-to-24-age group, 24 percent of Hispanic women and 23 percent of non-Hispanic white men have never had sexual contact with another person, including intercourse, oral sex, anal sex, or a same-sex experience.

■ Slightly fewer than half (46 to 49 percent) of 15-to-17-year-olds have never had sexual contact with another person.

Men and women are about equally likely to engage in sexual activities

(percent of people aged 15 to 44 who have engaged in selected sexual activities with an opposite-sex partner in their lifetime, by sex, 2002)

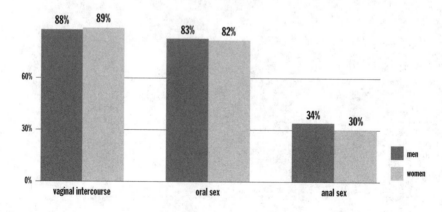

Table 3.13 Sexual Experience of Women Aged 15 to 24, 2002

(total number of women aged 15 to 24, and percent distribution by type of sexual contact ever experienced, by selected characteristics, 2002; numbers in thousands)

| | total | | opposite-sex sexual contact | | | | | | any sexual experience with female | no sexual contact with another person |
| | | | | | oral | | | | | |
	number	percent	any	vaginal intercourse	any oral	gave	received	anal		
Total women aged 15 to 24	**19,674**	**100.0%**	**77.3%**	**70.2%**	**68.6%**	**59.8%**	**64.9%**	**20.3%**	**12.4%**	**21.9%**
Aged 15 to 19	9,834	100.0	63.3	53.0	54.3	43.6	49.6	10.9	10.6	35.5
Aged 15 to 17	5,819	100.0	49.8	38.7	42.0	30.4	38.0	5.6	8.4	48.6
Aged 18 to 19	4,015	100.0	82.9	73.8	72.3	62.7	66.7	18.7	13.8	16.5
Aged 20 to 24	9,840	100.0	91.3	87.3	83.1	76.3	80.3	29.6	14.2	8.2
Aged 20 to 21	4,005	100.0	86.4	80.7	80.6	74.2	77.6	26.0	13.0	12.4
Aged 22 to 24	5,834	100.0	94.7	91.9	84.9	77.7	82.1	32.1	15.0	5.3
Race and Hispanic origin										
Black, non-Hispanic	2,805	100.0	80.3	75.9	67.5	42.3	65.6	14.7	10.2	18.6
Hispanic	3,153	100.0	75.3	70.2	59.8	49.9	54.5	16.9	9.1	23.5
White, non-Hispanic	12,007	100.0	77.9	69.6	73.3	68.2	69.9	23.5	14.2	21.4

Note: The questions about same-sex sexual contact in the National Survey of Family Growth were worded differently for men and women. Women were asked whether they had ever had a sexual experience of any kind with another female. Men were asked whether they had performed any of four specific sexual acts with another male. The question asked of women may have elicited more "yes" answers than the questions asked of men.

Source: National Center for Health Statistics, Sexual Behavior and Selected Health Measures: Men and Women 15–44 Years of Age, United States, 2002, Advance Data, No. 362, 2005; Internet site http://www.cdc.gov/nchs/nsfg.htm

Table 3.14 Sexual Experience of Men Aged 15 to 24, 2002

(total number of men aged 15 to 24, and percent distribution by type of sexual contact ever experienced, by selected characteristics, 2002; numbers in thousands)

| | total | | opposite-sex sexual contact | | | | | | any sexual experience with male | no sexual contact with another person |
	number	percent	any	vaginal intercourse	any oral	gave	received	anal		
						oral				
Total men aged 15 to 24	**20,091**	**100.0%**	**77.4%**	**68.1%**	**68.5%**	**55.4%**	**65.6%**	**21.7%**	**5.0%**	**21.9%**
Aged 15 to 19	10,208	100.0	63.9	49.1	55.2	38.8	51.5	11.2	4.5	35.4
Aged 15 to 17	5,748	100.0	53.2	36.3	44.0	28.2	40.3	8.1	3.9	46.1
Aged 18 to 19	4,460	100.0	77.7	65.5	69.5	52.4	66.0	15.2	5.1	21.6
Aged 20 to 24	9,883	100.0	91.4	87.6	82.3	72.5	80.0	32.6	5.5	7.9
Aged 20 to 21	3,921	100.0	90.4	85.5	83.2	72.5	80.2	30.6	2.7	9.0
Aged 22 to 24	5,963	100.0	92.1	89.0	81.7	72.6	80.0	34.0	7.4	7.2
Race and Hispanic origin										
Black, non-Hispanic	2,550	100.0	83.5	76.9	68.5	37.7	67.8	24.5	5.7	15.4
Hispanic	3,579	100.0	82.9	77.7	66.6	53.3	63.2	28.4	5.4	16.5
White, non-Hispanic	12,311	100.0	76.5	64.9	70.7	61.0	67.7	19.6	4.6	22.8

Note: The questions about same-sex sexual contact in the National Survey of Family Growth were worded differently for men and women. Women were asked whether they had ever had a sexual experience of any kind with another female. Men were asked whether they had performed any of four specific sexual acts with another male. The question asked of women may have elicited more "yes" answers than the questions asked of men.
Source: National Center for Health Statistics, Sexual Behavior and Selected Health Measures: Men and Women 15–44 Years of Age, United States, 2002, Advance Data, No. 362, 2005; Internet site http://www.cdc.gov/nchs/nsfg.htm

Table 3.15 Sexual Experience of Women Aged 15 to 44, 2002

(total number of women aged 15 to 44, and percent distribution by type of sexual contact ever experienced, by selected characteristics, 2002; numbers in thousands)

	total		opposite-sex sexual contact				any same-sex sexual contact
	number	percent	any	vaginal intercourse	oral sex	anal sex	
Total women aged 15 to 44	**61,561**	**100.0%**	**91.7%**	**89.2%**	**82.0%**	**30.0%**	**11.2%**
Aged 15 to 19	9,834	100.0	63.3	53.0	54.3	10.9	10.6
Aged 20 to 24	9,840	100.0	91.3	87.3	83.0	29.6	14.2
Aged 25 to 29	9,249	100.0	97.5	97.2	87.8	32.8	14.1
Aged 30 to 34	10,272	100.0	98.2	98.1	89.3	37.8	9.1
Aged 35 to 39	10,853	100.0	99.0	98.7	88.2	34.3	12.3
Aged 40 to 44	11,512	100.0	98.7	98.6	88.0	33.8	7.8
Race and Hispanic origin							
Black, non-Hispanic	8,250	100.0	92.7	91.0	74.8	21.5	10.6
Hispanic	9,107	100.0	90.1	88.1	68.4	22.7	6.5
White, non-Hispanic	39,498	100.0	92.4	89.7	87.9	34.2	12.6
Marital status							
Currently married	28,327	100.0	100.0	100.0	89.9	32.2	7.2
Currently cohabiting	5,570	100.0	100.0	100.0	89.9	41.6	17.6
Never married, not cohabiting	21,568	100.0	76.2	69.2	67.0	20.0	13.5
Formerly married, not cohabiting	6,096	100.0	100.0	100.0	91.2	45.2	16.3

Source: National Center for Health Statistics, Sexual Behavior and Selected Health Measures: Men and Women 15–44 Years of Age, United States, 2002, Advance Data, No. 362, 2005; Internet site http://www.cdc.gov/nchs/nsfg.htm

Table 3.16   Sexual Experience of Men Aged 15 to 44, 2002

(total number of men aged 15 to 44, and percent distribution by type of sexual contact ever experienced, by selected characteristics, 2002; numbers in thousands)

| | total | | opposite-sex sexual contact | | | | any same-sex sexual contact |
	number	percent	any	vaginal intercourse	oral sex	anal sex	
Total men aged 15 to 44	**61,147**	**100.0%**	**90.8%**	**87.6%**	**83.0%**	**34.0%**	**6.0%**
Aged 15 to 19	10,208	100.0	63.9	49.1	55.1	11.2	4.5
Aged 20 to 24	9,883	100.0	91.4	87.6	82.2	32.6	5.5
Aged 25 to 29	9,226	100.0	95.3	95.3	88.7	36.5	5.7
Aged 30 to 34	10,138	100.0	97.4	96.9	90.3	41.1	6.2
Aged 35 to 39	10,557	100.0	98.2	98.1	91.1	42.1	8.0
Aged 40 to 44	11,135	100.0	98.3	98.1	90.3	39.9	6.0
Race and Hispanic origin							
Black, non-Hispanic	6,940	100.0	92.4	90.3	78.6	30.8	5.0
Hispanic	10,188	100.0	92.3	90.5	74.4	32.7	6.2
White, non-Hispanic	38,738	100.0	90.7	86.8	87.3	35.2	6.5
Marital status							
Currently married	25,808	100.0	100	100.0	91.6	38.4	3.4
Currently cohabiting	5,653	100.0	100	100.0	92.7	45.2	5.3
Never married, not cohabiting	25,412	100.0	77.9	70.0	70.1	23.8	8.6
Formerly married, not cohabiting	4,274	100.0	100	100.0	95.1	53.7	7.1

Source: National Center for Health Statistics, Sexual Behavior and Selected Health Measures: Men and Women 15–44 Years of Age, United States, 2002, Advance Data, No. 362, 2005; Internet site http://www.cdc.gov/nchs/nsfg.htm

Most Men Have a Long-Term Relationship with Their Sex Partner

Few say their last sexual partner was just a friend.

Most men are in a committed relationship with their sexual partner. Among men aged 15 to 44 who have had sexual intercourse in the past three months, the 57 percent majority is married to their partner. Another 32 percent are living with or going steady with their partner. Fewer than 10 percent say they and their last sexual partner were "just friends" or only going out once in a while.

Teenagers are most likely to have had only a casual relationship with their last sexual partner. Fourteen percent of men aged 15 to 19 say they and their last sexual partner were "just friends." Even among teens, however, most are in a committed relationship with their sex partner. Sixty-two percent of men aged 15 to 19 say they were going steady with their last sex partner.

■ Fundamentalist Protestants are just as likely as men raised without a religion to say their last sex partner was "just a friend."

Nearly 90 percent of men are in a committed relationship with their sex partner

(percent distribution of men aged 15 to 44 who have had sexual intercourse in the past three months, by relationship with last sexual partner, 2002)

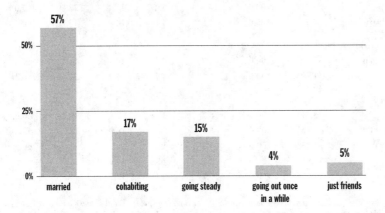

Table 3.17 Relationship between Men Aged 15 to 44 and Last Sexual Partner, 2002

(number of men aged 15 to 44 who have had sexual intercourse in the past three months and percent distribution by relationship with last sexual partner, by selected characteristics, 2002; numbers in thousands)

Men aged 15 to 44 who had sexual intercourse in past three months	total number	percent	just friends	going out once in a while	going steady	cohabiting	married	other
	43,599	100.0%	5.2%	4.3%	15.0%	17.2%	56.9%	1.4%
Age								
Aged 15 to 19	3,234	100.0	14.1	9.1	61.8	9.6	1.3	4.2
Aged 20 to 24	6,828	100.0	8.6	6.5	31.6	28.9	22.7	1.8
Aged 25 to 29	7,292	100.0	3.4	3.5	10.9	26.1	54.7	1.4
Aged 30 to 34	8,634	100.0	4.7	3.5	6.7	14.8	69.3	1.0
Aged 35 to 39	8,713	100.0	1.8	2.8	5.7	13.6	75.4	0.8
Aged 40 to 44	8,898	100.0	4.8	4.0	6.9	9.8	73.6	1.0
Age at first sexual intercourse								
Under age 16	14,880	100.0	8.1	4.6	16.1	22.8	46.3	2.1
Aged 16	7,636	100.0	5.9	5.3	16.8	18.0	53.2	0.9
Aged 17	6,988	100.0	3.1	6.0	16.9	16.7	56.1	1.2
Aged 18	4,676	100.0	3.6	4.5	18.7	15.5	56.8	–
Aged 19	2,158	100.0	5.6	3.4	12.2	16.6	61.5	–
Aged 20 or older	7,260	100.0	1.4	1.3	7.8	6.9	81.7	0.9
Race and Hispanic origin								
Black, non-Hispanic	5,221	100.0	8.6	3.8	23.2	21.8	40.9	1.7
Hispanic	7,549	100.0	4.7	6.2	11.4	22.4	53.0	2.3
White, non-Hispanic	27,552	100.0	4.8	4.1	14.7	14.7	60.7	1.0
Family structure at age 14								
Living with both parents	31,895	100.0	4.7	4.2	14.7	15.7	59.3	1.5
Other	11,704	100.0	6.5	4.7	15.9	21.6	50.1	1.1
Religion raised								
None	3,511	100.0	8.2	3.8	22.6	18.3	46.2	–
Fundamentalist Protestant	1,950	100.0	8.1	5.5	14.0	18.0	52.5	1.9
Other Protestant	19,433	100.0	5.2	3.7	14.1	15.2	60.9	1.0
Catholic	15,823	100.0	4.1	4.9	14.9	19.7	54.5	1.9
Other religion	2,775	100.0	5.7	5.8	12.5	15.6	59.4	–

Note: "Other" includes "just met" and other relationships. "–" means sample is too small to make a reliable estimate.
Source: National Center for Health Statistics, Fertility, Contraception, and Fatherhood: Data on Men and Women from Cycle 6 of the 2002 National Survey of Family Growth, Vital and Health Statistics, Series 23, No. 26, 2006; Internet site http://www.cdc.gov/nchs/nsfg.htm

Some Men Have Been Forced to Have Sex

The younger the age of the male at first sexual intercourse, the more likely he has ever been forced to have sex.

Women are not the only gender vulnerable to sexual predation. Men as well as women can be forced to have sex. Among men aged 18 to 44, a substantial 8 percent say they were forced to have sexual intercourse at some point in their life. Six percent were forced by a female to have sex, and 2 percent were forced to have sex by a male.

Men who first had sexual intercourse at age 14 or younger are most likely to have been forced to have sex at some point in their life. Fifteen percent of men aged 18 to 44 who first had sex at age 14 or younger have been forced to have sex. Among black men, 18 percent have been forced to have sex at some point in their life.

■ Among men forced to have sex, the largest share were pressured into it without threats of harm.

Blacks are most likely to report being forced to have sexual intercourse

(percent of men aged 18 to 44 who have ever been forced to have sexual intercourse, by race and Hispanic origin, 2002)

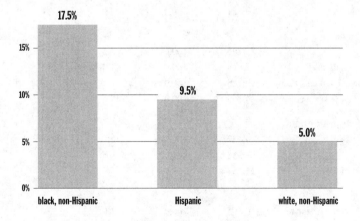

Table 3.18 Men Ever Forced to Have Sexual Intercourse, 2002

(total number of men aged 18 to 44, and percent ever forced to have sexual intercourse by a female or male, by selected characteristics, 2002; numbers in thousands)

	total		percent ever forced to have sexual intercourse		
	number	percent	total	by a female	by a male
Total men aged 18 to 44	**55,399**	**100.0%**	**7.6%**	**5.8%**	**2.0%**
Age					
Aged 18 to 19	4,460	100.0	4.2	3.7	0.8
Aged 20 to 24	9,883	100.0	9.0	7.4	1.7
Aged 25 to 29	9,226	100.0	8.7	6.2	2.9
Aged 30 to 34	10,138	100.0	6.8	5.2	2.1
Aged 35 to 39	10,557	100.0	8.6	6.6	2.1
Aged 40 to 44	11,135	100.0	6.4	4.7	1.7
Age at first sexual intercourse					
Never had sexual intercourse with female	3,956	100.0	3.0	0.0	3.0
Under age 15	9,378	100.0	14.5	11.9	3.5
Aged 15	6,952	100.0	7.9	6.4	1.8
Aged 16	9,002	100.0	7.0	5.1	1.9
Aged 17	8,161	100.0	9.0	7.7	1.3
Aged 18	5,890	100.0	5.5	4.2	1.3
Aged 19	2,938	100.0	4.1	3.4	–
Aged 20 or older	9,121	100.0	3.9	2.6	1.5
Marital status					
Currently married	25,795	100.0	5.3	4.6	0.7
Currently cohabiting	5,614	100.0	11.4	10.1	2.0
Never married, not cohabiting	19,725	100.0	9.1	5.8	3.5
Formerly married, not cohabiting	4,265	100.0	9.6	7.5	2.5
Race and Hispanic origin					
Black, non-Hispanic	6,127	100.0	17.5	15.1	2.8
Hispanic	9,336	100.0	9.5	7.9	2.0
White, non-Hispanic	35,154	100.0	5.0	3.4	1.8
Education					
Not a high school graduate	6,355	100.0	5.9	3.2	2.7
High school graduate or GED	15,659	100.0	8.3	6.6	2.0
Some college, no degree	13,104	100.0	11.5	9.3	2.5
Bachelor's degree or more	11,901	100.0	4.1	2.4	1.8

Note: Education categories include only people aged 22 to 44. "–" means sample is too small to make a reliable estimate.
Source: National Center for Health Statistics, Fertility, Contraception, and Fatherhood: Data on Men and Women from Cycle 6 of the 2002 National Survey of Family Growth, Vital and Health Statistics, Series 23, No. 26, 2006; Internet site http://www.cdc .gov/nchs/nsfg.htm

Table 3.19 Men Ever Forced to Have Sexual Intercourse by Type of Force Used, 2002

(percent of men aged 18 to 44 ever forced to have sexual intercourse by type of force used, 2002)

	men ever forced to have sexual intercourse		
	total	by a female	by a male
Men aged 18 to 44 ever forced to have sexual intercourse	**7.6%**	**5.8%**	**2.0%**
Pressured into it by her/his words or actions, but without threats of harm	5.2	4.1	1.3
Did what she/he said because she/he was bigger or grownup, and you were young	3.3	2.0	1.4
Given alcohol or drugs	2.4	2.0	0.5
Physically held down	2.4	1.7	0.7
Told that the relationship would end if you didn't have sex	1.6	1.4	0.3
Threatened with physical harm or injury	1.0	0.4	0.6
Physically hurt or injured	0.8	0.3	0.4

Source: National Center for Health Statistics, Fertility, Contraception, and Fatherhood: Data on Men and Women from Cycle 6 of the 2002 National Survey of Family Growth, Vital and Health Statistics, Series 23, No. 26, 2006; Internet site http://www.cdc .gov/nchs/nsfg.htm

Most Think It Is OK for Unmarried Adults to Have Sex

Most of those for whom religion is "very important" disapprove, however.

Americans think premarital sex is OK, within limits. Among 15-to-44-year-olds, 60 percent of men and 51 percent of women agree that premarital sex between unmarried 18–year-olds is all right. But only 20 percent of men and 13 percent of women say premarital sex is OK between 16-year-olds. Tolerance toward premarital sex tends to fall with age. Only 40 percent of women aged 35 to 44 think premarital sex between 18-year-olds is OK.

The younger the age at first sexual intercourse, the greater the tolerance for premarital sex. Among women aged 15 to 44 who first had sex before age 18, the 60 percent majority say premarital sex between 18-year-olds is OK. But among those who first had sex at ages 18 or older, only 40 percent say it is OK.

Religion plays a big role in attitudes toward premarital sex. Among people with no religion, 74 to 79 percent say premarital sex between 18-year-olds is OK. But among fundamentalist Protestants, only 29 to 34 percent approve.

■ Regardless of religion, a minority thinks premarital sex between 16-year-olds is all right.

Women for whom religion is very important are against premarital sex

(percent of women aged 15 to 44 who agree with the statement, "It is all right for unmarried 18-year-olds to have sexual relations if they have strong affection for one another," by importance of religion, 2002)

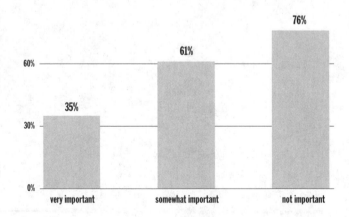

Table 3.20 Attitudes of People Aged 15 to 44 toward Sexual Activity by Age and Sex, 2002

(percent of people aged 15 to 44 agreeing with statement, by age and sex, 2002)

	percent agreeing	
	men	women
"It is all right for unmarried 18-year-olds to have sexual relations if they have strong affection for one another."		
Total aged 15 to 44	**59.7%**	**50.6%**
Aged 15 to 19	65.0	60.9
Aged 20 to 24	70.7	60.5
Aged 25 to 29	64.0	55.9
Aged 30 to 34	56.8	49.3
Aged 35 to 39	50.5	40.4
Aged 40 to 44	53.0	40.1
"It is all right for unmarried 16-year-olds to have sexual relations if they have strong affection for one another."		
Total aged 15 to 44	**19.9**	**13.4**
Aged 15 to 19	35.7	30.5
Aged 20 to 24	28.0	18.8
Aged 25 to 29	24.2	13.3
Aged 30 to 34	15.1	9.7
Aged 35 to 39	9.4	6.7
Aged 40 to 44	9.0	3.9

Source: National Center for Health Statistics, Fertility, Contraception, and Fatherhood: Data on Men and Women from Cycle 6 of the 2002 National Survey of Family Growth, Vital and Health Statistics, Series 23, No. 26, 2006; Internet site http://www.cdc .gov/nchs/nsfg.htm

Table 3.21 Attitudes of People Aged 15 to 44 toward Sexual Activity by Age at First Sexual Intercourse and Sex, 2002

(percent of people aged 15 to 44 agreeing with statement, by age at first sexual intercourse and sex, 2002)

	percent agreeing	
	men	women
"It is all right for unmarried 18-year-olds to have sexual relations if they have strong affection for one another."		
Total aged 15 to 44	**59.7%**	**50.6%**
Never had sexual intercourse	44.0	37.4
Had first sexual intercourse under age 18	67.6	60.1
Had first sexual intercourse at age 18 or older	51.3	40.4
"It is all right for unmarried 16-year-olds to have sexual relations if they have strong affection for one another."		
Total aged 15 to 44	**19.9**	**13.4**
Never had sexual intercourse	18.0	13.4
Had first sexual intercourse under age 18	28.0	22.1
Had first sexual intercourse at age 18 or older	16.3	9.9

Source: National Center for Health Statistics, Fertility, Contraception, and Fatherhood: Data on Men and Women from Cycle 6 of the 2002 National Survey of Family Growth, Vital and Health Statistics, Series 23, No. 26, 2006; Internet site http://www.cdc.gov/nchs/nsfg.htm

Table 3.22 Attitudes of People Aged 15 to 44 toward Sexual Activity by Marital Status and Sex, 2002

(percent of people aged 15 to 44 agreeing with statement, by marital status and sex, 2002)

	percent agreeing	
	men	women
"It is all right for unmarried 18-year-olds to have sexual relations if they have strong affection for one another."		
Total aged 15 to 44	**59.7%**	**50.6%**
Currently married	47.8	43.4
Currently cohabiting	76.0	67.6
Never married, not cohabiting	68.6	57.2
Formerly married, not cohabiting	57.7	45.1
"It is all right for unmarried 16-year-olds to have sexual relations if they have strong affection for one another."		
Total aged 15 to 44	**19.9**	**13.4**
Currently married	9.8	7.7
Currently cohabiting	20.1	20.2
Never married, not cohabiting	31.0	21.2
Formerly married, not cohabiting	14.2	6.0

Source: National Center for Health Statistics, Fertility, Contraception, and Fatherhood: Data on Men and Women from Cycle 6 of the 2002 National Survey of Family Growth, Vital and Health Statistics, Series 23, No. 26, 2006; Internet site http://www.cdc .gov/nchs/nsfg.htm

Table 3.23 Attitudes of People Aged 15 to 44 toward Sexual Activity by Current Religion and Sex, 2002

(percent of people aged 15 to 44 agreeing with statement, by current religion, importance of religion, and sex, 2002)

	percent agreeing	
	men	women
"It is all right for unmarried 18-year-olds to have sexual relations if they have strong affection for one another."		
Total aged 15 to 44	**59.7%**	**50.6%**
Current religion		
No religion	78.5	74.3
Fundamentalist Protestant	33.7	28.9
Other Protestant	49.0	42.5
Catholic	67.6	54.0
Other religion	55.8	63.2
Importance of religion		
Very important	39.4	34.5
Somewhat important	67.4	61.1
Not important	78.3	76.1
"It is all right for unmarried 16-year-olds to have sexual relations if they have strong affection for one another."		
Total aged 15 to 44	**19.9**	**13.4**
Current religion		
No religion	34.2	22.6
Fundamentalist Protestant	5.3	8.8
Other Protestant	14.9	10.0
Catholic	19.4	12.8
Other religion	20.7	24.6
Importance of religion		
Very important	11.2	7.1
Somewhat important	20.6	16.3
Not important	30.7	24.6

Source: National Center for Health Statistics, Fertility, Contraception, and Fatherhood: Data on Men and Women from Cycle 6 of the 2002 National Survey of Family Growth, Vital and Health Statistics, Series 23, No. 26, 2006; Internet site http://www.cdc.gov/nchs/nsfg.htm

Sexual Orientation

■ How many Americans are homosexual? Researchers have been trying to answer that question for years. The answer is elusive because some will not reveal their orientation and others are not sure.

■ Few say they are homosexual. When asked to identify their sexual orientation, 90 percent of men and women aged 18 to 44 say they are heterosexual. Only 2 percent of men and 1 percent of women say they are homosexual.

■ Most Americans say they are attracted only to the opposite sex. Ninety-two percent of men and 86 percent of women say they are attracted only to the opposite sex.

■ Homosexual experiences are not uncommon. Six percent of men and 11 percent of women aged 15 to 44 say they have engaged in sexual activity with a same-sex partner in their lifetime.

■ Sexually transmitted infections are commonplace. Homosexual women are least likely to have had a sexually transmitted infection. Homosexual men are most likely to have had an infection.

■ Americans are ambivalent about adoption by gays and lesbians. Among women aged 15 to 44, the 55 percent majority thinks they should have the right to adopt. Among men, a smaller 47 percent agree.

Only 2 Percent of Men Say They Are Homosexual

Among women, the proportion is just 1 percent.

When asked to identify their sexual orientation, 90 percent of men and women aged 18 to 44 say they are heterosexual. Four percent of men and women identify themselves as homosexual or bisexual. Another 4 percent say they are "something else," which may indicate that some respondents did not understand the terminology.

Self-identification as homosexual or bisexual does not vary much by age, race, or Hispanic origin. It is slightly more common in metropolitan areas than in nonmetropolitan areas. Among men who have ever had a sexual experience with another male, 43 percent identify themselves as homosexual or bisexual. Among women with a same-sex experience, the figure is 28 percent.

■ The incidence of homosexuality is probably greater than these numbers suggest because some are hesitant to identify their sexual orientation, even on a confidential government survey.

The proportion of men who say they are homosexual peaks at 5 percent among the never-married.

(percent of men aged 18 to 44 who identify themselves as homosexual, by marital status, 2002)

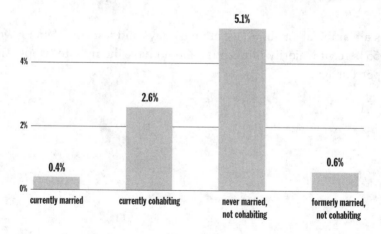

Table 4.1 Sexual Orientation by Sex and Age, 2002

(number of people aged 18 to 44 and percent distribution by sexual orientation, by sex and age, 2002; numbers in thousands)

	total		sexual orientation				
	number	percent	heterosexual	homosexual	bisexual	something else	did not report
Total men aged 18 to 44	**55,399**	**100.0%**	**90.2%**	**2.3%**	**1.8%**	**3.9%**	**1.8%**
Aged 18 to 19	4,460	100.0	91.3	1.7	1.4	3.5	2.1
Aged 20 to 24	9,883	100.0	91.0	2.3	2.0	3.5	1.3
Aged 25 to 29	9,226	100.0	87.3	2.8	0.9	5.7	3.3
Aged 30 to 34	10,138	100.0	91.1	2.0	1.7	4.0	1.2
Aged 35 to 44	21,692	100.0	90.3	2.4	2.2	3.5	1.6
Total women aged 18 to 44	**55,742**	**100.0**	**90.3**	**1.3**	**2.8**	**3.8**	**1.8**
Aged 18 to 19	4,015	100.0	84.2	0.9	7.4	5.7	1.9
Aged 20 to 24	9,840	100.0	90.0	0.8	3.5	4.4	1.3
Aged 25 to 29	9,249	100.0	89.9	1.5	2.8	2.8	3.1
Aged 30 to 34	10,272	100.0	91.2	1.3	2.1	3.8	1.6
Aged 35 to 44	22,365	100.0	91.4	1.5	2.0	3.5	1.6

Source: National Center for Health Statistics, Sexual Behavior and Selected Health Measures: Men and Women 15–44 Years of Age, United States, 2002, Advance Data, No. 362, 2005; Internet site http://www.cdc.gov/nchs/nsfg.htm

Table 4.2 Sexual Orientation by Sex and Marital Status, 2002

(number of people aged 18 to 44 and percent distribution by sexual orientation, by sex and marital status, 2002; numbers in thousands)

	total		sexual orientation				
	number	percent	heterosexual	homosexual	bisexual	something else	did not report
Total men aged 18 to 44	**55,399**	**100.0%**	**90.2%**	**2.3%**	**1.8%**	**3.9%**	**1.8%**
Currently married	25,795	100.0	93.8	0.4	1.3	3.1	1.5
Currently cohabiting	5,614	100.0	86.6	2.6	0.4	8.5	1.9
Never married, not cohabiting	19,725	100.0	86.4	5.1	2.7	3.9	1.9
Formerly married, not cohabiting	4,265	100.0	90.6	0.6	2.7	2.8	3.3
Total women aged 18 to 44	**55,742**	**100.0**	**90.3**	**1.3**	**2.8**	**3.8**	**1.8**
Currently married	28,323	100.0	93.5	0.8	1.3	2.9	1.5
Currently cohabiting	5,452	100.0	85.8	0.4	4.9	6.5	2.4
Never married, not cohabiting	15,871	100.0	87.1	2.5	4.0	4.2	2.3
Formerly married, not cohabiting	6,096	100.0	88.2	1.4	4.8	4.5	1.2

Source: National Center for Health Statistics, Sexual Behavior and Selected Health Measures: Men and Women 15–44 Years of Age, United States, 2002, Advance Data, No. 362, 2005; Internet site http://www.cdc.gov/nchs/nsfg.htm

Table 4.3 Sexual Orientation by Sex, Race, and Hispanic Origin, 2002

(number of people aged 18 to 44 and percent distribution by sexual orientation, by sex, race, and Hispanic origin, 2002; numbers in thousands)

	total		sexual orientation				
	number	percent	heterosexual	homosexual	bisexual	something else	did not report
Total men aged 18 to 44	**55,399**	**100.0%**	**90.2%**	**2.3%**	**1.8%**	**3.9%**	**1.8%**
Black, non-Hispanic	6,127	100.0	86.0	1.6	1.7	7.5	3.2
Hispanic	9,336	100.0	85.3	2.1	1.7	7.3	3.5
White, non-Hispanic	35,154	100.0	92.5	2.6	1.8	2.3	0.7
Total women aged 18 to 44	**55,742**	**100.0**	**90.3**	**1.3**	**2.8**	**3.8**	**1.8**
Black, non-Hispanic	7,399	100.0	87.1	1.5	2.9	6.5	2.0
Hispanic	8,194	100.0	87.5	0.8	1.5	6.1	4.1
White, non-Hispanic	35,936	100.0	92.3	1.3	3.0	2.3	1.2

Source: National Center for Health Statistics, Sexual Behavior and Selected Health Measures: Men and Women 15–44 Years of Age, United States, 2002, Advance Data, No. 362, 2005; Internet site http://www.cdc.gov/nchs/nsfg.htm

Table 4.4   Sexual Orientation by Sex and Metropolitan Residence, 2002

(number of people aged 18 to 44 and percent distribution by sexual orientation, by sex and metropolitan residence, 2002; numbers in thousands)

	total		sexual orientation				
	number	percent	heterosexual	homosexual	bisexual	something else	did not report
Total men aged 18 to 44	**55,399**	**100.0%**	**90.2%**	**2.3%**	**1.8%**	**3.9%**	**1.8%**
Central city of 12 largest metropolitan areas	7,713	100.0	86.3	3.0	2.7	5.6	2.5
Central city of other metropolitan areas	13,067	100.0	87.8	3.9	2.1	4.4	1.7
Suburb of 12 largest metropolitan areas	12,397	100.0	93.7	1.6	1.1	1.9	1.7
Suburb of other metropolitan areas	11,895	100.0	91.9	1.9	0.8	3.9	1.4
Nonmetropolitan area	10,326	100.0	89.7	1.0	2.8	4.5	2.0
Total women aged 18 to 44	**55,742**	**100.0**	**90.3**	**1.3**	**2.8**	**3.8**	**1.8**
Central city of 12 largest metropolitan areas	7,671	100.0	86.4	2.1	3.7	5.7	2.1
Central city of other metropolitan areas	13,017	100.0	89.5	1.1	3.2	3.5	2.6
Suburb of 12 largest metropolitan areas	12,599	100.0	92.1	1.9	2.4	2.0	1.7
Suburb of other metropolitan areas	12,863	100.0	92.4	0.8	2.6	3.4	0.8
Nonmetropolitan area	9,593	100.0	89.5	0.8	2.4	5.5	1.9

Source: National Center for Health Statistics, Sexual Behavior and Selected Health Measures: Men and Women 15–44 Years of Age, United States, 2002, Advance Data, No. 362, 2005; Internet site http://www.cdc.gov/nchs/nsfg.htm

Table 4.5 Sexual Orientation by Sex and Number of Opposite-Sex Partners, 2002

(number of people aged 18 to 44 and percent distribution by sexual orientation, by sex and number of opposite-sex partners, 2002; numbers in thousands)

	total		sexual orientation				
	number	percent	heterosexual	homosexual	bisexual	something else	did not report
Total men aged 18 to 44	**55,399**	**100.0%**	**90.2%**	**2.3%**	**1.8%**	**3.9%**	**1.8%**
No opposite-sex partners	4,243	100.0	74.5	9.7	1.5	7.3	7.1
One	6,211	100.0	90.5	3.2	1.9	3.4	1.1
Two to four	12,481	100.0	90.3	2.4	2.1	3.9	1.3
Five or more	30,853	100.0	92.1	1.1	1.7	3.8	1.4
Total women aged 18 to 44	**55,742**	**100.0**	**90.3**	**1.3**	**2.8**	**3.8**	**1.8**
No opposite-sex partners	3,175	100.0	79.6	3.5	1.2	6.0	9.7
One	11,941	100.0	91.8	1.9	0.8	3.5	2.1
Two to four	16,648	100.0	91.2	1.2	2.7	3.8	1.2
Five or more	23,038	100.0	90.9	0.8	4.0	3.6	0.7

Source: National Center for Health Statistics, Sexual Behavior and Selected Health Measures: Men and Women 15–44 Years of Age, United States, 2002, Advance Data, No. 362, 2005; Internet site http://www.cdc.gov/nchs/nsfg.htm

Table 4.6 Sexual Orientation by Sex, Sexual Attraction, and Sexual Experience, 2002

(number of people aged 18 to 44 and percent distribution by sexual orientation, by sex, sexual attraction, and sexual experience, 2002; numbers in thousands)

	total		sexual orientation				
	number	percent	heterosexual	homosexual	bisexual	something else	did not report
TOTAL MEN AGED 18 TO 44	**55,399**	**100.0%**	**90.2%**	**2.3%**	**1.8%**	**3.9%**	**1.8%**
Sexual attraction							
Only to opposite sex	50,846	100.0	91.3	1.7	1.4	3.5	2.1
Mostly to opposite sex	2,126	100.0	91.0	2.3	2.0	3.5	1.3
All other	2,375	100.0	87.3	2.8	0.9	5.7	3.3
Ever had sexual experience with male							
No	51,914	100.0	92.9	0.7	0.9	3.7	1.9
Yes	3,433	100.0	49.1	26.9	16.1	7.0	1.0
TOTAL WOMEN AGED 18 TO 44	**55,742**	**100.0**	**90.3**	**1.3**	**2.8**	**3.8**	**1.8**
Sexual attraction							
Only to opposite sex	47,431	100.0	84.2	0.9	7.4	5.7	1.9
Mostly to opposite sex	5,617	100.0	90.0	0.8	3.5	4.4	1.3
All other	2,635	100.0	89.9	1.5	2.8	2.8	3.1
Ever had sexual experience with female							
No	49,268	100.0	93.6	0.5	0.5	3.5	1.8
Yes	6,415	100.0	65.1	7.3	20.2	5.9	1.5

Source: National Center for Health Statistics, Sexual Behavior and Selected Health Measures: Men and Women 15–44 Years of Age, United States, 2002, Advance Data, No. 362, 2005; Internet site http://www.cdc.gov/nchs/nsfg.htm

More than Nine out of Ten Men Are Attracted Only to the Opposite Sex

Among women, the proportion is slightly lower.

Few men and women say they are attracted to same-sex partners. Only 1.5 to 2.2 percent of men and women aged 18 to 44 say they are attracted mostly or only to the same sex. Another 1 to 2 percent say they are attracted to both sexes. Four percent of men and 10 percent of women say they are attracted mostly to the opposite sex. Ninety-two percent of men and 86 percent of women say they are attracted only to the opposite sex.

Those who have never married and are not cohabiting are most likely to say they are attracted to same-sex partners. Seven percent of never-married men and 5 percent of never-married women are attracted to both sexes, mostly the same sex, or only the same sex.

■ Sexual attraction appears not to be an either-or situation, with a substantial percentage of Americans having some attraction to the opposite sex.

Many men who have had a sexual experience with another man say they are attracted only to the opposite sex

(percent distribution of men aged 18 to 44 who have ever had a sexual experience with a male, by sexual attraction, 2002)

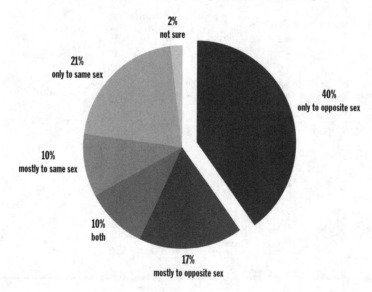

2%
not sure

21%
only to same sex

10%
mostly to same sex

10%
both

17%
mostly to opposite sex

40%
only to opposite sex

Table 4.7 Sexual Attraction by Sex and Age, 2002

(number of people aged 18 to 44 and percent distribution by sexual attraction, by sex and age, 2002; numbers in thousands)

	total		sexual attraction					
	number	percent	only opposite sex	mostly opposite sex	both	mostly same sex	only same sex	not sure
Total men aged 18 to 44	**55,399**	**100.0%**	**92.2%**	**3.9%**	**1.0%**	**0.7%**	**1.5%**	**0.7%**
Aged 18 to 19	4,460	100.0	93.8	3.4	1.7	–	–	–
Aged 20 to 24	9,883	100.0	91.2	5.0	0.7	0.8	1.3	1.0
Aged 25 to 29	9,226	100.0	92.6	3.7	0.8	0.9	1.3	0.9
Aged 30 to 34	10,138	100.0	92.5	3.8	0.6	0.5	2.0	0.6
Aged 35 to 44	21,692	100.0	92.1	3.5	1.3	0.7	1.8	0.6
Total women aged 18 to 44	**55,742**	**100.0**	**85.7**	**10.2**	**1.9**	**0.8**	**0.7**	**0.8**
Aged 18 to 19	4,015	100.0	80.1	12.8	4.9	–	–	0.8
Aged 20 to 24	9,840	100.0	82.5	13.3	2.3	0.3	0.5	1.0
Aged 25 to 29	9,249	100.0	82.1	13.5	2.4	0.7	0.6	0.8
Aged 30 to 34	10,272	100.0	86.6	9.8	1.9	0.5	0.4	0.7
Aged 35 to 44	22,365	100.0	89.2	7.1	1.1	1.0	1.0	0.6

Note: "–" means sample is too small to make a reliable estimate.
Source: National Center for Health Statistics, Sexual Behavior and Selected Health Measures: Men and Women 15–44 Years of Age, United States, 2002, Advance Data, No. 362, 2005; Internet site http://www.cdc.gov/nchs/nsfg.htm

Table 4.8 Sexual Attraction by Sex and Marital Status, 2002

(number of people aged 18 to 44 and percent distribution by sexual attraction, by sex and marital status, 2002; numbers in thousands)

	total		sexual attraction					
	number	percent	only opposite sex	mostly opposite sex	both	mostly same sex	only same sex	not sure
Total men aged 18 to 44	**55,399**	**100.0%**	**92.2%**	**3.9%**	**1.0%**	**0.7%**	**1.5%**	**0.7%**
Currently married	25,795	100.0	96.3	2.8	0.3	–	0.3	0.3
Currently cohabiting	5,614	100.0	92.8	6.4	–	–	–	–
Never married, not cohabiting	19,725	100.0	86.6	4.8	1.8	1.7	3.6	1.5
Formerly married, not cohabiting	4,265	100.0	92.5	2.7	2.3	0.9	0.8	0.9
Total women aged 18 to 44	**55,742**	**100.0**	**85.7**	**10.2**	**1.9**	**0.8**	**0.7**	**0.8**
Currently married	28,323	100.0	90.7	6.9	1.4	0.2	0.2	0.6
Currently cohabiting	5,452	100.0	77.8	16.2	2.6	–	0.8	1.9
Never married, not cohabiting	15,871	100.0	80.6	13.2	2.2	1.7	1.5	0.8
Formerly married, not cohabiting	6,096	100.0	82.9	11.8	3.1	1.0	0.8	0.5

Note: "–" means sample is too small to make a reliable estimate.
Source: National Center for Health Statistics, Sexual Behavior and Selected Health Measures: Men and Women 15–44 Years of Age, United States, 2002, Advance Data, No. 362, 2005; Internet site http://www.cdc.gov/nchs/nsfg.htm

Table 4.9 Sexual Attraction by Sex, Race, and Hispanic Origin, 2002

(number of people aged 18 to 44 and percent distribution by sexual attraction, by sex, race, and Hispanic origin, 2002; numbers in thousands)

	total		sexual attraction					
	number	percent	only opposite sex	mostly opposite sex	both	mostly same sex	only same sex	not sure
Total men aged 18 to 44	**55,399**	**100.0%**	**92.2%**	**3.9%**	**1.0%**	**0.7%**	**1.5%**	**0.7%**
Black, non-Hispanic	6,127	100.0	91.5	3.4	1.6	0.7	1.4	1.6
Hispanic	35,154	100.0	89.5	6.1	1.4	0.8	1.1	1.1
White, non-Hispanic	9,336	100.0	93.0	3.3	0.8	0.7	1.8	0.4
Total women aged 18 to 44	**55,742**	**100.0**	**85.7**	**10.2**	**1.9**	**0.8**	**0.7**	**0.8**
Black, non-Hispanic	7,399	100.0	90.1	5.3	1.8	1.0	1.0	0.9
Hispanic	35,936	100.0	89.2	7.4	1.2	–	0.6	1.4
White, non-Hispanic	8,194	100.0	84.5	11.6	2.0	0.8	0.7	0.9

Note: "–" means sample is too small to make a reliable estimate.
Source: National Center for Health Statistics, Sexual Behavior and Selected Health Measures: Men and Women 15–44 Years of Age, United States, 2002, Advance Data, No. 362, 2005; Internet site http://www.cdc.gov/nchs/nsfg.htm

Table 4.10 Sexual Attraction by Sex and Metropolitan Residence, 2002

(number of people aged 18 to 44 and percent distribution by sexual attraction, by sex and metropolitan residence, 2002; numbers in thousands)

	total		sexual attraction					
	number	percent	only opposite sex	mostly opposite sex	both	mostly same sex	only same sex	not sure
Total men aged 18 to 44	**55,399**	**100.0%**	**92.2%**	**3.9%**	**1.0%**	**0.7%**	**1.5%**	**0.7%**
Central city of 12 largest metropolitan areas	7,713	100.0	87.2	6.7	1.7	1.1	2.6	0.6
Central city of other metropolitan areas	13,067	100.0	89.9	4.0	0.9	1.4	2.8	0.9
Suburb of 12 largest metropolitan areas	12,397	100.0	92.7	4.0	1.2	0.4	1.0	0.8
Suburb of other metropolitan areas	11,895	100.0	95.6	2.4	0.5	–	1.1	–
Nonmetropolitan area	10,326	100.0	94.4	3.1	0.8	0.4	–	1.1
Total women aged 18 to 44	**55,742**	**100.0**	**85.7**	**10.2**	**1.9**	**0.8**	**0.7**	**0.8**
Central city of 12 largest metropolitan areas	7,671	100.0	81.4	12.0	1.4	2.0	1.5	1.7
Central city of other metropolitan areas	13,017	100.0	83.6	11.9	2.2	0.7	0.8	0.9
Suburb of 12 largest metropolitan areas	12,599	100.0	86.6	9.8	1.4	0.7	0.8	0.8
Suburb of other metropolitan areas	12,863	100.0	87.1	9.3	2.6	0.4	–	0.3
Nonmetropolitan area	9,593	100.0	88.9	7.8	2.0	0.4	0.4	–

Note: "–" means sample is too small to make a reliable estimate.
Source: National Center for Health Statistics, Sexual Behavior and Selected Health Measures: Men and Women 15–44 Years of Age, United States, 2002, Advance Data, No. 362, 2005; Internet site http://www.cdc.gov/nchs/nsfg.htm

Table 4.11 Sexual Attraction by Sex, Sexual Orientation, and Sexual Experience, 2002

(number of people aged 18 to 44 and percent distribution by sexual orientation, by sex, sexual orientation, and sexual experience, 2002; numbers in thousands)

	total		sexual attraction					
	number	percent	only opposite sex	mostly opposite sex	both	mostly same sex	only same sex	not sure
TOTAL MEN AGED 18 TO 44	**55,399**	**100.0%**	**92.2%**	**3.9%**	**1.0%**	**0.7%**	**1.5%**	**0.7%**
Sexual orientation								
Heterosexual	49,902	100.0	95.8	3.3	–	–	0.2	0.4
Homosexual	1,266	100.0	23.2	–	–	19.0	54.8	0.7
Bisexual	1,000	100.0	27.6	25.7	32.0	10.8	–	4.0
Something else	2,177	100.0	78.8	8.6	3.7	0.6	2.5	5.8
Did not report	1,003	100.0	93.7	2.7	–	–	0.9	2.7
Ever had sexual experience with male								
Yes	3,433	100.0	39.7	16.8	10.0	10.3	21.2	2.1
No	51,914	100.0	95.7	3.0	0.4	0.1	0.2	0.6
TOTAL WOMEN AGED 18 TO 44	**55,742**	**100.0**	**85.7**	**10.2**	**1.9**	**0.8**	**0.7**	**0.8**
Sexual orientation								
Heterosexual	50,295	100.0	89.7	9.5	0.4	–	0.1	0.3
Homosexual	725	100.0	28.4	–	–	21.9	40.1	4.6
Bisexual	1,564	100.0	5.5	32.1	50.5	9.8	–	–
Something else	2,101	100.0	71.1	14.0	3.1	3.0	1.4	7.3
Did not report	998	100.0	77.8	–	–	–	–	6.3
Ever had sexual experience with female								
Yes	6,415	100.0	36.6	38.9	12.2	6.1	4.9	1.4
No	49,268	100.0	92.1	6.4	–	0.1	0.2	0.7

Note: "–" means sample is too small to make a reliable estimate.
Source: National Center for Health Statistics, Sexual Behavior and Selected Health Measures: Men and Women 15–44 Years of Age, United States, 2002, Advance Data, No. 362, 2005; Internet site http://www.cdc.gov/nchs/nsfg.htm

Six Percent of Men Have Had Oral or Anal Sex with Another Male

Among women, 11 percent have had a same-sex experience.

When the National Survey of Family Growth asked Americans about their sexual experiences, respondents could answer anonymously through computer-aided interviewing techniques. Even so, statistics based on the answers provided may be lowball estimates of the incidence of homosexuality because of the hesitancy of respondents to admit to same-sex experiences.

Six percent of men and 11 percent of women aged 15 to 44 say they have engaged in sexual activity with a same-sex partner in their lifetime. The larger number of women involved in same-sex activity is most likely due to differences in the way the survey asked men and women to report same-sex activity. Men were asked whether they had engaged in specific sex acts with another man, while women were asked about sexual experiences of any kind with another woman. The proportion of men who report same-sex activity peaks at 18 percent among those aged 30 to 44 who had never married and were not cohabiting.

■ Only 3 to 4 percent of men and women aged 15 to 44 have engaged in sexual activity with a same-sex partner in the past year.

Men living in central cities of large metropolitan areas are most likely to have had same-sex experiences

(percent of men aged 15 to 44 who have had oral or anal sex with same-sex partner in lifetime, by metropolitan residence, 2002)

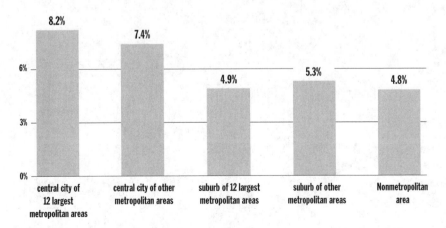

Table 4.12 Lifetime Same-Sex Sexual Activity by Age and Sex, 2002

(total number of people aged 15 to 44 and percent reporting any sexual activity with same-sex partners in their lifetime, by age and sex, 2002; numbers in thousands)

	men					women		
	total		any oral or anal sex	anal sex	oral sex	total		any same-sex experience
	number	percent				number	percent	
Total aged 15 to 44	**61,147**	**100.0%**	**6.0%**	**3.7%**	**5.7%**	**61,561**	**100.0%**	**11.2%**
Aged 15 to 19	10,208	100.0	4.5	3.2	4.1	9,834	100.0	10.6
Aged 15	1,930	100.0	2.2	1.7	2.2	1,819	100.0	7.2
Aged 16	1,998	100.0	3.1	2.2	3.1	1,927	100.0	13.1
Aged 17	1,820	100.0	6.6	4.7	6.3	2,073	100.0	5.1
Aged 18	2,392	100.0	4.3	2.9	3.7	2,035	100.0	13.7
Aged 19	2,067	100.0	6.0	4.5	5.5	1,980	100.0	13.9
Aged 20 to 24	9,883	100.0	5.5	3.4	5.0	9,840	100.0	14.2
Aged 20 to 21	3,921	100.0	2.7	2.1	2.3	4,005	100.0	13.0
Aged 22 to 24	5,963	100.0	7.4	4.3	6.8	5,834	100.0	15.0
Aged 25 to 29	9,226	100.0	5.7	4.2	5.2	9,249	100.0	14.1
Aged 30 to 44	31,830	100.0	6.7	3.8	6.6	32,638	100.0	9.7

Note: The questions about same-sex sexual contact in the National Survey of Family Growth were worded differently for men and women. Women were asked whether they had ever had a sexual experience of any kind with another female. Men were asked whether they had performed any of four specific sexual acts with another male. The question asked of women may have elicited more "yes" answers than the questions asked of men.

Source: National Center for Health Statistics, Sexual Behavior and Selected Health Measures: Men and Women 15–44 Years of Age, United States, 2002, Advance Data, No. 362, 2005; Internet site http://www.cdc.gov/nchs/nsfg.htm

Table 4.13 Lifetime Same-Sex Sexual Activity by Marital Status and Sex, 2002

(total number of people aged 15 to 44 and percent reporting any sexual activity with same-sex partners in their lifetime, by marital status, age and sex, 2002; numbers in thousands)

	men					women		
	total		any oral or anal sex	anal sex	oral sex	total		any same-sex experience
	number	percent				number	percent	
Total aged 15 to 44	**61,147**	**100.0%**	**6.0%**	**3.7%**	**5.7%**	**61,561**	**100.0%**	**11.2%**
Currently married	25,808	100.0	3.4	1.0	3.2	28,327	100.0	7.2
Aged 15 to 29	5,737	100.0	2.6	1.4	2.1	7,246	100.0	10.8
Aged 30 to 44	20,070	100.0	3.6	0.9	3.5	21,081	100.0	5.9
Currently cohabiting	5,653	100.0	5.3	2.1	4.8	5,570	100.0	17.6
Aged 15 to 29	3,154	100.0	5.3	2.8	4.3	3,281	100.0	18.9
Aged 30 to 44	2,499	100.0	5.4	1.3	5.4	2,289	100.0	15.8
Never married, not cohabiting	25,412	100.0	8.6	6.8	8.3	21,568	100.0	13.5
Aged 15 to 19	9,948	100.0	4.2	3.2	3.9	9,048	100.0	9.6
Aged 20 to 24	6,900	100.0	5.9	3.6	5.6	5,681	100.0	14.7
Aged 25 to 29	3,047	100.0	11.5	9.6	10.8	2,640	100.0	17.0
Aged 30 to 44	5,518	100.0	18.4	15.7	18.1	4,199	100.0	18.0
Formerly married, not cohabiting	4,274	100.0	7.1	3.8	7.1	6,096	100.0	16.3
Aged 15 to 29	532	100.0	6.9	5.7	6.9	1,027	100.0	18.1
Aged 30 to 44	3,742	100.0	7.1	3.5	7.1	5,069	100.0	15.9

Note: The questions about same-sex sexual contact in the National Survey of Family Growth were worded differently for men and women. Women were asked whether they had ever had a sexual experience of any kind with another female. Men were asked whether they had performed any of four specific sexual acts with another male. The question asked of women may have elicited more "yes" answers than the questions asked of men.

Source: National Center for Health Statistics, Sexual Behavior and Selected Health Measures: Men and Women 15–44 Years of Age, United States, 2002, Advance Data, No. 362, 2005; Internet site http://www.cdc.gov/nchs/nsfg.htm

Table 4.14 Lifetime Same-Sex Sexual Activity by Race, Hispanic Origin, and Sex, 2002

(total number of people aged 15 to 44 and percent reporting any sexual activity with same-sex partners in their lifetime, by race, Hispanic origin, and sex, 2002; numbers in thousands)

	men					women		
	total		any oral or anal sex	anal sex	oral sex	total		any same-sex experience
	number	percent				number	percent	
Total aged 15 to 44	**61,147**	**100.0%**	**6.0%**	**3.7%**	**5.7%**	**61,561**	**100.0%**	**11.2%**
Black, non-Hispanic	6,940	100.0	5.0	4.4	4.4	8,250	100.0	10.6
Hispanic	10,188	100.0	6.2	4.0	5.7	9,107	100.0	6.5
White, non-Hispanic	38,738	100.0	6.5	3.7	6.3	39,498	100.0	12.6

Note: The questions about same-sex sexual contact in the National Survey of Family Growth were worded differently for men and women. Women were asked whether they had ever had a sexual experience of any kind with another female. Men were asked whether they had performed any of four specific sexual acts with another male. The question asked of women may have elicited more "yes"answers than the questions asked of men.
Source: National Center for Health Statistics, Sexual Behavior and Selected Health Measures: Men and Women 15–44 Years of Age, United States, 2002, Advance Data, No. 362, 2005; Internet site http://www.cdc.gov/nchs/nsfg.htm

Table 4.15 Lifetime Same-Sex Sexual Activity by Education and Sex, 2002

(total number of people aged 15 to 44 and percent reporting any sexual activity with same-sex partners in their lifetime, by education and sex, 2002; numbers in thousands)

	men					women		
	total		any oral or anal sex	anal sex	oral sex	total		any same-sex experience
	number	percent				number	percent	
Total aged 15 to 44	**61,147**	**100.0%**	**6.0%**	**3.7%**	**5.7%**	**61,561**	**100.0%**	**11.2%**
Not a high school graduate	6,355	100.0	4.6	3.1	4.1	5,627	100.0	9.5
High school grad. or GED	15,659	100.0	6.0	3.4	5.8	14,264	100.0	12.2
Some college, no degree	13,104	100.0	6.7	4.2	6.5	14,279	100.0	12.0
Bachelor's degree or more	11,901	100.0	6.6	4.2	6.5	13,551	100.0	10.6

Note: Numbers will not add to total because education categories include only people aged 22 to 44. The questions about same-sex sexual contact in the National Survey of Family Growth were worded differently for men and women. Women were asked whether they had ever had a sexual experience of any kind with another female. Men were asked whether they had performed any of four specific sexual acts with another male. The question asked of women may have elicited more "yes" answers than the questions asked of men.
Source: National Center for Health Statistics, Sexual Behavior and Selected Health Measures: Men and Women 15–44 Years of Age, United States, 2002, Advance Data, No. 362, 2005; Internet site http://www.cdc.gov/nchs/nsfg.htm

Table 4.16 Lifetime Same-Sex Sexual Activity by Metropolitan Residence and Sex, 2002

(total number of people aged 15 to 44 and percent reporting any sexual activity with same-sex partners in their lifetime, by metropolitan residence and sex, 2002; numbers in thousands)

	men					women		
	total		any oral or anal sex	anal sex	oral sex	total		any same-sex experience
	number	percent				number	percent	
Total aged 15 to 44	**61,147**	**100.0%**	**6.0%**	**3.7%**	**5.7%**	**61,561**	**100.0%**	**11.2%**
Central city of 12 largest metropolitan areas	8,313	100.0	8.2	6.2	7.6	8,538	100.0	14.1
Central city of other metropolitan areas	14,191	100.0	7.4	5.2	7.2	14,082	100.0	12.7
Suburb of 12 largest metropolitan areas	13,844	100.0	4.9	2.5	4.8	13,981	100.0	9.6
Suburb of other metropolitan areas	13,415	100.0	5.3	2.9	4.6	14,079	100.0	11.4
Nonmetropolitan area	11,384	100.0	4.8	2.3	4.7	10,880	100.0	8.9

Note: The questions about same-sex sexual contact in the National Survey of Family Growth were worded differently for men and women. Women were asked whether they had ever had a sexual experience of any kind with another female. Men were asked whether they had performed any of four specific sexual acts with another male. The question asked of women may have elicited more "yes" answers than the questions asked of men.
Source: National Center for Health Statistics, Sexual Behavior and Selected Health Measures: Men and Women 15–44 Years of Age, United States, 2002, Advance Data, No. 362, 2005; Internet site http://www.cdc.gov/nchs/nsfg.htm

Table 4.17 Lifetime Same-Sex Sexual Activity by Number of Opposite-Sex Partners, 2002

(total number of people aged 15 to 44 and percent reporting any sexual activity with same-sex partners in their lifetime, by number of opposite-sex partners in lifetime and sex, 2002; numbers in thousands)

	men					women		
	total		any oral or anal sex	anal sex	oral sex	total		any same-sex experience
	number	percent				number	percent	
Total aged 15 to 44	**61,147**	**100.0%**	**6.0%**	**3.7%**	**5.7%**	**61,561**	**100.0%**	**11.2%**
No opposite-sex partners	2,031	100.0	14.8	15.5	16.2	1,439	100.0	6.3
One	3,712	100.0	6.2	5.5	6.0	8,407	100.0	2.2
Two	2,700	100.0	6.7	5.6	6.8	4,310	100.0	6.5
Three to six	10,793	100.0	5.8	3.5	5.7	14,504	100.0	7.9
Seven to fourteen	9,221	100.0	6.6	2.1	6.1	7,833	100.0	15.7
Fifteen or more	11,340	100.0	5.9	3.0	5.6	4,579	100.0	31.5

Note: Numbers will not add to total because question was asked only of people aged 25 to 44. The questions about same-sex sexual contact in the National Survey of Family Growth were worded differently for men and women. Women were asked whether they had ever had a sexual experience of any kind with another female. Men were asked whether they had performed any of four specific sexual acts with another male. The question asked of women may have elicited more "yes" answers than the questions asked of men.
Source: National Center for Health Statistics, Sexual Behavior and Selected Health Measures: Men and Women 15–44 Years of Age, United States, 2002, Advance Data, No. 362, 2005; Internet site http://www.cdc.gov/nchs/nsfg.htm

Table 4.18 Past Year Same-Sex Sexual Activity by Age and Sex, 2002

(total number of people aged 15 to 44 and percent reporting any sexual activity with same-sex partners in the past 12 months, by age and sex, 2002; numbers in thousands)

	men total		any same-sex sexual contact in past year	women total		any same-sex sexual contact in past year
	number	percent		number	percent	
Total aged 15 to 44	**61,147**	**100.0%**	**2.9%**	**61,561**	**100.0%**	**4.4%**
Aged 15 to 19	10,208	100.0	2.4	9,834	100.0	7.7
Aged 20 to 24	9,883	100.0	3.0	9,840	100.0	5.8
Aged 25 to 29	9,226	100.0	2.6	9,249	100.0	3.6
Aged 30 to 34	10,138	100.0	3.3	10,272	100.0	3.0
Aged 35 to 39	10,557	100.0	2.9	10,853	100.0	4.5
Aged 40 to 44	11,135	100.0	3.0	11,512	100.0	2.4

Note: The questions about same-sex sexual contact in the National Survey of Family Growth were worded differently for men and women. Women were asked whether they had ever had a sexual experience of any kind with another female. Men were asked whether they had performed any of four specific sexual acts with another male. The question asked of women may have elicited more "yes" answers than the questions asked of men.
Source: National Center for Health Statistics, Sexual Behavior and Selected Health Measures: Men and Women 15–44 Years of Age, United States, 2002, Advance Data, No. 362, 2005; Internet site http://www.cdc.gov/nchs/nsfg.htm

Table 4.19 Past Year Same-Sex Sexual Activity by Metropolitan Residence and Sex, 2002

(total number of people aged 15 to 44 and percent reporting any sexual activity with same-sex partners in the past 12 months, by metropolitan residence and sex, 2002; numbers in thousands)

	men total		any same-sex sexual contact in past year	women total		any same-sex sexual contact in past year
	number	percent		number	percent	
Total aged 15 to 44	**61,147**	**100.0%**	**2.9%**	**61,561**	**100.0%**	**4.4%**
Central city of 12 largest metropolitan areas	8,313	100.0	4.8	8,538	100.0	5.6
Central city of other metropolitan areas	14,191	100.0	4.7	14,082	100.0	5.2
Suburb of 12 largest metropolitan areas	13,844	100.0	1.8	13,981	100.0	4.5
Suburb of other metropolitan areas	13,415	100.0	2.2	14,079	100.0	3.8
Nonmetropolitan area	11,384	100.0	1.5	10,880	100.0	3.3

Note: The questions about same-sex sexual contact in the National Survey of Family Growth were worded differently for men and women. Women were asked whether they had ever had a sexual experience of any kind with another female. Men were asked whether they had performed any of four specific sexual acts with another male. The question asked of women may have elicited more "yes" answers than the questions asked of men.
Source: National Center for Health Statistics, Sexual Behavior and Selected Health Measures: Men and Women 15–44 Years of Age, United States, 2002, Advance Data, No. 362, 2005; Internet site http://www.cdc.gov/nchs/nsfg.htm

Among Women, Homosexuals Are Least Likely to Have Had a Sexually Transmitted Infection

Among men, homosexuals are most likely to have had an infection.

Sexually transmitted infections are commonplace among the nation's young and middle-aged adults. Seventeen percent of sexually experienced women aged 15 to 44 have had a sexually transmitted infection (excluding HIV). Among homosexual women, however, only 7.5 percent have had a sexually transmitted infection.

Men are less likely than women to have had a sexually transmitted infection, with only 7 percent reporting it. In contrast to women, homosexual men are most likely to have had an infection, with 19 percent reporting it.

■ The more sexual partners, the greater the likelihood of having a sexually transmitted infection.

Among women, bisexuals are most likely to have had a sexually transmitted infection

(percent of women aged 15 to 44 who have ever had a sexually transmitted infection, by sexual orientation, 2002)

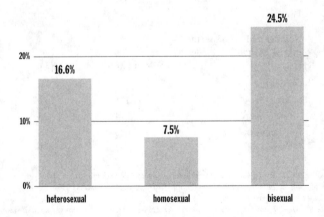

Table 4.20 Women Reporting Any Sexually Transmitted Infection except HIV by Sexual Orientation, 2002

(number of sexually experienced women aged 15 to 44 and percent reporting any sexually transmitted infection except HIV, by sexual orientation, attraction, and experience, 2002; numbers in thousands)

	number	percent reporting sexually transmitted infection, except HIV
Total sexually experienced women aged 15 to 44	**55,553**	**16.8%**
Sexual orientation		
Heterosexual	49,929	16.6
Homosexual	743	7.5
Bisexual	1,857	24.5
Something else	2,274	19.0
Did not report	750	9.9
Sexual attraction		
Only to opposite sex	47,155	15.6
Mostly to opposite sex	5,823	25.9
All other	2,414	17.4
Ever had sexual experience with same-sex partner		
No	48,651	15.3
Yes	6,902	26.8
Number and sex of partners in past 12 months		
None	3,668	12.0
Opposite sex only		
One	41,119	16.0
Two or more	7,814	22.3
Any same sex	2,686	20.5
Did not report	267	6.0

Note: Sexual experience includes any sexual contact with another person, including oral sex, anal sex, or vaginal intercourse. Sexually transmitted infections include genital herpes, genital warts, pelvic inflammatory disease, or syphilis in lifetime, and gonorrhea or chlamydia if treated in past 12 months.
Source: National Center for Health Statistics, Sexual Behavior and Selected Health Measures: Men and Women 15–44 Years of Age, United States, 2002, Advance Data, No. 362, 2005; Internet site http://www.cdc.gov/nchs/nsfg.htm

Table 4.21 Men Reporting Any Sexually Transmitted Infection except HIV by Sexual Orientation, 2002

(number of sexually experienced men aged 15 to 44 and percent reporting any sexually transmitted infection except HIV, by sexual orientation, attraction, and experience, 2002; numbers in thousands)

	number	percent reporting sexually transmitted infection, except HIV
Total sexually experienced men aged 15 to 44	**54,773**	**7.4%**
Sexual orientation		
Heterosexual	49,587	6.8
Homosexual	1,291	19.3
Bisexual	1,015	17.8
Something else	2,105	9.8
Did not report	775	3.9
Sexual attraction		
Only to opposite sex	50,510	6.7
Mostly to opposite sex	2,133	12.9
All other	2,074	18.3
Ever had sexual experience with same-sex partner		
No	51,114	6.6
Yes	3,659	17.3
Number and sex of partners in past 12 months		
None	3,839	5.3
Opposite sex only		
One	38,052	6.2
Two or more	10,770	9.3
Any same sex	1,634	25.7
Did not report	1,615	4.5

Note: Sexual experience includes any sexual contact with another person, including oral sex, anal sex, or vaginal intercourse. Sexually transmitted infections include genital herpes, genital warts, or syphilis in lifetime, and gonorrhea or chlamydia if treated in past 12 months.
Source: National Center for Health Statistics, Sexual Behavior and Selected Health Measures: Men and Women 15–44 Years of Age, United States, 2002, Advance Data, No. 362, 2005; Internet site http://www.cdc.gov/nchs/nsfg.htm

Most Women Think Adoption by Homosexuals Is OK

Men are less likely to approve.

Americans are ambivalent about adoption by gays and lesbians. Among women aged 15 to 44, the 55 percent majority thinks homosexuals should have the right to adopt. Among men, however, a smaller 47 percent agree.

Attitudes toward gay and lesbian adoption vary by demographic characteristic. Those most supportive are young adults, the childless, non-Hispanic whites, college graduates, and those for whom religion is not important. Not surprisingly, 70 to 84 percent of people who identify themselves as homosexual or bisexual think gay and lesbian adoption is OK.

Fundamentalist Protestants are least supportive of gay and lesbian adoption. Only 15 percent of men who identify themselves as fundamentalist Protestant think gays and lesbians should have the right to adopt. Among their female counterparts, a larger 33 percent are supportive. In contrast, among men and women with no religion, 64 to 77 percent think gays and lesbians should have the right to adopt.

■ As younger adults are more supportive of gay and lesbian adoption, attitudes may be shifting toward greater tolerance.

Religious beliefs play a big role in men's attitude toward gay adoption

(percent of men aged 15 to 44 who agree with the statement,
"Gay and lesbian adults should have the right to adopt," by current religion, 2002

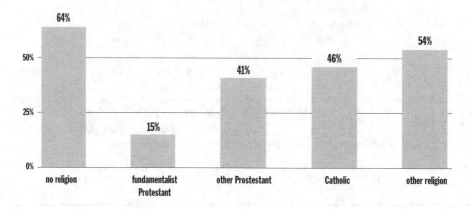

Table 4.22 Attitude toward Gay and Lesbian Adoption by Sex, 2002

"Gay and lesbian adults should have the right to adopt."

(percent of people aged 15 to 44 agreeing with statement, by selected characateristics and sex, 2002)

	percent agreeing	
	men	women
Total aged 15 to 44	**46.9%**	**55.4%**
Aged 15 to 24	56.3	63.8
Aged 25 to 29	47.5	59.1
Aged 30 to 44	40.8	49.3
Marital status		
Currently married	37.3	46.8
Currently cohabiting	48.2	60.6
Never married, not cohabiting	56.6	65.3
Formerly married, not cohabiting	46.3	56.1
Number of children ever borne or fathered		
None	54.5	66.3
One or more	38.3	47.6
Race and Hispanic origin		
Black, non-Hispanic	41.8	45.5
Hispanic	37.2	46.7
White, non-Hispanic	49.6	59.1
Education		
Not a high school graduate	28.4	41.3
High school graduate or GED	37.7	47.3
Some college, no degree	45.9	53.8
Bachelor's degree or more	56.3	61.2
Current religion		
No religion	64.2	77.2
Fundamentalist Protestant	14.6	33.0
Other Protestant	41.1	47.6
Catholic	46.2	58.1
Other religion	54.2	73.1
Importance of religion		
Very important	31.7	39.8
Somewhat important	50.4	66.4
Not important	63.4	78.2
Sexual orientation		
Heterosexual	46.2	54.7
Homosexual or bisexual	70.4	83.8
Something else or did not report	43.2	45.8

Source: National Center for Health Statistics, Fertility, Contraception, and Fatherhood: Data on Men and Women from Cycle 6 of the 2002 National Survey of Family Growth, Vital and Health Statistics, Series 23, No. 26, 2006; Internet site http://www.cdc .gov/nchs/nsfg.htm

5

AIDS and STDs

■ Sexually transmitted diseases have been plaguing humans throughout most of history, with medical science playing catch-up as new diseases emerge. Great progress has been made in reducing the lethality of HIV over the past decade, but risky behavior still makes many vulnerable to contracting the virus.

■ Nearly one million people in the United States have developed AIDS since the disease was first recognized in the early 1980s. Males aged 13 or older account for 80 percent of AIDS victims. Sixty percent of those with AIDS were diagnosed between the ages of 30 and 44.

■ Since the early 1980s, more than one-half million people have died of AIDS. Blacks and Hispanics account for 56 percent of AIDS deaths.

■ An AIDS diagnosis is no longer a death sentence. Among people diagnosed with AIDS in 2000, fully 83 percent were alive three years later. HIV once ranked among the top ten causes of death in the United States, but by 2003 it had fallen to 18th place.

■ The distribution of AIDS differs greatly by state. Half of all Americans living with AIDS reside in just five states: New York, California, Florida, Texas, and New Jersey.

■ HIV testing is common among young and middle-aged adults. Among women aged 15 to 44, the 55 percent majority have had an HIV test at some point in their life, and 16 percent have been tested in the past year.

■ Sexually transmitted infections are common, and ever changing. As one disease is conquered, others appear. Seventeen percent of sexually experienced women aged 15 to 44 say they have had a sexually transmitted infection at some point in their life.

AIDS Cases in the United States Are Approaching 1 Million

Minorities account for the majority of AIDS cases.

Nearly one million people in the United States have developed AIDS since the disease was first recognized in the early 1980s. Eighty percent of victims were males aged 13 or older, 19 percent females aged 13 or older, and just 1 percent children under age 13. The 30-to-44 age group accounts for 60 percent of AIDS cases.

By race and Hispanic origin, blacks account for the largest share of AIDS victims—just over 40 percent of the total through 2004. Non-Hispanic whites are close behind at just under 40 percent. Another 19 percent of those with AIDS are Hispanic.

Among men with AIDS, male-to-male sexual contact accounts for 58 percent of cases. Injection drug use is second, accounting for another 23 percent.

■ Among women with AIDS, heterosexual contact explains 56 percent of cases, and injection drug use accounts for another 41 percent.

AIDS hits certain age groups much harder than others

(percent distribution of cumulative AIDS cases, by age at diagnosis, through 2004)

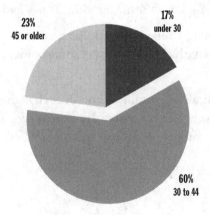

23%
45 or older

17%
under 30

60%
30 to 44

Table 5.1 Cumulative Number of AIDS Cases by Sex and Age, through 2004

(cumulative number and percent distribution of AIDS cases by sex and age at diagnosis, through 2004)

	number	percent distribution
Total cases	**944,306**	**100.0%**
Sex		
Males aged 13 or older	756,399	80.1
Females aged 13 or older	178,463	18.9
Children under age 13	9,443	1.0
Age		
Under age 13	9,443	1.0
Aged 13 to 14	959	0.1
Aged 15 to 19	4,936	0.5
Aged 20 to 24	34,164	3.6
Aged 25 to 29	114,642	12.1
Aged 30 to 34	195,404	20.7
Aged 35 to 39	208,199	22.0
Aged 40 to 44	161,964	17.2
Aged 45 to 49	99,644	10.6
Aged 50 to 54	54,869	5.8
Aged 55 to 59	29,553	3.1
Aged 60 to 64	16,119	1.7
Aged 65 or older	14,410	1.5

Note: Total includes cases in U.S. dependencies and possessions.
Source: Centers for Disease Control and Prevention, HIV/AIDS Surveillance Report, 2004, Vol. 16, 2005; Internet site http://www.cdc.gov/hiv/topics/surveillance/resources/reports/2004report/default.htm

Table 5.2 Cumulative Number of AIDS Cases by Race and Hispanic Origin, through 2004

(cumulative number and percent distribution of AIDS cases by race and Hispanic origin, through 2004)

	number	percent distribution
Total cases	**944,306**	**100.0%**
American Indian	3,084	0.3
Asian	7,317	0.8
Black, non-Hispanic	379,278	40.2
Hispanic	177,164	18.8
White, non-Hispanic	375,155	39.7

Note: Total includes cases in U.S. dependencies and possessions. Numbers will not add to total because not all races are shown.
Source: Centers for Disease Control and Prevention, HIV/AIDS Surveillance Report, 2004, Vol. 16, 2005; Internet site http://www.cdc.gov/hiv/topics/surveillance/resources/reports/2004report/default.htm

Table 5.3 Cumulative Number of AIDS Cases by Region, through 2004

(cumulative number and percent distribution of AIDS cases by region, through 2004)

	number	percent distribution
Total cases	**944,306**	**100.0%**
Northeast	289,792	30.7
Midwest	93,701	9.9
South	343,449	36.4
West	187,730	19.9
U.S. dependencies, possessions	29,634	3.1

Source: Centers for Disease Control and Prevention, HIV/AIDS Surveillance Report, 2004, Vol. 16, 2005; Internet site http://www.cdc.gov/hiv/topics/surveillance/resources/reports/2004report/default.htm

---

Table 5.4 Cumulative Number of AIDS Cases by Sex and Transmission Category, through 2004

(cumulative number and percent distribution of AIDS cases by sex and transmission category, through 2004)

	total	percent distribution
Males, aged 13 or older	**756,399**	**100.0%**
Male-to-male sexual contact	441,380	58.4
Injection drug use	176,162	23.3
Male-to-male sexual contact and injection drug use	64,833	8.6
Heterosexual contact	59,939	7.9
Other	14,085	1.9
Females, aged 13 or older	**178,463**	**100.0**
Heterosexual contact	99,175	55.6
Injection drug use	72,651	40.7
Other	6,636	3.7
Children under age 13*	**9,443**	**100.0**
Perinatal	8,779	93.0
Other	664	7.0

* At diagnosis
Note: "Other" includes hemophilia, blood transfusion, and not identified.
Source: Centers for Disease Control and Prevention, HIV/AIDS Surveillance Report, 2004, Vol. 16, 2005; Internet site http://www.cdc.gov/hiv/topics/surveillance/resources/reports/2004report/default.htm

AIDS Deaths Exceed Half a Million

Non-Hispanic whites account for the largest share of AIDS deaths.

Since AIDS was first recognized in the early 1980s, 529,113 people have died of the disease. Males aged 13 or older account for 83 percent of the deaths, 16 percent have been females aged 13 or older, and 1 percent have been children under age 13.

Non-Hispanic whites account for the largest share of AIDS deaths—43 percent through 2004. Blacks are close behind at 38 percent, and Hispanics account for 18 percent of deaths. Asians and American Indians combined account for less than 1 percent of AIDS deaths.

Among men who have died from AIDS, 58 percent were infected through male-to-male sexual contact and another 25 percent through injection drug use. Nearly half (49 percent) of the women who have died from AIDS were infected through injection drug use, and almost as many (47 percent) through heterosexual contact.

■ Fewer than 10 percent of AIDS deaths have occurred in the Midwest, while nearly one-third have occurred in the Northeast.

Blacks and Hispanics account for more than half of AIDS deaths

(percent distribution of cumulative deaths of people with AIDS, by race and Hispanic origin, through 2004)

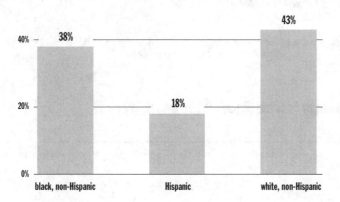

Table 5.5 AIDS Deaths by Sex and Age, through 2004

(cumulative number and percent distribution of deaths of people with AIDS by sex and age at diagnosis, through 2004)

	number	percent distribution
Total AIDS deaths	**529,113**	**100.0%**
Sex		
Males aged 13 or older	438,701	82.9
Females aged 13 or older	84,897	16.0
Children under age 13*	5,515	1.0
Age		
Under age 13	5,094	1.0
Aged 13 to 14	266	0.1
Aged 15 to 19	1,055	0.2
Aged 20 to 24	8,808	1.7
Aged 25 to 29	44,516	8.4
Aged 30 to 34	96,357	18.2
Aged 35 to 39	116,206	22.0
Aged 40 to 44	100,633	19.0
Aged 45 to 49	67,842	12.8
Aged 50 to 54	39,936	7.5
Aged 55 to 59	22,452	4.2
Aged 60 to 64	12,946	2.4
Aged 65 or older	13,004	2.5

* At diagnosis
Source: Centers for Disease Control and Prevention, HIV/AIDS Surveillance Report, 2004, Vol. 16, 2005; Internet site http://www.cdc.gov/hiv/topics/surveillance/resources/reports/2004report/default.htm

Table 5.6 AIDS Deaths by Race and Hispanic Origin, through 2004

(cumulative number and percent distribution of deaths of people with AIDS by race and Hispanic origin, through 2004)

	number	percent distribution
Total AIDS deaths	**529,113**	**100.0%**
American Indian	1,578	0.3
Asian	3,272	0.6
Black, non-Hispanic	201,045	38.0
Hispanic	93,163	17.6
White, non-Hispanic	229,220	43.3

Note: Numbers will not add to total because not all races are shown.
Source: Centers for Disease Control and Prevention, HIV/AIDS Surveillance Report, 2004, Vol. 16, 2005; Internet site http://www.cdc.gov/hiv/topics/surveillance/resources/reports/2004report/default.htm

Table 5.7 AIDS Deaths by Region, through 2004

(cumulative number and percent distribution of deaths of people with AIDS by region, through 2004)

	number	percent distribution
Total AIDS deaths	**529,113**	**100.0%**
Northeast	169,693	32.1
Midwest	50,333	9.5
South	181,690	34.3
West	108,183	20.4
U.S. dependencies, possessions	19,214	3.6

Source: Centers for Disease Control and Prevention, HIV/AIDS Surveillance Report, 2004, Vol. 16, 2005; Internet site http://www.cdc.gov/hiv/topics/surveillance/resources/reports/2004report/default.htm

Table 5.8 AIDS Deaths by Sex and Transmission Category, through 2004

(cumulative number and percent distribution of deaths of people with AIDS by sex and transmission category, through 2004)

	total	percent distribution
Deaths of males, aged 13 or older	**438,701**	**100.0%**
Male-to-male sexual contact	256,053	58.4
Injection drug use	109,070	24.9
Male-to-male sexual contact and injection drug use	39,467	9.0
Heterosexual contact	24,268	5.5
Other	9,843	2.2
Deaths of females, aged 13 or older	**84,897**	**100.0**
Injection drug use	41,178	48.5
Heterosexual contact	39,576	46.6
Other	4,142	4.9
Deaths of children under age 13*	**5,515**	**100.0**
Perinatal	4,982	90.3
Other	533	9.7

* At diagnosis
Note: "Other" includes hemophilia, blood transfusion, and not identified.
Source: Centers for Disease Control and Prevention, HIV/AIDS Surveillance Report, 2004, Vol. 16, 2005; Internet site http://www.cdc.gov/hiv/topics/surveillance/resources/reports/2004report/default.htm

The AIDS Survival Rate Is above 80 Percent

After three years, more than 80 percent of those diagnosed with AIDS are still alive.

Among people diagnosed with AIDS in 2000, fully 90 percent were alive one year later. Eighty-three percent were still alive three years later. The AIDS survival rate does not vary much by sex, but it falls with age. More than 90 percent of people under age 20 who were diagnosed with AIDS in 2000 were still alive three years later, but only 61 percent of those aged 65 or older were still alive.

There are few differences in the survival rate by race and Hispanic origin. Survival is more variable by transmission category. Only 78 percent of men with AIDS who became infected through injection drug use were alive after 36 months compared with 87 percent of men with AIDS who became infected through male-to-male sexual contact.

■ Women with AIDS who became infected through injection drug use also have a lower survival rate than those who became infected through sexual contact.

Survival rate does not differ much by race and Hispanic origin

(percent of people diagnosed with AIDS in 2000 who were still alive after 36 months, by race and Hispanic origin)

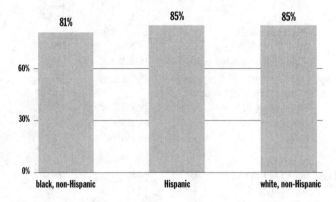

Table 5.9   Three-Year Survival Rate after an AIDS Diagnosis by Sex and Age

(percentage of people surviving for more than 12 and 36 months after an AIDS diagnosis in 2000, by sex and age)

	percent surviving after	
	12 months	36 months
Total people diagnosed with AIDS in 2000	**90%**	**83%**
Males aged 13 or older	90	84
Females aged 13 or older	91	82
Age at diagnosis		
Under age 13	96	95
Aged 13 to 14	100	93
Aged 15 to 19	98	93
Aged 20 to 24	95	89
Aged 25 to 29	94	89
Aged 30 to 34	94	88
Aged 35 to 39	92	86
Aged 40 to 44	90	83
Aged 45 to 49	88	79
Aged 50 to 54	86	76
Aged 55 to 59	84	75
Aged 60 to 64	79	70
Aged 65 or older	73	61

Source: Centers for Disease Control and Prevention, HIV/AIDS Surveillance Report, 2004, Vol. 16, 2005; Internet site http://www.cdc.gov/hiv/topics/surveillance/resources/reports/2004report/default.htm

Table 5.10   Three-Year Survival Rate after an AIDS Diagnosis by Race and Hispanic Origin

(percentage of people surviving for more than 12 and 36 months after an AIDS diagnosis in 2000, by race and Hispanic origin)

	percent surviving after	
	12 months	36 months
Total people diagnosed with AIDS in 2000	**90%**	**83%**
American Indian	92	85
Asian	91	88
Black, non-Hispanic	90	81
Hispanic	91	85
White, non-Hispanic	91	85

Source: Centers for Disease Control and Prevention, HIV/AIDS Surveillance Report, 2004, Vol. 16, 2005; Internet site http://www.cdc.gov/hiv/topics/surveillance/resources/reports/2004report/default.htm

Table 5.11 Three-Year Survival Rate after an AIDS Diagnosis by Transmission Category

(percentage of people surviving for more than 12 and 36 months after an AIDS diagnosis in 2000, by transmission category)

	percent surviving after	
	12 months	36 months
Total people diagnosed with AIDS in 2000	**90%**	**83%**
Males, aged 13 or older	**90**	**84**
Male-to-male sexual contact	92	87
Injection drug use	87	78
Male-to-male sexual contact and injection drug use	92	83
Heterosexual contact	91	84
Other	87	81
Females, aged 13 or older	**91**	**82**
Injection drug use	89	77
Heterosexual contact	92	85
Other	90	82
Children under age 13*	**96**	**95**
Perinatal	95	94
Other	100	100

* At diagnosis
Note: "Other" includes hemophilia, blood transfusion, and not identified.
Source: Centers for Disease Control and Prevention, HIV/AIDS Surveillance Report, 2004, Vol. 16, 2005; Internet site http://www.cdc.gov/hiv/topics/surveillance/resources/reports/2004report/default.htm

The HIV Death Rate Has Plummeted among Men Since 1990

The death rate rose among black women, however.

The death rate among males due to human immunodeficiency virus (HIV) fell 60 percent between 1990 and 2002 as new drug treatments turned infection from a death sentence to a manageable chronic condition. The male death rate from HIV fell from 18.5 to 7.4 deaths per 100,000 population during those years. The death rate fell the most among young and middle-aged men and rose among men aged 65 or older. The death rate fell for both white and black males, although the decline was larger for whites.

In contrast to the decline in the HIV death rate among males, the rate among females rose 14 percent between 1990 and 2002, from 2.2 to 2.5 per 100,000 population. While the rate was down 18 percent among white females during those years, it rose 33 percent among black females.

■ HIV once ranked among the top ten causes of death in the United States, but by 2003 it had fallen to 18th place.

The HIV death rate has fallen among males, regardless of race

(percent change in number of deaths per 100,000 population from HIV, by sex and race, 1990–2002)

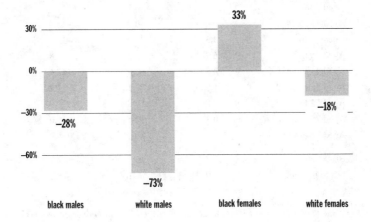

Table 5.12 Death Rate from Human Immunodeficiency Virus (HIV) Disease by Sex and Race, 1990 and 2002

(number of deaths due to human immunodeficiency virus (HIV) per 100,000 population by sex, age, and race, 1990 and 2002; percent change in rate, 1990–2002)

	2002	1990	percent change
Total males	**7.4**	**18.5**	**−60.0%**
Under age 1	–	2.4	–
Aged 1 to 4	–	0.8	–
Aged 5 to 14	–	0.3	–
Aged 15 to 24	0.4	2.2	−81.8
Aged 25 to 34	5.9	34.5	−82.9
Aged 35 to 44	18.8	50.2	−62.5
Aged 45 to 54	17.7	29.1	−39.2
Aged 55 to 64	8.5	12.0	−29.2
Aged 65 to 74	3.9	3.7	5.4
Aged 75 to 84	1.4	1.1	27.3
Aged 85 or older	–	–	–
Black male	33.3	46.3	−28.1
White male	4.3	15.7	−72.6
Total females	**2.5**	**2.2**	**13.6**
Under age 1	–	3.0	–
Aged 1 to 4	–	0.8	–
Aged 5 to 14	–	0.2	–
Aged 15 to 24	0.4	0.7	−42.9
Aged 25 to 34	3.3	4.9	−32.7
Aged 35 to 44	6.7	5.2	28.8
Aged 45 to 54	4.8	1.9	152.6
Aged 55 to 64	1.9	1.1	72.7
Aged 65 to 74	0.8	0.8	0.0
Aged 75 to 84	0.3	0.4	−25.0
Aged 85 or older	–	–	–
Black female	13.4	10.1	32.7
White female	0.9	1.1	−18.2

Note: "–" means sample is too small to make a reliable estimate.
Source: Bureau of the Census, Statistical Abstract of the United States: 2006; Internet site http://www.census.gov/prod/www/ statistical-abstract.html; calculations by New Strategist

Table 5.13 Deaths by Cause, 2003

(number and percent distribution of deaths by cause, 2003)

		number	percent distribution
All causes		**2,448,288**	**100.0%**
1.	Diseases of the heart	685,089	28.0
2.	Malignant neoplasms (cancer)	556,902	22.7
3.	Cerebrovascular diseases	157,689	6.4
4.	Chronic lower respiratory disease	126,382	5.2
5.	Accidents (unintentional injuries)	109,277	4.5
6.	Diabetes mellitus	74,219	3.0
7.	Influenza and pneumonia	65,163	2.7
8.	Alzheimer's disease	63,457	2.6
9.	Nephritis, nephrotic syndrome, nephrosis	42,453	1.7
10.	Septicemia	34,069	1.4
11.	Suicide	31,484	1.3
12.	Chronic liver disease and cirrhosis	27,503	1.1
13.	Essential (primary) hypertension and hypertensive renal disease	21,940	0.9
14.	Parkinson's disease	17,997	0.7
15.	Homicide	17,732	0.7
16.	Pneumonitis due to solids and liquids	17,335	0.7
17.	Perinatal conditions	14,378	0.6
18.	**Human immunodeficiency virus (HIV)**	**13,658**	**0.6**
	All other causes	371,561	15.2

Source: National Center for Health Statistics, Deaths: Final Data for 2003, National Vital Statistics Reports, Vol. 54, No. 13, 2006; Internt site http://www.cdc.gov/nchs/deaths.htm; calculations by New Strategist

Many People Live with AIDS

Sixty-four percent of those living with AIDS are black or Hispanic.

More than 400,000 Americans were living with AIDS in 2004, according to the Centers for Disease Control and Prevention. More than three out of four were males aged 13 or older, 23 percent were females aged 13 or older, and less than 1 percent were children under age 13. Seventy-three percent of those living with AIDS were aged 35 to 54.

Blacks and Hispanics account for the majority of people living with AIDS, while non-Hispanic whites are just 35 percent of the total. Most men living with AIDS were infected by male-to-male sexual contact. In contrast, most women living with AIDS were infected through heterosexual contact.

■ Twenty-one percent of men and 34 percent of women living with AIDS were infected through injection drug use.

Non-Hispanic whites are a minority of those living with AIDS

(percent distribution of people living with AIDS by race and Hispanic origin, 2004)

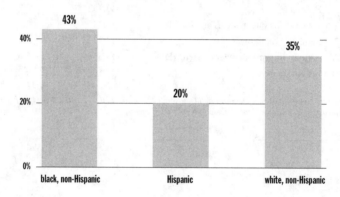

Table 5.14 People Living with AIDS by Sex and Age, 2004

(number and percent distribution of people living with AIDS by sex and age, 2004)

	number	percent distribution
Total people living with AIDS	**415,193**	**100.0%**
Sex		
Males aged 13 or older	317,698	76.5
Females aged 13 or older	93,566	22.5
Children under age 13*	3,927	0.9
Age		
Under age 13	1,695	0.4
Aged 13 to 14	776	0.2
Aged 15 to 19	2,043	0.5
Aged 20 to 24	4,942	1.2
Aged 25 to 29	13,721	3.3
Aged 30 to 34	33,669	8.1
Aged 35 to 39	68,389	16.5
Aged 40 to 44	95,874	23.1
Aged 45 to 49	81,636	19.7
Aged 50 to 54	56,336	13.6
Aged 55 to 59	30,033	7.2
Aged 60 to 64	14,228	3.4
Aged 65 or older	11,850	2.9

* At diagnosis
Note: Numbers may not sum to total because total includes people of unknown sex.
Source: Centers for Disease Control and Prevention, HIV/AIDS Surveillance Report, 2004, Vol. 16, 2005; Internet site http://www.cdc.gov/hiv/topics/surveillance/resources/reports/2004report/default.htm

Table 5.15 People Living with AIDS by Race and Hispanic Origin, 2004

(number and percent distribution of people living with AIDS by race and Hispanic origin, 2004)

	number	percent distribution
Total people living with AIDS	**415,193**	**100.0%**
American Indian	1,506	0.4
Asian	4,045	1.0
Black, non-Hispanic	178,233	42.9
Hispanic	84,001	20.2
White, non-Hispanic	145,935	35.1

Note: Numbers will not add to total because not all races are shown.
Source: Centers for Disease Control and Prevention, HIV/AIDS Surveillance Report, 2004, Vol. 16, 2005; Internet site http:// www.cdc.gov/hiv/topics/surveillance/resources/reports/2004report/default.htm

Table 5.16 People Living with AIDS by Sex and Transmission Category, 2004

(number and percent distribution of people aged 13 or older living with AIDS by sex and transmission category, 2004)

	number	percent distribution
Males, aged 13 or older living with AIDS	**317,698**	**100.0%**
Male-to-male sexual contact	185,326	58.3
Injection drug use	67,091	21.1
Heterosexual contact	35,671	11.2
Male-to-male sexual contact and injection drug use	25,367	8.0
Other	4,242	1.3
Females, aged 13 or older living with AIDS	**93,566**	**100.0**
Heterosexual contact	59,599	63.7
Injection drug use	31,472	33.6
Other	2,494	2.7

Note: "Other" includes hemophilia, blood transfusion, and not identified.
Source: Centers for Disease Control and Prevention, HIV/AIDS Surveillance Report, 2004, Vol. 16, 2005; Internet site http:// www.cdc.gov/hiv/topics/surveillance/resources/reports/2004report/default.htm

New York State Has Largest Number of People Living with AIDS

Nearly one-third of Americans living with AIDS are residents of New York or California.

The distribution of AIDS differs greatly by state. New York has the largest number of people living with AIDS, and it also has the largest number of cumulative AIDS cases since the disease was first recognized in the early 1980s. The more than 166,000 New Yorkers who had been diagnosed with AIDS through 2004 account for 19 percent of all AIDS cases in the United States. California ranks second with more than 135,000 AIDS cases through 2004. In North Dakota, in contrast, only 131 people have been diagnosed with AIDS over the years.

Among the 50 states, New York had the highest rate of new AIDS cases reported—39.7 cases per 100,000 population in 2004. Florida, Maryland, Louisiana, and New Jersey round out the top five. The rate of AIDS cases reported in 2004 was lowest in Montana, at just 0.8 cases per 100,000 population.

Of the more than 400,000 people living with AIDS in the United States, 70,133 live in New York State (17 percent). Half of all Americans living with AIDS reside in just five states: New York, California, Florida, Texas, and New Jersey.

■ North Dakota has the fewest number of people living with AIDS, just 66 in 2004.

Fifty-four percent of those living with AIDS reside in just five states

(percent distribution of people living with AIDS, by state, for the top five states, 2004)

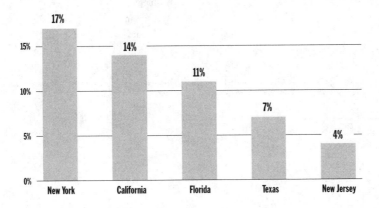

Table 5.17 Cumulative Number of AIDS Cases by State, through 2004

(cumulative number and percent distribution of AIDS cases by state, through 2004)

	number	percent distribution		number	percent distribution
Total cases	**888,795**	**100.0%**	Missouri	10,265	1.2%
Alabama	7,744	0.9	Montana	353	0.0
Alaska	597	0.1	Nebraska	1,329	0.1
Arizona	9,320	1.0	Nevada	5,190	0.6
Arkansas	3,487	0.4	New Hampshire	997	0.1
California	135,221	15.2	New Jersey	47,224	5.3
Colorado	8,141	0.9	New Mexico	2,396	0.3
Connecticut	13,890	1.6	New York	166,814	18.8
Delaware	3,302	0.4	North Carolina	14,078	1.6
District of Columbia	16,259	1.8	North Dakota	131	0.0
Florida	96,712	10.9	Ohio	13,655	1.5
Georgia	28,248	3.2	Oklahoma	4,381	0.5
Hawaii	2,770	0.3	Oregon	5,557	0.6
Idaho	560	0.1	Pennsylvania	30,526	3.4
Illinois	31,020	3.5	Rhode Island	2,413	0.3
Indiana	7,569	0.9	South Carolina	12,089	1.4
Iowa	1,565	0.2	South Dakota	226	0.0
Kansas	2,579	0.3	Tennessee	11,126	1.3
Kentucky	4,241	0.5	Texas	64,479	7.3
Louisiana	16,066	1.8	Utah	2,209	0.2
Maine	1,056	0.1	Vermont	445	0.1
Maryland	27,550	3.1	Virginia	15,740	1.8
Massachusetts	18,339	2.1	Washington	11,046	1.2
Michigan	13,631	1.5	West Virginia	1,375	0.2
Minnesota	4,415	0.5	Wisconsin	4,217	0.5
Mississippi	6,032	0.7	Wyoming	220	0.0

Source: Centers for Disease Control and Prevention, HIV/AIDS Surveillance Report, 2004, Vol. 16, 2005; Internet site http://www.cdc.gov/hiv/topics/surveillance/resources/reports/2004report/default.htm

Table 5.18 Number and Rate of Reported AIDS Cases by State in 2004

(number of AIDS cases reported and rate per 100,000 population, by state, 2004)

	number	rate		number	rate
Total cases	**43,653**	**14.9**	Missouri	394	6.8
Alabama	466	10.3	Montana	7	0.8
Alaska	55	8.4	Nebraska	69	3.9
Arizona	563	9.8	Nevada	305	13.1
Arkansas	185	6.7	New Hampshire	42	3.2
California	4,679	13	New Jersey	1,848	21.2
Colorado	338	7.3	New Mexico	183	9.6
Connecticut	643	18.4	New York	7,641	39.7
Delaware	157	18.9	North Carolina	1,137	13.3
District of Columbia	992	179.2	North Dakota	17	2.7
Florida	5,822	33.5	Ohio	665	5.8
Georgia	1,640	18.6	Oklahoma	195	5.5
Hawaii	136	10.8	Oregon	281	7.8
Idaho	22	1.6	Pennsylvania	1,629	13.1
Illinois	1,679	13.2	Rhode Island	132	12.2
Indiana	396	6.3	South Carolina	759	18.1
Iowa	64	2.2	South Dakota	12	1.6
Kansas	116	4.2	Tennessee	774	13.1
Kentucky	251	6.1	Texas	3,298	14.7
Louisiana	1,010	22.4	Utah	79	3.3
Maine	60	4.6	Vermont	17	2.7
Maryland	1,451	26.1	Virginia	796	10.7
Massachusetts	564	8.8	Washington	444	7.2
Michigan	655	6.5	West Virginia	93	5.1
Minnesota	218	4.3	Wisconsin	177	3.2
Mississippi	479	16.5	Wyoming	18	3.6

Source: Centers for Disease Control and Prevention, HIV/AIDS Surveillance Report, 2004, Vol. 16, 2005; Internet site http://www.cdc.gov/hiv/topics/surveillance/resources/reports/2004report/default.htm

Table 5.19 People Living with AIDS by State, 2004

(number and percent distribution of people living with AIDS by state, 2004)

	number	percent distribution		number	percent distribution
Total living with AIDS	**404,206**	**100.0%**	Missouri	5,021	1.2%
Alabama	3,352	0.8	Montana	175	0.0
Alaska	300	0.1	Nebraska	638	0.2
Arizona	4,068	1.0	Nevada	2,649	0.7
Arkansas	2,036	0.5	New Hampshire	535	0.1
California	56,988	14.1	New Jersey	17,408	4.3
Colorado	3,741	0.9	New Mexico	1,161	0.3
Connecticut	6,472	1.6	New York	70,133	17.4
Delaware	1,639	0.4	North Carolina	7,245	1.8
District of Columbia	9,036	2.2	North Dakota	66	0.0
Florida	45,140	11.2	Ohio	6,722	1.7
Georgia	14,245	3.5	Oklahoma	1,943	0.5
Hawaii	1,271	0.3	Oregon	2,541	0.6
Idaho	277	0.1	Pennsylvania	15,308	3.8
Illinois	15,418	3.8	Rhode Island	1,165	0.3
Indiana	3,731	0.9	South Carolina	6,554	1.6
Iowa	749	0.2	South Dakota	112	0.0
Kansas	1,147	0.3	Tennessee	5,753	1.4
Kentucky	2,354	0.6	Texas	29,891	7.4
Louisiana	7,472	1.8	Utah	1,121	0.3
Maine	501	0.1	Vermont	233	0.1
Maryland	13,045	3.2	Virginia	7,916	2.0
Massachusetts	8,254	2.0	Washington	5,136	1.3
Michigan	5,697	1.4	West Virginia	662	0.2
Minnesota	2,059	0.5	Wisconsin	1,942	0.5
Mississippi	3,078	0.8	Wyoming	102	0.0

Source: Centers for Disease Control and Prevention, HIV/AIDS Surveillance Report, 2004, Vol. 16, 2005; Internet site http://www.cdc.gov/hiv/topics/surveillance/resources/reports/2004report/default.htm

Having Multiple Sex Partners Increases HIV Risk

Though few admit to engaging in HIV risk behavior, many men and women have had sex with partners who have had sex with others recently.

Few people admit to engaging in HIV risk behavior, but many men and women have sex partners who have recently had sex with others, potentially exposing them to the HIV virus. Among unmarried women aged 15 to 44, only 4 percent say they have engaged in HIV risk behavior in the past year. (Risk behavior is defined as injecting drugs without a prescription, giving or receiving drugs or money in exchange for sex, or having sex with a partner who was infected with HIV.) But 20 percent of women say their male partner had sex with other people around the same time as with the respondent, which might mean they have been exposed to the virus.

Among unmarried men aged 15 to 44, the proportions are similar. Fewer than 5 percent admit to injecting drugs or exchanging sex for drugs or money, and only 1 percent say they had sex with an HIV-infected partner. But 23 percent of unmarried men say their female partner had sex with others around the same time as with the respondent.

Those most likely to admit to HIV risk behavior are those who have had the largest number of sexual partners. To make matters worse, more than half of those with three or more partners in the past year say their partner had sex with others at the same time as with them.

■ The younger the age at first sexual intercourse, the more likely a woman is to have engaged in HIV risk behavior in the past year.

The more sex partners, the greater the exposure to HIV

(percent of unmarried men aged 15 to 44 who have had sex in the past 12 months whose female partner had sex with others around the same time as with the respondent, by number of female partners in past year, 2002)

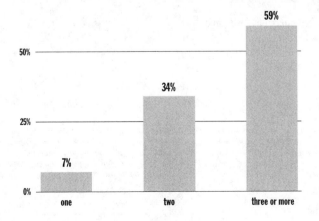

Table 5.20 HIV Risk Behavior among Women and Their Partners, 2002

(number of total and unmarried women aged 15 to 44 who have had at least one male sexual partner in the past 12 months, percent of women who engaged in HIV risk behavior and percent of male partners who did, by selected characteristics, 2002; numbers in thousands)

	number	woman engaged in HIV risk behavior	injected drugs without prescription	had sex with a male	had sex with other people around same time as with respondent
			male partner engaged in HIV risk behavior		
TOTAL WOMEN AGED 15 TO 44	**50,823**	**2.8%**	**3.6%**	**2.8%**	**10.4%**
Currently married	27,480	1.9	2.3	1.6	2.4
Currently cohabiting	5,308	3.5	5.2	2.2	8.6
Never married, not cohabiting	13,356	3.4	4.5	5.1	23.1
Formerly married, not cohabiting	4,679	5.9	6.6	3.9	24.5
UNMARRIED WOMEN AGED 15 TO 44	**23,343**	**4.0**	**5.1**	**4.2**	**20.0**
Aged 15 to 19	5,030	3.2	5.7	5.1	20.4
Aged 20 to 24	6,140	3.1	3.3	4.6	20.6
Aged 25 to 29	3,723	4.8	4.4	3.1	22.9
Aged 30 to 44	8,450		6.2	3.9	18.1
Race and Hispanic origin					
Black, non-Hispanic	4,691	7.4	8.7	4.9	24.6
Hispanic	3,447	3.3	4.0	4.3	13.9
White, non-Hispanic	13,457	2.9	3.8	3.6	20.1
Education					
Not a high school graduate	2,297	4.8	7.9	4.2	14.0
High school graduate or GED	5,096	4.3	4.7	4.0	19.8
Some college, no degree	4,613	5.1	6.8	4.6	24.0
Bachelor's degree or more	3,615	1.8	1.7	3.1	19.2
Number of male partners in past 12 months					
One	15,534	2.4	3.9	3.2	8.4
Two	4,186	5.4	4.9	6.5	36.5
Three or more	3,624	8.9	10.1	5.6	51.6
Age at first sexual intercourse with male					
Never had sexual intercourse	1,213	2.6	4.7	6.3	6.8
Under age 15	4,597	6.9	7.8	5.3	26.7
Aged 15 to 17	11,389	2.9	3.9	3.2	20.3
Aged 18 to 19	4,019	4.3	5.7	5.4	18.9
Aged 20 or older	2,125	3.0	4.6	3.9	13.9

Note: Sexual partner is defined as any partner with whom respondent had sexual contact, including vaginal intercourse, oral sex, or anal sex. HIV risk behavior is defined as injecting drugs without a prescription, giving or receiving drugs or money in exchange for sex, or having sex with a male partner who was infected with HIV. Education categories include only people aged 22 to 44. Source: National Center for Health Statistics, Fertility, Family Planning, and Reproductive Health of U.S. Women: Data from the 2002 National Survey of Family Growth, Vital and Health Statistics, Series 23, No. 25, 2005; Internet site http://www.cdc.gov/nchs/nsfg.htm

Table 5.21 HIV Risk Behavior among Men, 2002

(number of total and unmarried men aged 15 to 44, and percent engaging in HIV risk behavior in the past 12 months, by selected characteristics, 2002; numbers in thousands)

	number	injection drug use or drugs/money in exchange for sex	sex with infected partner
TOTAL MEN AGED 15 TO 44	**61,147**	**3.4%**	**0.8%**
Currently married	25,808	1.8	0.3
Currently cohabiting	5,653	4.2	2.5
Never married, not cohabiting	25,412	4.1	0.9
Formerly married, not cohabiting	4,274	5.9	1.0
UNMARRIED MEN AGED 15 TO 44	**35,340**	**4.5**	**1.2**
Aged 15 to 19	10,166	2.3	–
Aged 20 to 24	8,366	4.2	1.0
Aged 25 to 29	5,048	3.4	0.8
Aged 30 to 44	11,760	6.8	2.4
Race and Hispanic origin			
Black, non-Hispanic	4,753	9.0	1.1
Hispanic	5,839	4.3	1.2
White, non-Hispanic	21,555	3.7	1.1
Education			
Not a high school graduate	2,976	4.4	1.5
High school graduate or GED	7,225	6.4	0.8
Some college, no degree	6,717	5.9	1.7
Bachelor's degree or more	4,562	4.7	3.5
Number of female partners in past 12 months			
None	3,710	3.2	2.5
One	14,679	3.0	1.1
Two	4,369	5.3	–
Three or more	5,690	11.8	1.5
Any oral or anal sex with male partner			
Yes	2,791	17.8	9.1
No	32,498	3.4	0.5
Self report of any sexually transmitted disease			
Yes	2,384	18.9	9.0
No	32,955	3.4	0.6

Note: Education categories include only people aged 22 to 44. "–" means sample is too small to make a reliable estimate.
Source: National Center for Health Statistics, Fertility, Contraception, and Fatherhood: Data on Men and Women from Cycle 6 of the 2002 National Survey of Family Growth, Vital and Health Statistics, Series 23, No. 26, 2006; Internet site http://www.cdc .gov/nchs/nsfg.htm

Table 5.22 HIV Risk Behavior among Men's Sexual Partners, 2002

(number of total and unmarried men aged 15 to 44 who have had sex with a male or female partner in the past 12 months, and percent with partners engaging in HIV risk behavior, by selected characteristics, 2002; numbers in thousands)

	number	partner injected drugs without presscription	female partner had sex with other people around same time as with respondent
TOTAL MEN AGED 15 TO 44	**50,913**	**2.9%**	**13.0%**
Currently married	24,871	2.0	2.7
Currently cohabiting	5,416	5.1	11.0
Never married, not cohabiting	16,938	3.4	27.0
Formerly married, not cohabiting	3,689	3.2	25.7
UNMARRIED MEN			
AGED 15 TO 44	**26,042**	**3.7**	**23.3**
Aged 15 to 19	5,535	2.8	21.1
Aged 20 to 24	6,823	2.3	25.1
Aged 25 to 29	4,031	5.5	24.5
Aged 30 to 44	9,653	4.6	22.7
Race and Hispanic origin			
Black, non-Hispanic	4,001	4.6	29.4
Hispanic	4,395	3.4	21.6
White, non-Hispanic	15,830	4.8	22.1
Education			
Not a high school graduate	2,366	6.6	22.0
High school graduate or GED	6,055	3.0	25.7
Some college, no degree	5,588	4.8	26.2
Bachelor's degree or more	3,353	4.0	21.4
Number of female partners in past 12 months			
One	14,679	2.9	7.1
Two	4,369	2.5	33.8
Three or more	5,690	6.0	58.5
Age at first sexual intercourse with female			
Never had sexual intercourse	1,736	2.8	11.7
Under age 15	5,638	5.6	31.8
Aged 15 to 17	12,604	3.8	23.8
Aged 18 to 19	3,927	1.7	16.1
Aged 20 or older	2,137	2.9	17.9
Any oral or anal sex with male partner			
Yes	2,472	11.3	45.5
No	23,570	3.0	21.9
Self report of any sexually transmitted disease			
Yes	2,094	13.4	36.8
No	23,948	2.9	22.2

Note: Sexual partner is defined as any partner with whom respondent had sexual contact, including vaginal intercourse, oral sex, or anal sex. Education categories include only people aged 22 to 44.
Source: National Center for Health Statistics, Fertility, Contraception, and Fatherhood: Data on Men and Women from Cycle 6 of the 2002 National Survey of Family Growth, Vital and Health Statistics, Series 23, No. 26, 2006; Internet site http://www.cdc .gov/nchs/nsfg.htm

Most People Aged 15 to 44 Have Been Tested for HIV

Women are more likely than men to have been tested.

HIV testing is common among young and middle-aged adults. Among women aged 15 to 44, the 55 percent majority have had an HIV test and 16 percent have been tested in the past year. Among men in the age group, 47 percent have ever been tested, and 14 percent have had a test in the past year. Many women are tested for HIV during pregnancy.

Blacks are more likely than Hispanics or non-Hispanic whites to have been tested for HIV. From 24 to 25 percent of blacks aged 15 to 44 have been tested for HIV in the past year versus only 12 to 13 percent of non-Hispanic whites. Among Hispanics, 16 percent of men and 21 percent of women have been tested for HIV in the past year.

■ Men and women with multiple sex partners in the past year, and those who have been treated for a sexually transmitted infection, are most likely to have been tested for HIV.

HIV testing peaks in the 25-to-29 age group

(percent of people aged 15 to 44 who have been tested for HIV in the past 12 months, by age, 2002)

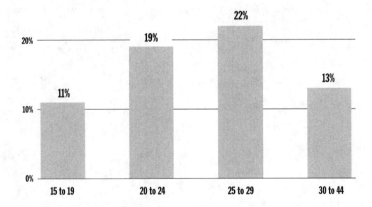

Table 5.23 HIV Testing by Sex and Age, 2002

(total number of people aged 15 to 44 and percent who have been tested for HIV in lifetime and in past year, by sex and age, 2002; numbers in thousands)

	number	ever had HIV test	had HIV test in past 12 months
Total aged 15 to 44	**122,708**	**50.7%**	**15.1%**
Aged 15 to 19	20,042	18.7	10.5
Aged 20 to 24	19,723	44.3	19.1
Aged 25 to 29	18,475	60.8	21.8
Aged 30 to 44	64,467	59.8	13.3
Total men	**61,147**	**46.6**	**14.2**
Aged 15 to 19	10,208	15.7	9.5
Aged 20 to 24	9,883	39.2	17.2
Aged 25 to 29	9,226	53.4	19.5
Aged 30 to 44	31,830	56.8	13.3
Total women	**61,561**	**54.9**	**15.9**
Aged 15 to 19	9,834	21.8	11.6
Aged 20 to 24	9,840	49.4	21.0
Aged 25 to 29	9,249	68.1	24.1
Aged 30 to 44	32,638	62.8	13.4

Source: National Center for Health Statistics, HIV Testing in the United States, 2002, Advance Data, No. 363, 2005; Internet site http://www.cdc.gov/nchs/products/pubs/pubd/ad/361-370/ad363.htm

Table 5.24 HIV Testing by Sex and Marital Status, 2002

(total number of people aged 15 to 44 and percent who have been tested for HIV in lifetime and in past year, by sex and marital status, 2002; numbers in thousands)

	number	ever had HIV test	had HIV test in past 12 months
Total aged 15 to 44	**122,708**	**50.7%**	**15.1%**
Never married, not cohabiting	46,981	36.8	15.1
Currently married	54,134	57.4	12.8
Currently cohabiting	11,223	62.2	18.9
Formerly married, not cohabiting	10,370	67.3	22.5
Total men	**61,147**	**46.6**	**14.2**
Never married, not cohabiting	25,412	36.1	15.4
Currently married	25,808	51.8	11.4
Currently cohabiting	5,653	58.0	15.9
Formerly married, not cohabiting	4,274	62.4	22.2
Total women	**61,561**	**54.9**	**15.9**
Never married, not cohabiting	21,568	37.6	14.8
Currently married	28,327	62.5	14.2
Currently cohabiting	5,570	66.4	21.9
Formerly married, not cohabiting	6,096	70.8	22.6

Source: National Center for Health Statistics, HIV Testing in the United States, 2002, Advance Data, No. 363, 2005; Internet site http://www.cdc.gov/nchs/products/pubs/pubd/ad/361-370/ad363.htm

Table 5.25 HIV Testing by Sex, Race, and Hispanic Origin, 2002

(total number of people aged 15 to 44 and percent who have been tested for HIV in lifetime and in past year, by sex, race, and Hispanic origin, 2002; numbers in thousands)

	number	ever had HIV test	had HIV test in past 12 months
Total aged 15 to 44	**122,708**	**50.7%**	**15.1%**
Black, non-Hispanic	15,190	61.4	24.2
Hispanic	19,295	50.2	18.1
White, non-Hispanic	78,237	49.2	12.5
Other, non-Hispanic	9,986	47.9	15.7
Total men	**61,147**	**46.6**	**14.2**
Black, non-Hispanic	6,940	56.5	23.7
Hispanic	10,188	44.7	15.6
White, non-Hispanic	38,738	45.8	12.4
Other, non-Hispanic	5,280	43.2	12.3
Total women	**61,561**	**54.9**	**15.9**
Black, non-Hispanic	8,250	65.4	24.6
Hispanic	9,107	56.3	20.8
White, non-Hispanic	39,498	52.5	12.5
Other, non-Hispanic	4,706	53.2	19.6

Source: National Center for Health Statistics, HIV Testing in the United States, 2002, Advance Data, No. 363, 2005; Internet site http://www.cdc.gov/nchs/products/pubs/pubd/ad/361-370/ad363.htm

Table 5.26 HIV Testing by Sex and Education, 2002

(total number of people aged 15 to 44 and percent who have been tested for HIV in lifetime and in past year, by sex and education, 2002; numbers in thousands)

	number	ever had HIV test	had HIV test in past 12 months
Total aged 15 to 44	**122,708**	**50.7%**	**15.1%**
Not a high school graduate	11,982	55.7	16.1
High school graduate or GED	29,923	58.8	16.4
Some college, no degree	27,382	61.6	17.4
Bachelor's degree or more	25,452	57.1	12.9
Total men	**61,147**	**46.6**	**14.2**
Not a high school graduate	6,355	47.4	11.9
High school graduate or GED	15,659	54.2	16.5
Some college, no degree	13,104	59.2	17.7
Bachelor's degree or more	11,901	54.0	11.2
Total women	**61,561**	**54.9**	**15.9**
Not a high school graduate	5,627	65.0	20.7
High school graduate or GED	14,264	64.0	16.4
Some college, no degree	14,279	63.8	17.0
Bachelor's degree or more	13,551	59.8	14.4

Note: Education categories include only people aged 22 to 44.
Source: National Center for Health Statistics, HIV Testing in the United States, 2002, Advance Data, No. 363, 2005; Internet site http://www.cdc.gov/nchs/products/pubs/pubd/ad/361-370/ad363.htm

Table 5.27 HIV Testing by Sex, Region, and Metropolitan Residence, 2002

(total number of people aged 15 to 44 and percent who have been tested for HIV in lifetime and in past year, by sex, region, and metropolitan residence, 2002; numbers in thousands)

	number	ever had HIV test	had HIV test in past 12 months
Total aged 15 to 44	**122,708**	**50.7%**	**15.1%**
Northeast	18,065	51.6	14.5
Midwest	26,866	46.6	12.5
South	47,481	52.4	16.5
West	30,295	51.3	15.5
Metropolitan, central city	59,537	51.4	14.4
Metropolitan, suburban	40,907	53.3	17.9
Nonmetropolitan	22,264	44.2	11.8
Total men	**61,147**	**46.6**	**14.2**
Northeast	8,361	47.2	13.2
Midwest	12,766	44.6	13.1
South	24,543	46.3	14.8
West	15,477	48.5	14.9
Metropolitan, central city	29,364	46.7	13.9
Metropolitan, suburban	20,399	49.3	16.1
Nonmetropolitan	11,384	41.6	11.7
Total women	**61,561**	**54.9**	**15.9**
Northeast	9,704	55.3	15.6
Midwest	14,100	48.4	12.0
South	22,939	58.9	18.2
West	14,818	54.3	16.2
Metropolitan, central city	30,172	56.1	14.8
Metropolitan, suburban	20,508	57.2	19.7
Nonmetropolitan	10,880	47.0	11.8

Source: National Center for Health Statistics, HIV Testing in the United States, 2002, Advance Data, No. 363, 2005; Internet site http://www.cdc.gov/nchs/products/pubs/pubd/ad/361-370/ad363.htm

Table 5.28 HIV Testing by Sex, Opposite-Sex Partners, and Treatment for Sexually Transmitted Disease, 2002

(total number of people aged 15 to 44 and percent who have been tested for HIV in lifetime and in past year, by sex, number of opposite-sex sexual partners in past year, and treatment for sexually transmitted disease (STD) in past year, 2002; numbers in thousands)

	number	ever had HIV test	had HIV test in past 12 months
Total people aged 15 to 44	**122,708**	**50.7%**	**15.1%**
No opposite-sex partners in past year	21,638	29.2	8.5
One opposite-sex partner	80,274	55.1	14.5
Two opposite-sex partners	9,581	53.7	21.7
Three or more opposite-sex partners	10,514	59.5	26.6
Treated for STD in past year	3,650	74.1	38.5
Not treated for STD in past year	118,549	50.0	14.4
Total men	**61,147**	**46.6**	**14.2**
No opposite-sex partners in past year	11,180	31.2	10.1
One opposite-sex partner	38,318	49.3	12.8
Two opposite-sex partners	4,894	46.3	19.6
Three or more opposite-sex partners	6,333	57.9	25.8
Treated for STD in past year	1,575	76.1	44.3
Not treated for STD in past year	59,303	45.8	13.4
Total women	**61,561**	**54.9**	**15.9**
No opposite-sex partners in past year	10,459	27.0	6.8
One opposite-sex partner	41,956	60.4	16.1
Two opposite-sex partners	4,687	61.6	23.9
Three or more opposite-sex partners	4,181	61.9	27.9
Treated for STD in past year	2,075	72.6	34.1
Not treated for STD in past year	59,246	54.2	15.3

Note: STD means sexually transmitted disease.
Source: National Center for Health Statistics, HIV Testing in the United States, 2002, Advance Data, No. 363, 2005; Internet site http://www.cdc.gov/nchs/products/pubs/pubd/ad/361-370/ad363.htm

Many Women Report Having Had a Sexually Transmitted Infection

Seventeen percent of women have had a sexually transmitted infection, excluding HIV.

Sexually transmitted infections are common, and ever changing. As one disease is conquered, others appear. Syphilis is much less common today than it was a few decades ago, and gonorrhea has also seen its peak. But chlamydia, genital herpes, and genital warts are on the rise. Women account for the majority of cases of chlamydia and gonorrhea, while men account for most cases of syphilis.

Seventeen percent of sexually experienced women aged 15 to 44 say they have had a sexually transmitted infection at some point in their life. Only 7 percent of men say they have had a sexually transmitted infection. A substantial 13 percent of women aged 15 to 44 have received counseling, testing, or treatment for a sexually transmitted infection in the past year, the figure peaking at 22 percent among women aged 20 to 24. Among men, 10 percent have received advice about sexually transmitted infections from a medical care provider in the past year, and 12 percent have gotten advice about HIV.

■ The rate of reported cases of chlamydia and gonorrhea peaks among teenage girls aged 15 to 19.

Many women have been counseled, tested, or treated for a sexually transmitted infection in the past year

(percent of women aged 15 to 44 who have received counseling, testing, or treatment for a sexually transmitted infection in the past year, by age, 2002)

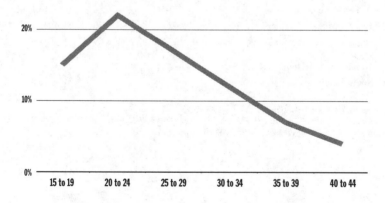

Table 5.29 Reported Cases of Nationally Notifiable Sexually Transmitted Diseases, 1950 to 2004

(number of cases of nationally notifiable sexually transmitted diseases reported by state health departments to the federal government and rate per 100,000 population, 1950 to 2004)

	chlamydia	gonorrhea	syphilis (all stages)	chancroid
2004	929,462	330,132	33,401	30
2000	709,452	363,136	31,618	78
1990	323,663	690,042	135,590	4,212
1980	–	1,004,029	68,832	788
1970	–	600,072	91,382	1,416
1960	–	258,933	122,538	1,680
1950	–	286,746	217,558	4,977
Rate per 100,000 population				
2004	319.6	113.5	11.5	0.0
2000	251.4	128.7	11.2	0.0
1990	160.2	276.4	54.3	1.7
1980	–	445.1	30.5	0.3
1970	–	297.2	45.3	0.7
1960	–	145.4	68.8	0.9
1950	–	192.5	146.0	3.3

Note: "–" means not reported.
Source: Centers for Disease Control and Prevention, Sexually Transmitted Disease Surveillance, 2004; Internet site http://www .cdc.gov/std/stats/toc2004.htm

Table 5.30 Initial Doctor Visits for Sexually Transmitted Diseases and Conditions, 1970 to 2004

(number of initial doctor visits for sexually transmitted diseases and conditions, 1970 to 2004)

	genital herpes	genital warts	vaginal trichomoniasis	other vaginitis	pelvic inflammatory disease
2004	269,000	316,000	221,000	3,602,000	132,000
2000	179,000	220,000	222,000	3,470,000	254,000
1990	172,000	275,000	213,000	4,474,000	358,000
1980	57,000	218,000	358,000	1,670,000	423,000
1970	17,000	119,000	529,000	1,500,000	–

Note: "–" means data not available.
Source: Centers for Disease Control and Prevention, Sexually Transmitted Disease Surveillance, 2004; Internet site http://www .cdc.gov/std/stats/toc2004.htm

Table 5.31 Reported Cases of Nationally Notifiable Sexually Transmitted Diseases by Sex, 2004

(number and percent distribution of reported cases of nationally notifiable sexually transmitted diseases, by sex, 2004)

	total	female	male
Chlamydia	929,462	716,675	210,396
Gonorrhea	330,132	172,142	157,303
Primary syphilis	2,269	241	2,026
Secondary syphilis	5,711	1,014	4,696
Latent syphilis	25,068	9,227	15,773
Neurosyphilis	833	182	650
Chancroid	30	9	19
Percent distribution			
Chlamydia	100.0%	77.1%	22.6%
Gonorrhea	100.0	52.1	47.6
Primary syphilis	100.0	10.6	89.3
Secondary syphilis	100.0	17.8	82.2
Latent syphilis	100.0	36.8	62.9
Neurosyphilis	100.0	21.8	78.0
Chancroid	100.0	30.0	63.3

Note: Numbers may not add to total because of unknown sex.
*Source: Centers for Disease Control and Prevention, Sexually Transmitted Disease Surveillance, 2004; Internet site http://www
.cdc.gov/std/stats/toc2004.htm; calculations by New Strategist*

Table 5.32 Women Reporting Any Sexually Transmitted Infection except HIV, 2002

(number of sexually experienced women aged 15 to 44 and percent reporting any sexually transmitted infection except HIV, by selected characteristics, 2002; numbers in thousands)

	number	percent reporting sexually transmitted infection, except HIV
Total sexually experienced women aged 15 to 44	**55,553**	**16.8%**
Aged 15 to 19	6,169	10.5
Aged 20 to 24	8,888	13.4
Aged 25 to 29	8,875	16.5
Aged 30 to 34	9,931	18.6
Aged 35 to 44	21,690	19.2
Marital status		
Currently married	27,785	17.0
Currently cohabiting	5,460	17.6
Never married, not cohabiting	16,290	14.0
Formerly married, not cohabiting	8,017	22.5
Race and Hispanic origin		
Black, non-Hispanic	7,499	18.5
Hispanic	7,835	13.1
White, non-Hispanic	36,251	17.2
Metropolitan residence		
Central city of 12 largest metropolitan areas	7,632	17.7
Central city of other metropolitan areas	12,849	19.0
Suburb of 12 largest metropolitan areas	12,301	13.3
Suburb of other metropolitan areas	12,821	19.4
Nonmetropolitan area	9,951	14.1

Note: Sexual experience includes any sexual contact with another person, including oral sex, anal sex, and vaginal intercourse. Sexually transmitted infections include genital herpes, genital warts, pelvic inflammatory disease, and syphilis in lifetime and treatment for gonorrhea or chlamydia in the past 12 months.
Source: National Center for Health Statistics, Sexual Behavior and Selected Health Measures: Men and Women 15–44 Years of Age, United States, 2002, Advance Data, No. 362, 2005; Internet site http://www.cdc.gov/nchs/nsfg.htm

Table 5.33   Men Reporting Any Sexually Transmitted Infection except HIV, 2002

(number of sexually experienced men aged 15 to 44 and percent reporting any sexually transmitted infection except HIV, by selected characteristics, 2002; numbers in thousands)

	number	percent reporting sexually transmitted infection, except HIV
Total sexually experienced men aged 15 to 44	**54,773**	**7.4%**
Aged 15 to 19	6,568	3.2
Aged 20 to 24	8,886	7.1
Aged 25 to 29	8,713	4.8
Aged 30 to 34	9,739	9.3
Aged 35 to 44	20,867	9.0
Marital status		
Currently married	25,079	6.9
Currently cohabiting	5,455	5.5
Never married, not cohabiting	20,053	7.6
Formerly married, not cohabiting	4,186	11.4
Race and Hispanic origin		
Black, non-Hispanic	6,247	10.0
Hispanic	8,983	6.8
White, non-Hispanic	35,247	7.3
Metropolitan residence		
Central city of 12 largest metropolitan areas	7,520	9.3
Central city of other metropolitan areas	13,082	8.5
Suburb of 12 largest metropolitan areas	12,340	7.6
Suburb of other metropolitan areas	11,828	6.2
Nonmetropolitan area	10,003	5.4

Note: Sexual experience includes any sexual contact with another person, including oral sex, anal sex, or vaginal intercourse. Sexually transmitted infections include genital herpes, genital warts, or syphilis in lifetime, and treatment for gonorrhea or chlamydia in the past 12 months.
Source: National Center for Health Statistics, Sexual Behavior and Selected Health Measures: Men and Women 15-44 Years of Age, United States, 2002, Advance Data, No. 362, 2005; Internet site http://www.cdc.gov/nchs/nsfg.htm

Table 5.34 Reported Cases of Chlamydia by Age and Sex, 2004

(number and rate per 100,000 population of reported cases of chlamydia, by age and sex, 2004)

	total		female		male	
	number	rate per 100,000	number	rate per 100,000	number	rate per 100,000
Total cases reported in 2004	**929,462**	**319.6**	**718,527**	**486.2**	**210,935**	**147.5**
Aged 10 to 14	14,817	69.9	13,646	132.0	1,172	10.8
Aged 15 to 19	323,246	1,578.5	275,036	2,761.5	48,209	458.3
Aged 20 to 24	344,159	1,660.4	264,749	2,630.7	79,410	744.7
Aged 25 to 29	137,041	714.9	97,667	1,039.5	39,374	402.9
Aged 30 to 34	56,759	274.1	37,406	364.8	19,353	185.2
Aged 35 to 39	26,486	123.7	15,839	148.3	10,647	99.3
Aged 40 to 44	13,626	59.3	7,229	62.6	6,397	56.1
Aged 45 to 54	9,251	22.7	4,649	22.4	4,602	23.0
Aged 55 to 64	1,885	6.8	892	6.2	993	7.4
Aged 65 or older	755	2.1	420	2.0	335	2.2

Note: Numbers may not add to total because cases among people under age 10 are not shown and because of proration of unknown age/sex.
Source: Centers for Disease Control and Prevention, Sexually Transmiitted Disease Surveillance, 2004; Internet site http://www .cdc.gov/std/stats/toc2004.htm; calculations by New Strategist

Table 5.35 Reported Cases of Chlamydia by Race and Hispanic Origin, 2004

(number and rate per 100,000 population of reported cases of chlamydia, by race and Hispanic origin, 2004)

	number	rate per 100,000
Total cases reported in 2004	**929,462**	**319.6**
American Indian	16,741	705.8
Asian	15,034	133.7
Black, non-Hispanic	420,546	1,209.4
Hispanic	164,182	436.1
White, non-Hispanic	272,560	143.6

Note: Numbers may not add to total because cases among people of unknown race/Hispanic origin are prorated and Colorado, the District of Columbia, Hawaii, and New Jersey did not report cases.
Source: Centers for Disease Control and Prevention, Sexually Transmitted Disease Surveillance, 2004; Internet site http://www .cdc.gov/std/stats/toc2004.htm; calculations by New Strategist

Table 5.36 Reported Cases of Gonorrhea by Age and Sex, 2004

(number and rate per 100,000 population of reported cases of gonorrhea, by age and sex, 2004)

	total		female		male	
	number	rate per 100,000	number	rate per 100,000	number	rate per 100,000
Total cases reported in 2004	**330,132**	**113.5**	**172,509**	**116.7**	**157,623**	**110.2**
Aged 10 to 14	4,447	21.0	3,817	36.9	630	5.8
Aged 15 to 19	87,454	427.1	60,847	610.9	26,607	252.9
Aged 20 to 24	103,187	497.8	57,269	569.1	45,917	430.6
Aged 25 to 29	54,857	286.2	25,337	269.7	29,250	302.1
Aged 30 to 34	30,372	146.7	11,708	114.2	18,664	178.6
Aged 35 to 39	19,793	92.5	6,443	60.3	13,350	124.5
Aged 40 to 44	14,026	61.1	3,806	32.9	10,220	89.6
Aged 45 to 54	12,078	29.6	2,433	11.7	9,645	48.1
Aged 55 to 64	2,653	9.5	367	2.5	2,286	17.0
Aged 65 or older	745	2.1	130	0.6	615	4.1

Note: Numbers may not add to total because cases among people under age 10 are not shown and because of proration of unknown age/sex.
Source: Centers for Disease Control and Prevention, Sexually Transmitted Disease Surveillance, 2004; Internet site http://www.cdc.gov/std/stats/toc2004.htm

Table 5.37 Reported Cases of Gonorrhea by Race and Hispanic Origin, 2004

(number and rate per 100,000 population of reported cases of gonorrhea, by race and Hispanic origin, 2004)

	number	rate per 100,000
Total cases reported in 2004	**330,132**	**113.5**
American Indian	2,858	117.7
Asian	2,726	21.4
Black, non-Hispanic	229,843	629.6
Hispanic	28,455	71.3
White, non-Hispanic	66,250	33.3

Source: Centers for Disease Control and Prevention, Sexually Transmitted Disease Surveillance, 2004; Internet site http:// www.cdc.gov/std/stats/toc2004.htm; calculations by New Strategist

Table 5.38   Reported Cases of Primary and Secondary Syphilis by Age and Sex, 2004

(number and rate per 100,000 population of reported cases of primary and secondary syphilis, by age and sex, 2004)

	total		female		male	
	number	rate per 100,000	number	rate per 100,000	number	rate per 100,000
Total cases reported in 2004	**7,975**	**2.8**	**1,254**	**0.9**	**6,721**	**4.7**
Aged 10 to 14	9	0.0	7	0.1	2	0.0
Aged 15 to 19	339	1.7	148	1.5	191	1.8
Aged 20 to 24	1,029	5.0	294	3.0	735	7.0
Aged 25 to 29	1,125	5.9	182	2.0	943	9.7
Aged 30 to 34	1,282	6.2	166	1.6	1,116	10.8
Aged 35 to 39	1,467	6.9	154	1.5	1,313	12.4
Aged 40 to 44	1,344	5.9	146	1.3	1,198	10.6
Aged 45 to 54	1,035	2.6	120	0.6	915	4.6
Aged 55 to 64	281	1.0	32	0.2	249	1.9
Aged 65 or older	55	0.2	1	0.0	54	0.4

Note: Numbers may not add to total because cases among people under age 10 are not shown and because of proration of unknown age/sex.
Source: Centers for Disease Control and Prevention, Sexually Transmitted Disease Surveillance, 2004; Internet site http://www.cdc.gov/std/stats/toc2004.htm; calculations by New Strategist

Table 5.39   Reported Cases of Primary and Secondary Syphilis by Race and Hispanic Origin, 2004

(number and rate per 100,000 population of reported cases of primary and secondary syphilis, by race and Hispanic origin, 2004)

	number	rate per 100,000
Total cases reported in 2004	**7,975**	**2.8**
American Indian	77	3.2
Asian	153	1.2
Black, non-Hispanic	3,263	9.0
Hispanic	1,278	3.2
White, non-Hispanic	3,203	1.6

Source: Centers for Disease Control and Prevention, Sexually Transmitted Disease Surveillance, 2004; Internet site http://www.cdc.gov/std/stats/toc2004.htm; calculations by New Strategist

Table 5.40 Women Receiving Testing or Treatment for Sexually Transmitted Diseases, 2002

(total number of women aged 15 to 44 and percent receiving counseling, testing, or treatment for a sexually trans-mitted disease in the past 12 months from a medical care provider, by selected characteristics, 2002; numbers in thousands)

	number	percent receiving counseling, testing, or treatment for a sexually transmitted disease
Total women aged 15 to 44	**61,561**	**12.6%**
Aged 15 to 19	9,834	15.2
Aged 20 to 24	9,840	22.3
Aged 25 to 29	9,249	16.6
Aged 30 to 34	10,272	12.2
Aged 35 to 39	10,853	6.9
Aged 40 to 44	11,512	4.4
Marital status		
Currently married	28,327	8.1
Currently cohabiting	5,570	20.3
Never married, not cohabiting	21,568	15.9
Formerly married, not cohabiting	6,096	14.4
Children ever borne		
None	25,622	14.4
One	11,193	14.6
Two	13,402	10.2
Three or more	11,343	9.3
Race and Hispanic origin		
Black, non-Hispanic	8,587	16.1
Hispanic	9,107	12.5
White, non-Hispanic	40,420	12.0

Source: National Center for Health Statistics, Use of Contraception and Use of Family Planning Services in the United States: 1982–2002, Advance Data, No. 350, 2004; Internet site http://www.cdc.gov/nchs/nsfg.htm

Table 5.41 Treatment for Pelvic Inflammatory Disease, 2002

(total number of women aged 15 to 44 and percent ever receiving treatment for pelvic inflammatory disease, by selected characteristics, 2002; numbers in thousands)

	number	percent treated
Total women aged 15 to 44	**61,561**	**5.1%**
Aged 15 to 19	9,834	1.2
Aged 20 to 24	9,840	3.9
Aged 25 to 29	9,249	5.3
Aged 30 to 34	10,272	5.5
Aged 35 to 39	10,853	5.8
Aged 40 to 44	11,512	8.0
Race and Hispanic origin		
Black, non-Hispanic	8,250	6.7
Hispanic	9,107	5.7
White, non-Hispanic	39,498	4.6
Marital status		
Currently married	28,327	5.7
Currently cohabiting	5,570	6.4
Never married, not cohabiting	21,568	3.2
Formerly married, not cohabiting	6,096	7.4
Number of male partners in lifetime		
None	7,371	0.6
One	13,374	3.3
Two or three	12,794	4.3
Four to nine	18,773	5.8
Ten or more	9,248	10.7
Age at first sexual intercourse with male		
Under age 15	8,074	9.6
Aged 15 to 17	25,033	5.4
Aged 18 to 19	11,136	5.0
Aged 20 or older	9,946	3.9

Source: National Center for Health Statistics, Fertility, Family Planning, and Reproductive Health of U.S. Women: Data from the 2002 National Survey of Family Growth, Vital and Health Statistics, Series 23, No. 25, 2005; Internet site http://www.cdc.gov/nchs/nsfg.htm

Table 5.42   Men Receiving Advice from Medical Providers about Sexually Transmitted Diseases or HIV, 2002

(total number of men aged 15 to 44 and percent receiving advice from a medical care provider about sexually transmitted diseases or human immunodeficiency virus in the past 12 months, by selected characteristics, 2002; numbers in thousands)

	number	percent receiving advice about STD	percent receiving advice about HIV
Total men aged 15 to 44	**61,147**	**10.4%**	**12.3%**
Aged 15 to 19	10,208	17.2	19.2
Aged 20 to 24	9,883	16.3	17.2
Aged 25 to 29	9,226	10.8	11.1
Aged 30 to 44	31,830	6.3	8.9
Marital status			
Currently married	25,808	5.5	6.6
Currently cohabiting	5,653	8.2	11.4
Never married, not cohabiting	25,412	16.1	18.4
Formerly married, not cohabiting	4,274	9.5	11.1
Number of biological children			
None	32,593	13.3	15.2
One	10,457	7.9	9.3
Two	9,829	7.0	8.6
Three or more	8,269	6.6	8.8
Race and Hispanic origin			
Black, non-Hispanic	6,940	19.1	23.5
Hispanic	10,188	16.2	17.1
White, non-Hispanic	38,738	7.8	9.2

Source: National Center for Health Statistics, Fertility, Contraception, and Fatherhood: Data on Men and Women from Cycle 6 of the 2002 National Survey of Family Growth, Vital and Health Statistics, Series 23, No. 26, 2006; Internet site http://www .cdc.gov/nchs/nsfg.htm

6

Cohabitation and Marriage

■ Marriage has become less important, while cohabitation and divorce have become commonplace. These changes have affected some demographic segments much more than others.

■ Many women have cohabited. Twenty-eight percent of women aged 15 to 44 lived with an opposite-sex partner before their first marriage. The figure rises with age to a peak of 44 percent among women aged 30 to 34.

■ Cohabitors are uncertain of future plans with their partner. Only 48 percent of men and 45 percent of women aged 15 to 44 who are currently cohabiting feel "almost certain" they will marry their partner.

■ Older boomers are most likely to divorce. The probability of divorce is greatest for men born between 1945 and 1949 and women born between 1950 and 1954—in other words, the oldest boomers.

■ Marriage at a young age usually results in divorce. Sixty-three percent of women who married for the first time before age 18 have seen their marriage end. Among women who first married at age 23 or older, only 22 percent have divorced.

■ Men care more about marriage than women. Two-thirds of men aged 15 to 44 agree with the statement, "It is better to get married than to go through life being single." Only 51 percent of their female counterparts agree.

Half of Women Aged 15 to 44 Have Cohabited

Only 9 percent of women in the age group are currently cohabiting.

Cohabitation has become commonplace among younger generations of Americans. Fully 50 percent of women aged 15 to 44 have ever lived with an opposite-sex partner outside of marriage. The proportion peaks at more than 60 percent among women aged 25 to 39. Only 9 percent of women in the 15 to 44 age group are currently cohabiting, however, with the figure peaking at 16 percent in the 20-to-24 age group.

A slightly smaller 49 percent of men aged 15 to 44 have ever cohabited. As with their female counterparts, only 9 percent of men are currently cohabiting. The percentage of men currently cohabiting peaks at 18 percent in the 25-to-29 age group.

Most cohabitations end in marriage, but many of those marriages dissolve. Fifty-two percent of women who have ever cohabited say their first cohabitation ended in marriage, but only 34 percent of those marriages are still intact. Another 35 percent of first cohabitations ended without marriage. Thirteen percent of first cohabitations are continuing.

■ Cohabitation is most common among the least-educated men and women.

Mamy cohabitations end in separation

(percent distribution of women aged 15 to 44 who have ever cohabited, by status of first cohabitation, 2002)

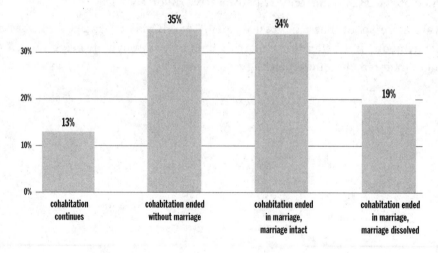

Table 6.1 Cohabitation Experience of Women, 2002

(total number of women aged 15 to 44, and percent who have ever cohabited or are currently cohabiting, by selected characteristics, 2002; numbers in thousands)

	total		ever cohabited	currently cohabiting
	number	percent		
Total women aged 15 to 44	**61,561**	**100.0%**	**50.0%**	**9.1%**
Aged 15 to 19	9,834	100.0	11.7	5.6
Aged 20 to 24	9,840	100.0	43.1	15.7
Aged 25 to 29	9,249	100.0	60.9	12.9
Aged 30 to 34	10,272	100.0	63.2	7.9
Aged 35 to 39	10,853	100.0	61.3	6.7
Aged 40 to 44	11,512	100.0	57.4	6.6
Number of children ever borne				
None	25,622	100.0	31.8	8.9
One	11,193	100.0	63.1	10.7
Two	13,402	100.0	61.4	6.1
Three or more	11,343	100.0	64.9	11.2
Race and Hispanic origin				
Black, non-Hispanic	8,250	100.0	51.1	9.6
Hispanic	9,107	100.0	48.8	13.4
White, non-Hispanic	39,498	100.0	50.5	7.9
Education				
Not a high school graduate	5,627	100.0	69.4	17.2
High school graduate or GED	14,264	100.0	68.5	11.3
Some college, no degree	14,279	100.0	58.3	7.6
Bachelor's degree or more	13,551	100.0	46.3	5.4
Family structure at age 14				
Living with both parents	43,921	100.0	45.5	7.4
Other	17,640	100.0	61.3	13.2

Note: Education categories include only people aged 22 to 44.
Source: National Center for Health Statistics, Fertility, Family Planning, and Reproductive Health of U.S. Women: Data from the 2002 National Survey of Family Growth, Vital and Health Statistics, Series 23, No. 25, 2005; Internet site http://www .cdc.gov/nchs/nsfg.htm

Table 6.2 Cohabitation Experience of Men, 2002

(total number of men aged 15 to 44, and percent who have ever cohabited or are currently cohabiting, by selected characteristics, 2002; numbers in thousands)

	total		ever cohabited	currently cohabiting
	number	percent		
Total men aged 15 to 44	**61,147**	**100.0%**	**48.8%**	**9.2%**
Aged 15 to 19	10,208	100.0	5.5	1.9
Aged 20 to 24	9,883	100.0	33.9	13.4
Aged 25 to 29	9,226	100.0	58.5	17.8
Aged 30 to 34	10,138	100.0	62.3	9.6
Aged 35 to 39	10,557	100.0	64.7	8.2
Aged 40 to 44	11,135	100.0	66.5	6.0
Number of biological children				
None	32,593	100.0	32.6	7.9
One	10,457	100.0	68.4	13.7
Two	9,829	100.0	63.0	7.9
Three or more	8,269	100.0	71.2	10.7
Race and Hispanic origin				
Black, non-Hispanic	6,940	100.0	52.6	10.0
Hispanic	10,188	100.0	47.3	14.0
White, non-Hispanic	38,738	100.0	49.4	7.9
Education				
Not a high school graduate	6,355	100.0	67.2	16.6
High school graduate or GED	15,659	100.0	66.6	12.3
Some college, no degree	13,104	100.0	55.0	9.8
Bachelor's degree or more	11,901	100.0	54.0	7.0
Family structure at age 14				
Living with both parents	45,166	100.0	46.5	8.4
Other	15,981	100.0	55.5	11.7

Note: Education categories include only people aged 22 to 44.
Source: National Center for Health Statistics, Fertility, Contraception, and Fatherhood: Data on Men and Women from Cycle 6 of the 2002 National Survey of Family Growth, Vital and Health Statistics, Series 23, No. 26, 2006; Internet site http://www.cdc.gov/nchs/nsfg.htm

Table 6.3 Status of First Cohabitation among Ever-Cohabiting Women, 2002

(total number of women aged 15 to 44 who have ever cohabited, and percent distribution by status of first cohabitation, 2002; numbers in thousands)

	total		first cohabitation continues	first cohabitation ended without marriage	first cohabitation ended in marriage, and marriage is intact	first cohabitation ended in marriage, and marriage dissolved
	number	percent				
Women aged 15 to 44 who have ever cohabited	**30,795**	**100.0%**	**13.2%**	**34.5%**	**33.6%**	**18.7%**
Aged 15 to 24	5,396	100.0	35.2	40.3	18.4	6.2
Aged 25 to 29	5,637	100.0	16.2	37.9	34.3	11.7
Aged 30 to 34	6,495	100.0	6.8	39.6	35.3	18.3
Aged 35 to 39	6,656	100.0	7.3	30.5	37.7	24.5
Aged 40 to 44	6,611	100.0	5.1	25.8	39.6	29.5
Number of children ever borne						
None	8,143	100.0	23.7	43.2	22.6	10.5
One	7,061	100.0	13.4	36.7	32.8	17.1
Two	8,231	100.0	7.3	27.3	42.4	23.0
Three or more	7,360	100.0	8.2	30.7	36.8	24.4
Race and Hispanic origin						
Black, non-Hispanic	4,217	100.0	15.3	46.3	23.9	14.5
Hispanic	4,442	100.0	22.9	29.4	31.1	16.5
White, non-Hispanic	19,952	100.0	10.6	31.9	36.9	20.6
Education						
Not a high school graduate	3,903	100.0	14.4	36.1	28.1	21.5
High school graduate or GED	9,774	100.0	10.1	35.4	31.4	23.1
Some college, no degree	8,318	100.0	8.8	34.0	36.4	20.8
Bachelor's degree or more	6,279	100.0	10.7	30.5	45.3	13.5
Family structure at age 14						
Living with both parents	19,983	100.0	12.4	31.3	37.2	19.0
Other	10,811	100.0	14.7	40.3	26.9	18.1

Note: Education categories include only people aged 22 to 44.
Source: National Center for Health Statistics, Fertility, Family Planning, and Reproductive Health of U.S. Women: Data from the 2002 National Survey of Family Growth, Vital and Health Statistics, Series 23, No. 25, 2005; Internet site http://www .cdc.gov/nchs/nsfg.htm

More than One-Fourth of 15-to-44-Year-Olds Cohabited before Their First Marriage

The likelihood of cohabitation before first marriage rises with age.

Twenty-eight percent of women aged 15 to 44 lived with an opposite-sex partner outside of marriage before their first marriage. The figure rises with age to a peak of 44 percent among women aged 30 to 34. Among men also, 28 percent cohabited before their first marriage, the figure rising above 40 percent for those aged 30 or older.

Only 7 percent of women and 4 percent of men cohabited after their first marriage. The proportion rises to 19 and 13 percent, respectively, among women and men aged 40 to 44. The more children they have, the more likely men and women are to have cohabited after the first marriage ended. Fifteen percent of women and 11 percent of men with three or more children have lived with an opposite sex partner after their first marriage ended.

■ Cohabitation before first marriage is most common among non-Hispanic whites.

The likelihood of cohabitation before first marriage peaks among women aged 30 to 34

(percent of women aged 15 to 44 who cohabited before their first marriage, by age, 2002)

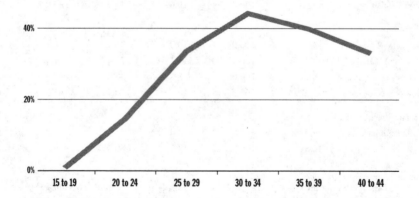

Table 6.4 Cohabitation Experience Relative to First Marriage among Women, 2002

(total number of women aged 15 to 44, and percent distribution by cohabitation experience relative to first marriage, 2002; numbers in thousands)

| | total | | never cohabited | ever cohabited | | |
	number	percent		never married	before first marriage	after first marriage
Total women aged 15 to 44	**61,561**	**100.0%**	**50.0%**	**15.1%**	**28.1%**	**6.9%**
Aged 15 to 19	9,834	100.0	88.3	10.9	0.8	0.1
Aged 20 to 24	9,840	100.0	56.9	28.2	14.6	0.3
Aged 25 to 29	9,249	100.0	39.1	25.0	33.6	2.4
Aged 30 to 34	10,272	100.0	36.8	13.6	44.2	5.4
Aged 35 to 39	10,853	100.0	38.7	10.4	39.8	11.1
Aged 40 to 44	11,512	100.0	42.6	5.2	33.0	19.3
Number of children ever borne						
None	25,622	100.0	68.2	17.0	13.1	1.7
One	11,193	100.0	36.9	20.4	36.4	6.3
Two	13,402	100.0	38.6	9.7	41.5	10.3
Three or more	11,343	100.0	35.1	11.9	37.9	15.1
Race and Hispanic origin						
Black, non-Hispanic	8,250	100.0	48.9	24.1	22.2	4.8
Hispanic	9,107	100.0	51.2	18.8	24.7	5.3
White, non-Hispanic	39,498	100.0	49.5	12.0	30.6	8.0
Education						
Not a high school graduate	5,627	100.0	30.7	24.4	36.1	8.8
High school graduate or GED	14,264	100.0	31.5	17.5	37.1	13.9
Some college, no degree	14,279	100.0	41.8	13.3	36.4	8.6
Bachelor's degree or more	13,551	100.0	53.7	10.5	32.1	3.8

Note: Education categories include only people aged 22 to 44.
Source: National Center for Health Statistics, Fertility, Family Planning, and Reproductive Health of U.S. Women: Data from the 2002 National Survey of Family Growth, Vital and Health Statistics, Series 23, No. 25, 2005; Internet site http://www .cdc.gov/nchs/nsfg.htm

Table 6.5 Cohabitation Experience Relative to First Marriage among Men, 2002

(total number of men aged 15 to 44, and percent distribution by cohabitation experience relative to first marriage, 2002; numbers in thousands)

| | total | | never cohabited | ever cohabited | | |
	number	percent		never married	before first marriage	after first marriage
Total men aged 15 to 44	**61,147**	**100.0%**	**51.2%**	**16.5%**	**28.3%**	**4.0%**
Aged 15 to 19	10,208	100.0	94.5	5.1	0.4	0.0
Aged 20 to 24	9,883	100.0	66.1	27.5	6.3	–
Aged 25 to 29	9,226	100.0	41.5	29.8	27.6	1.1
Aged 30 to 34	10,138	100.0	37.7	17.5	42.4	2.4
Aged 35 to 39	10,557	100.0	35.4	12.8	46.2	5.6
Aged 40 to 44	11,135	100.0	33.5	8.9	44.3	13.3
Number of biological children						
None	32,593	100.0	67.4	19.4	12.3	0.9
One	10,457	100.0	31.6	20.3	42.6	5.5
Two	9,829	100.0	37.0	8.9	46.9	7.2
Three or more	8,269	100.0	28.8	9.5	51.3	10.5
Race and Hispanic origin						
Black, non-Hispanic	6,940	100.0	47.4	21.7	28.0	3.0
Hispanic	10,188	100.0	52.8	20.2	24.2	2.8
White, non-Hispanic	38,738	100.0	50.6	14.6	30.1	4.7
Education						
Not a high school graduate	6,355	100.0	32.8	24.9	36.8	5.6
High school graduate or GED	15,659	100.0	33.4	19.3	39.0	8.2
Some college, no degree	13,104	100.0	45.0	19.2	31.3	4.5
Bachelor's degree or more	11,901	100.0	46.0	13.5	38.9	1.7

Note: Education categories include only people aged 22 to 44. "–" means sample is too small to make a reliable estimate.
Source: National Center for Health Statistics, Fertility, Contraception, and Fatherhood: Data on Men and Women from Cycle 6 of the 2002 National Survey of Family Growth, Vital and Health Statistics, Series 23, No. 26, 2006; Internet site http://www.cdc.gov/nchs/nsfg.htm

Most Think It Is OK for Couples to Live Together without Marrying

Fewer than half of cohabiters think they will marry their partner.

Only 48 percent of men and 45 percent of women aged 15 to 44 who are currently cohabiting feel "almost certain" they will marry their partner. At times, the gap between men's and women's future plans are considerable. Among black cohabitors, for example, only 39 percent of women think they will marry their partner compared with 53 percent of men. Among those for whom religion is not important, only 41 percent of women say it is "almost certain" they will marry their partner versus 52 percent of men.

Few men and women in the 15-to-44 age group think cohabitation is wrong. Just 32 percent of men and 35 percent of women agree with the statement, "A young couple should not live together unless they are married." Only among fundamentalist Protestants and men and women for whom religion is "very" important does the majority agree that cohabitation is wrong.

■ Attitudes toward living together outside of marriage have changed dramatically over the past few decades.

Fundamentalist Protestants are most likely to disapprove of cohabitation

(percent of people who agree with the statement, "A young couple should not live together unless they are married," by current religion and sex, 2002)

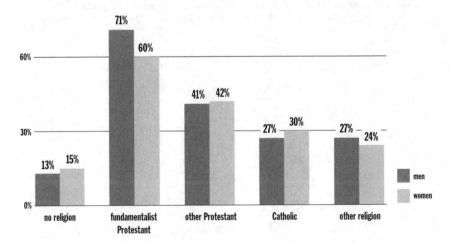

Table 6.6 Attitude of Cohabitors toward Marriage with Partner, 2002

"What is the chance that you and your partner will marry each other?"

(percent of cohabitors aged 15 to 44 who responded "almost certain" to statement, by selected characteristics and sex, 2002)

	percent responding "almost certain"	
	men	women
Total cohabitors aged 15 to 44	**48.1%**	**45.4%**
Aged 15 to 24	42.5	47.6
Aged 25 to 29	49.2	50.9
Aged 30 to 44	50.9	40.5
Race and Hispanic origin		
Black, non-Hispanic	52.9	39.3
Hispanic	39.7	33.7
White, non-Hispanic	52.4	52.3
Education		
High school graduate or less	43.2	40.7
Some college or more	54.8	51.2
Importance of religion		
Very important	54.8	48.5
Somewhat important	35.7	45.9
Not important	51.7	41.0

Source: National Center for Health Statistics, Fertility, Contraception, and Fatherhood: Data on Men and Women from Cycle 6 of the 2002 National Survey of Family Growth, Vital and Health Statistics, Series 23, No. 26, 2006; Internet site http://www.cdc.gov/nchs/nsfg.htm

Table 6.7 Attitude toward Cohabition by Sex, 2002

"A young couple should not live together unless they are married."

(percent of people aged 15 to 44 who agree with statement, by selected characateristics and sex, 2002)

	percent agreeing	
	men	women
Total aged 15 to 44	**32.1%**	**34.7%**
Aged 15 to 19	32.3	36.1
Aged 20 to 24	27.5	29.8
Aged 25 to 29	32.0	32.9
Aged 30 to 34	32.7	32.1
Aged 35 to 39	35.3	36.3
Aged 40 to 44	32.1	39.9
Marital status		
Currently married	39.7	39.8
Currently cohabiting	14.4	15.9
Never married, not cohabiting	28.4	33.9
Formerly married, not cohabiting	30.3	31.2
Race and Hispanic origin		
Black, non-Hispanic	37.7	43.5
Hispanic	40.1	40.0
White, non-Hispanic	27.9	31.1
Education		
Not a high school graduate	36.3	42.0
High school graduate or GED	34.3	33.0
Some college, no degree	32.9	37.0
Bachelor's degree or more	28.3	32.0
Current religion		
No religion	13.2	14.8
Fundamentalist Protestant	71.0	59.9
Other Protestant	41.0	41.7
Catholic	27.4	30.3
Other religion	27.4	23.5
Importance of religion		
Very important	54.9	50.7
Somewhat important	22.3	21.9
Not important	12.3	13.9

Source: National Center for Health Statistics, Fertility, Contraception, and Fatherhood: Data on Men and Women from Cycle 6 of the 2002 National Survey of Family Growth, Vital and Health Statistics, Series 23, No. 26, 2006; Internet site http://www.cdc .gov/nchs/nsfg.htm

Age at First Marriage Varies Widely by Education

Only 38 percent of female college graduates are married by age 25.

Among women aged 15 to 44, the probability that they will marry for the first time by age 18 is just 5 percent. The chances surpass 50 percent by age 25. Eighty-two percent of women have married for the first time by age 35. Among men aged 15 to 44, the probability of first marriage is lower at every age because men marry at a later age than women.

The more educated the woman, the older she is at marriage. Among women who do not have a college degree, most marry for the first time by age 25. Among those with a college degree, only 38 percent have married by age 25. But college women eventually catch up and even surpass less-educated women. Eighty-three percent of college graduates have married for the first time by age 35 compared with only 73 percent of those who did not graduate from high school.

Overall, 58 percent of women and 51 percent of men aged 15 to 44 have ever married. Blacks are much less likely to have married than Hispanics or non-Hispanic whites. Among black men aged 15 to 44, only 42 percent have ever married compared with 50 percent of Hispanics and 53 percent of non-Hispanic whites. Among women, only 39 percent of blacks have ever married compared with 63 percent of non-Hispanic whites.

■ Differences in marriage rates create differences in lifestyles by race and Hispanic origin.

The probability of marriage is lower for blacks than for Hispanics or non-Hispanic whites

(percent probability that a woman aged 15 to 44 will be married for the first time by age 35, by race and Hispanic origin, 2002)

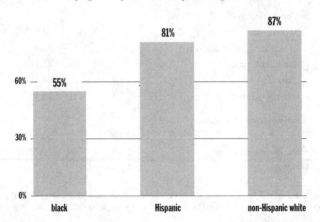

Table 6.8 Probability of First Marriage among Women by Age, 2002

(total number of women aged 15 to 44 and percent probablility that a woman will marry by specified age, 2002; numbers in thousands)

	total		percent probability of woman marrying for the first time by specified age				
	number	percent	age 18	age 20	age 25	age 30	age 35
Total women aged 15 to 44	**61,561**	**100.0%**	**5.0%**	**17.0%**	**51.0%**	**73.0%**	**82.0%**
Aged 15 to 24	19,674	100.0	2.0	10.0	–	–	–
Aged 25 to 29	9,249	100.0	4.0	14.0	47.0	–	–
Aged 30 to 34	10,272	100.0	4.0	15.0	47.0	72.0	–
Aged 35 to 39	10,853	100.0	7.0	20.0	54.0	73.0	81.0
Aged 40 to 44	11,512	100.0	10.0	24.0	61.0	79.0	85.0
Number of children ever borne							
None	25,622	100.0	5.0	16.0	52.0	75.0	83.0
One or more	35,938	100.0	6.0	19.0	48.0	69.0	76.0
Race and Hispanic origin							
Black, non-Hispanic	8,250	100.0	2.0	8.0	31.0	49.0	55.0
Hispanic	9,107	100.0	9.0	23.0	53.0	73.0	81.0
White, non-Hispanic	39,498	100.0	5.0	17.0	55.0	78.0	87.0
Education							
Not a high school graduate	5,627	100.0	17.0	33.0	55.0	69.0	73.0
High school grad. or GED	14,264	100.0	8.0	26.0	59.0	74.0	81.0
Some college, no degree	14,279	100.0	4.0	16.0	56.0	78.0	85.0
Bachelor's degree or more	13,551	100.0	1.0	4.0	38.0	70.0	83.0
Family structure at age 14							
Living with both parents	43,921	100.0	5.0	16.0	52.0	75.0	83.0
Other	17,640	100.0	6.0	19.0	48.0	69.0	76.0

Note: Education categories include only people aged 22 to 44. "–" means not applicable.
Source: National Center for Health Statistics, Fertility, Family Planning, and Reproductive Health of U.S. Women: Data from the 2002 National Survey of Family Growth, Vital and Health Statistics, Series 23, No. 25, 2005; Internet site http://www .cdc.gov/nchs/nsfg.htm

Table 6.9 Probability of First Marriage among Men by Age, 2002

(total number of men aged 15 to 44 and percent probablility that a man will marry by specified age, 2002; numbers in thousands)

	total		percent probability of woman marrying for the first time by specified age				
	number	percent	age 18	age 20	age 25	age 30	age 35
Total men aged 15 to 44	**61,147**	**100.0%**	**2.0%**	**7.0%**	**36.0%**	**61.0%**	**75.0%**
Aged 15 to 24	20,091	100.0	1.0	3.0	–	–	–
Aged 25 to 29	9,226	100.0	1.0	5.0	31.0	–	–
Aged 30 to 34	10,138	100.0	1.0	6.0	37.0	62.0	–
Aged 35 to 39	10,557	100.0	1.0	6.0	34.0	57.0	73.0
Aged 40 to 44	11,135	100.0	5.0	16.0	43.0	67.0	78.0
First birth timing relative to first marriage							
Before first marriage	9,656	100.0	0.0	5.0	30.0	50.0	66.0
Same month or later than first marriage	18,898	100.0	5.0	17.0	61.0	90.0	98.0
Race and Hispanic origin							
Black, non-Hispanic	6,940	100.0	0.0	5.0	25.0	47.0	65.0
Hispanic	10,188	100.0	2.0	9.0	39.0	62.0	75.0
White, non-Hispanic	38,738	100.0	1.0	7.0	36.0	64.0	77.0
Education							
Not a high school graduate	6,355	100.0	5.0	14.0	41.0	62.0	71.0
High school grad. or GED	15,659	100.0	3.0	12.0	42.0	63.0	78.0
Some college, no degree	13,104	100.0	0.0	5.0	37.0	61.0	69.0
Bachelor's degree or more	11,901	100.0	0.0	1.0	24.0	60.0	78.0
Family structure at age 14							
Living with both parents	45,166	100.0	1.0	6.0	35.0	62.0	76.0
Other	15,981	100.0	2.0	10.0	37.0	60.0	73.0

Note: Education categories include only people aged 22 to 44. "–" means not applicable.
Source: National Center for Health Statistics, Fertility, Contraception, and Fatherhood: Data on Men and Women from Cycle 6 of the 2002 National Survey of Family Growth, Vital and Health Statistics, Series 23, No. 26, 2006; Internet site http://www.cdc .gov/nchs/nsfg.htm

Table 6.10 Marriage and Cohabitation Experience of Women, 2002

(total number of women aged 15 to 44, and percent who have ever cohabited or been married, by selected characteristics, 2002; numbers in thousands)

	total number	total percent	ever married or cohabited	ever married
Total women aged 15 to 44	**61,561**	**100.0%**	**73.3%**	**58.2%**
Aged 15 to 19	9,834	100.0	13.3	2.4
Aged 20 to 24	9,840	100.0	55.5	27.3
Aged 25 to 29	9,249	100.0	85.2	60.2
Aged 30 to 34	10,272	100.0	91.2	77.6
Aged 35 to 39	10,853	100.0	93.7	83.3
Aged 40 to 44	11,512	100.0	95.1	89.9
Number of children ever borne				
None	25,622	100.0	41.8	24.8
One	11,193	100.0	91.4	71.1
Two	13,402	100.0	97.8	88.1
Three or more	11,343	100.0	97.7	85.9
Race and Hispanic origin				
Black, non-Hispanic	8,250	100.0	63.4	39.3
Hispanic	9,107	100.0	76.7	57.9
White, non-Hispanic	39,498	100.0	74.8	62.8
Education				
Not a high school graduate	5,627	100.0	92.2	67.8
High school graduate or GED	14,264	100.0	92.5	75.0
Some college, no degree	14,279	100.0	88.4	75.1
Bachelor's degree or more	13,551	100.0	82.3	71.8
Family structure at age 14				
Living with both parents	43,921	100.0	73.2	61.1
Other	17,640	100.0	73.6	51.1

Note: Education categories include only people aged 22 to 44.
Source: National Center for Health Statistics, Fertility, Family Planning, and Reproductive Health of U.S. Women: Data from the 2002 National Survey of Family Growth, Vital and Health Statistics, Series 23, No. 25, 2005; Internet site http://www.cdc.gov/nchs/nsfg.htm

Table 6.11 Marriage and Cohabitation Experience of Men, 2002

(total number of men aged 15 to 44, and percent who have ever cohabited or been married, by selected characteristics, 2002; numbers in thousands)

	total		ever married or cohabited	ever married
	number	percent		
Total men aged 15 to 44	**61,147**	**100.0%**	**67.2%**	**50.7%**
Aged 15 to 19	10,208	100.0	5.8	0.7
Aged 20 to 24	9,883	100.0	44.2	16.8
Aged 25 to 29	9,226	100.0	79.6	49.8
Aged 30 to 34	10,138	100.0	87.6	70.1
Aged 35 to 39	10,557	100.0	91.1	78.2
Aged 40 to 44	11,135	100.0	92.3	83.4
Number of biological children				
None	32,593	100.0	39.7	20.3
One	10,457	100.0	96.7	76.3
Two	9,829	100.0	99.4	90.6
Three or more	8,269	100.0	99.8	90.3
Race and Hispanic origin				
Black, non-Hispanic	6,940	100.0	63.4	41.7
Hispanic	10,188	100.0	69.9	49.7
White, non-Hispanic	38,738	100.0	67.8	53.2
Education				
Not a high school graduate	6,355	100.0	88.4	63.5
High school graduate or GED	15,659	100.0	88.3	68.9
Some college, no degree	13,104	100.0	78.0	58.7
Bachelor's degree or more	11,901	100.0	81.8	68.3
Family structure at age 14				
Living with both parents	45,166	100.0	66.7	51.5
Other	15,981	100.0	68.6	48.2

Note: Education categories include only people aged 22 to 44.
Source: National Center for Health Statistics, Fertility, Contraception, and Fatherhood: Data on Men and Women from Cycle 6 of the 2002 National Survey of Family Growth, Vital and Health Statistics, Series 23, No. 26, 2006; Internet site http://www.cdc .gov/nchs/nsfg.htm

Many Women Are in a Second or Higher Marriage

Divorce is common among young and middle-aged adults.

Among women aged 15 to 44, nearly half—46 percent—are currently married. Thirty-eight percent are in their first marriage and 9 percent are in their second or higher marriage. The numbers are slightly lower for men aged 15 to 44, with 35 percent in their first marriage and 7 percent in their second or higher marriage.

The probability of being in a second or higher marriage rises steeply with age. Among women aged 40 to 44, fully 21 percent are in their second or higher marriage. The figure is 20 percent for men in the age group. Twenty-two percent of women and 21 percent of men aged 40 to 44 are currently separated or divorced.

College-educated men and women are much more likely to be in their first marriage than those with less education. Among college graduates aged 15 to 44, the 56 to 57 percent majority of men and women is in their first marriage. Among those who went no further than high school, only 40 to 41 percent are in their first marriage and 13 to 17 percent are in their second or higher marriage.

■ The lower incomes of the less educated makes marriage more stressful and leads to greater incidence of divorce.

Twenty-two percent of women aged 40 to 44 are currently divorced or separated

(percent distribution of women aged 40 to 44 by current marital status, 2002)

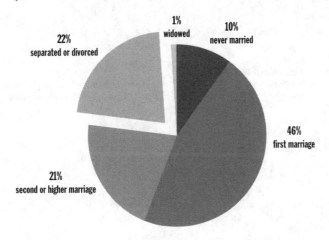

Table 6.12 Current Marital Status of Women, 2002

(total number of women aged 15 to 44, and percent distribution by current marital status, by selected characteristics, 2002; numbers in thousands)

	total		never	currently married			formerly married		
	number	percent	married	total	first marriage	second or higher marriage	separated	divorced	widowed
Total women aged 15 to 44	**61,561**	**100.0%**	**41.8%**	**46.0%**	**37.5%**	**8.5%**	**3.0%**	**8.7%**	**0.4%**
Aged 15 to 19	9,834	100.0	97.6	2.0	2.0	0.0	0.3	0.1	0.0
Aged 20 to 24	9,840	100.0	72.7	23.1	22.6	0.5	2.1	2.0	0.1
Aged 25 to 29	9,249	100.0	39.8	51.6	47.7	4.0	3.0	5.3	0.3
Aged 30 to 34	10,272	100.0	22.4	61.8	54.1	7.8	5.6	9.9	0.2
Aged 35 to 39	10,853	100.0	16.7	64.4	49.5	14.9	3.3	14.7	0.9
Aged 40 to 44	11,512	100.0	10.1	67.2	46.3	20.9	3.6	18.0	1.0
Number of children ever borne									
None	25,622	100.0	75.2	20.1	18.1	2.0	0.9	3.7	0.1
One	11,193	100.0	28.9	56.8	47.9	9.0	3.2	10.4	0.6
Two	13,402	100.0	11.9	70.2	57.4	12.8	4.8	12.5	0.7
Three or more	11,343	100.0	14.2	65.4	47.6	17.8	5.7	14.0	0.7
Race and Hispanic origin									
Black, non-Hispanic	8,250	100.0	60.7	25.8	22.0	3.8	4.6	8.5	0.4
Hispanic	9,107	100.0	42.1	45.4	39.5	5.9	5.5	6.1	0.8
White, non-Hispanic	39,498	100.0	37.2	50.8	40.3	10.5	2.1	9.6	0.3
Education									
Not a high school graduate	5,627	100.0	32.2	49.1	39.0	10.2	8.1	9.4	1.2
High school graduate or GED	14,264	100.0	25.1	56.7	39.8	17.0	3.8	13.6	0.8
Some college, no degree	14,279	100.0	24.9	57.4	47.2	10.2	3.8	13.4	0.5
Bachelor's degree or more	13,551	100.0	28.2	62.9	57.0	5.9	1.7	7.0	0.2
Family structure at age 14									
Living with both parents	43,921	100.0	39.0	49.3	41.2	8.1	2.9	8.5	0.5
Other	17,640	100.0	48.9	38.0	28.3	9.7	3.3	9.4	0.3

Note: Education categories include only people aged 22 to 44.
Source: National Center for Health Statistics, Fertility, Family Planning, and Reproductive Health of U.S. Women: Data from the 2002 National Survey of Family Growth, Vital and Health Statistics, Series 23, No. 25, 2005; Internet site http://www .cdc.gov/nchs/nsfg.htm

Table 6.13 Current Marital Status of Men, 2002

(total number of men aged 15 to 44, and percent distribution by current marital status, by selected characteristics, 2002; numbers in thousands)

| | total | | never married | currently married | | | formerly married | | |
	number	percent		total	first marriage	second or higher marriage	separated	divorced	widowed
Total men aged 15 to 44	**61,147**	**100.0%**	**49.4%**	**42.2%**	**35.0%**	**7.2%**	**1.7%**	**6.6%**	**0.1%**
Aged 15 to 19	10,208	100.0	99.3	0.4	0.4	0.0	–	0.0	0.0
Aged 20 to 24	9,883	100.0	83.2	15.4	15.4	0.0	1.2	–	0.0
Aged 25 to 29	9,226	100.0	50.3	45.3	44.4	0.9	1.3	3.2	0.0
Aged 30 to 34	10,138	100.0	29.9	60.6	52.0	8.6	2.4	6.9	–
Aged 35 to 39	10,557	100.0	21.8	65.5	53.8	11.7	2.2	10.3	–
Aged 40 to 44	11,135	100.0	16.6	62.9	43.1	19.8	2.8	17.7	–
Number of biological children									
None	32,593	100.0	79.7	16.8	15.0	1.8	0.6	2.8	–
One	10,457	100.0	23.7	61.5	50.5	11.0	3.4	11.4	–
Two	9,829	100.0	9.4	76.3	67.6	8.7	3.2	11.0	–
Three or more	8,269	100.0	9.7	77.3	55.5	21.8	2.4	10.5	–
Race and Hispanic origin									
Black, non-Hispanic	6,940	100.0	58.3	31.5	24.9	6.6	2.8	7.1	–
Hispanic	10,188	100.0	50.3	42.7	38.6	4.1	2.5	4.5	0.0
White, non-Hispanic	38,738	100.0	46.8	44.4	36.2	8.2	1.5	7.3	–
Education									
Not a high school graduate	6,355	100.0	36.5	53.2	41.6	11.6	3.6	6.7	–
High school graduate or GED	15,659	100.0	31.1	53.9	41.1	12.8	2.8	12.0	–
Some college, no degree	13,104	100.0	41.3	48.7	40.7	8.0	1.6	8.3	–
Bachelor's degree or more	11,901	100.0	31.7	61.7	56.6	5.1	1.0	5.6	–
Family structure at age 14									
Living with both parents	45,166	100.0	48.5	43.8	36.5	7.3	1.7	6.0	0.1
Other	15,981	100.0	51.8	37.8	30.9	6.9	1.9	8.4	–

Note: Education categories include only people aged 22 to 44. "–" means sample is too small to make a reliable estimate.
Source: National Center for Health Statistics, Fertility, Contraception, and Fatherhood: Data on Men and Women from Cycle 6 of the 2002 National Survey of Family Growth, Vital and Health Statistics, Series 23, No. 26, 2006; Internet site http://www.cdc.gov/nchs/nsfg.htm

Older Boomers Are Most Prone to Divorce

More than one-third of women born between 1950 and 1954 have divorced.

The divorce rate is higher for some birth cohorts than others. It peaks among men born between 1945 and 1949 and women born between 1950 and 1954—in other words, the oldest boomers.

Among women born between 1950 and 1954, fully 39 percent have ever divorced. This compares with a smaller 30 percent who have divorced among women born ten years earlier. For men born between 1945 and 1949, a substantial 40 percent have ever divorced compared with a 35 percent of their counterparts born in the previous five-year period. The probability of divorce appears to be somewhat lower for people born after the 1945-to-1954 period. The probability of making it to a 25th wedding anniversary has declined for both men and women because of rising divorce rates.

■ Government studies of divorce have consistently shown more divorce among older boomers. The Vietnam War and women's changing roles are two factors that may play a role in their higher divorce rate.

Fewer than half of women marrying in 1970–74 have celebrated their 25th wedding anniversary

(percent of women whose first marriage reached the 25th anniversary, by year of marriage, 2001)

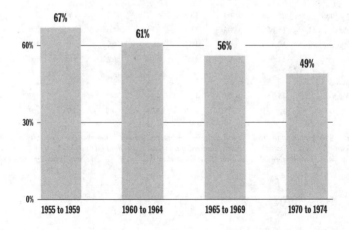

Table 6.14 Women's Marital History by Year of Birth, 1935–39 to 1975–79

(percent of women experiencing marital event by specified age and year of birth, 2001)

	year of birth								
	1935 to 1939	1940 to 1944	1945 to 1949	1950 to 1954	1955 to 1959	1960 to 1964	1965 to 1969	1970 to 1974	1975 to 1979
Percent ever married by age									
Aged 20	51.3%	46.2%	44.8%	40.5%	36.6%	30.2%	24.6%	21.9%	17.5%
Aged 25	82.5	79.0	78.7	70.1	66.0	59.5	54.8	53.4	–
Aged 30	88.7	87.6	85.4	80.7	78.1	74.4	74.3	–	–
Aged 35	91.1	90.5	88.3	86.2	84.5	83.0	–	–	–
Aged 40	92.2	92.2	90.9	89.1	87.7	–	–	–	–
Aged 45	93.8	93.9	92.1	90.6	–	–	–	–	–
Aged 50	94.5	94.6	93.0	–	–	–	–	–	–
Percent ever divorced by age									
Aged 20	2.5	1.9	1.7	2.1	3.0	2.7	1.8	2.1	1.1
Aged 25	5.8	7.0	9.4	10.8	11.8	11.5	9.9	9.7	–
Aged 30	11.6	14.1	18.9	21.6	21.3	19.4	16.9	–	–
Aged 35	16.9	21.6	27.9	28.9	27.3	26.0	–	–	–
Aged 40	22.7	26.9	33.2	35.2	31.7	–	–	–	–
Aged 45	25.4	29.9	36.7	38.8	–	–	–	–	–
Aged 50	27.2	32.6	39.0	–	–	–	–	–	–
Aged 55	28.9	34.1	–	–	–	–	–	–	–
Percent married two or more times by age									
Aged 25	3.4	3.9	3.8	3.8	5.0	4.2	4.4	3.7	–
Aged 30	6.4	7.8	10.3	11.1	11.7	10.8	9.8	–	–
Aged 35	11.5	12.9	16.6	17.4	17.7	16.1	–	–	–
Aged 40	15.2	16.9	22.3	23.1	21.7	–	–	–	–
Aged 45	18.7	20.7	25.4	26.6	–	–	–	–	–
Aged 50	21.1	23.2	28.5	–	–	–	–	–	–
Aged 55	22.8	24.9	–	–	–	–	–	–	–

Note: "–" means not applicable.
Source: Bureau of the Census, Number, Timing, and Duration of Marriages and Divorces: 2001, Current Population Reports, P70–97, 2005; Internet site http://www.census.gov/population/www/socdemo/marr-div.html

Table 6.15   Men's Marital History by Year of Birth, 1935–39 to 1975–79

(percent of men experiencing marital event by specified age and year of birth, 2001)

	year of birth								
	1935 to 1939	1940 to 1944	1945 to 1949	1950 to 1954	1955 to 1959	1960 to 1964	1965 to 1969	1970 to 1974	1975 to 1979
Percent ever married by age									
Aged 20	20.9%	24.1%	20.4%	23.0%	17.6%	15.8%	13.0%	11.0%	8.1%
Aged 25	66.6	70.0	66.6	59.2	49.9	45.0	40.6	39.4	–
Aged 30	85.3	85.3	79.7	74.0	68.8	65.6	65.2	–	–
Aged 35	89.4	89.6	86.2	81.7	78.5	76.6	–	–	–
Aged 40	91.0	91.4	89.6	85.9	83.6	–	–	–	–
Aged 45	92.8	92.7	91.5	88.2	–	–	–	–	–
Aged 50	94.1	94.0	93.1	–	–	–	–	–	–
Percent ever divorced by age									
Aged 20	0.7	0.6	0.6	1.3	1.0	0.6	1.1	1.0	0.5
Aged 25	4.0	5.9	5.8	7.2	5.4	6.1	7.0	5.8	–
Aged 30	8.5	13.3	15.6	17.8	14.7	13.8	13.1	–	–
Aged 35	15.2	21.9	25.3	26.2	20.8	19.9	–	–	–
Aged 40	22.7	27.4	31.0	31.4	26.2	–	–	–	–
Aged 45	27.4	31.5	36.3	34.7	–	–	–	–	–
Aged 50	30.2	34.7	39.7	–	–	–	–	–	–
Aged 55	32.0	37.3	–	–	–	–	–	–	–
Percent married two or more times by age									
Aged 25	1.7	2.3	1.8	2.5	2.0	1.8	3.0	1.9	–
Aged 30	5.5	6.9	8.1	8.4	6.0	6.7	7.5	–	–
Aged 35	10.7	13.0	15.1	16.5	12.0	11.0	–	–	–
Aged 40	15.5	19.7	22.4	21.7	16.8	–	–	–	–
Aged 45	21.7	24.2	26.4	25.4	–	–	–	–	–
Aged 50	26.0	27.2	29.5	–	–	–	–	–	–
Aged 55	26.8	30.2	–	–	–	–	–	–	–

Note: "–" means not applicable.
Source: Bureau of the Census, Number, Timing, and Duration of Marriages and Divorces: 2001, Current Population Reports, P70–97, 2005; Internet site http://www.census.gov/population/www/socdemo/marr-div.html

Table 6.16 Marital History of Women by Age, 2001

(number of women aged 15 or older and percent distribution by marital history and age, 2001; numbers in thousands)

	total	15–19	20–24	25–29	30–34	35–39	40–49	50–59	60–69	70+
Total women, number	113,777	9,764	9,518	9,239	10,211	11,110	22,036	16,626	10,956	14,318
Total women, percent	100.0%	100.0%	100.0%	100.0%	100.0%	100.0%	100.0%	100.0%	100.0%	100.0%
Never married	24.6	96.3	72.4	37.3	21.7	15.6	10.5	6.4	4.1	3.3
Ever married	75.4	3.7	27.6	62.7	78.3	84.4	89.5	93.6	95.9	96.7
Married once	58.7	3.6	26.5	57.3	67.3	66.8	65.1	65.2	72.9	77.8
Still married	40.7	3.1	22.6	47.1	56.2	53.0	48.8	46.4	47.5	29.8
Married twice	13.6	0.1	1.1	5.1	10.0	15.7	19.8	22.1	17.4	15.5
Still married	9.1	0.1	0.8	4.1	7.9	12.0	14.5	15.3	10.6	6.1
Married three or more times	3.1	0.0	0.0	0.3	1.0	1.8	4.6	6.3	5.6	3.5
Still married	1.9	0.0	0.0	0.2	0.8	1.5	3.3	4.1	3.1	1.1
Ever divorced	23.1	0.2	2.6	11.9	18.6	28.1	35.4	38.9	28.4	17.7
Currently divorced	10.8	0.0	1.6	7.4	9.3	13.7	16.8	17.9	12.6	6.5
Ever widowed	11.6	0.0	0.3	0.5	0.6	1.1	3.5	9.5	23.3	56.3
Currently widowed	10.2	0.0	0.3	0.4	0.4	0.6	2.4	7.1	19.7	52.6

Source: Bureau of the Census, Number, Timing, and Duration of Marriages and Divorces: 2001, Current Population Reports, P70–97, 2005; Internet site http://www.census.gov/population/www/socdemo/marr-div.html

Table 6.17 Marital History of Men by Age, 2001

(number of men aged 15 or older and percent distribution by marital history and age, 2001; numbers in thousands)

	total	15–19	20–24	25–29	30–34	35–39	40–49	50–59	60–69	70+
Total men, number	105,850	10,186	9,465	9,177	10,069	10,704	21,202	15,694	9,558	9,795
Total men, percent	100.0%	100.0%	100.0%	100.0%	100.0%	100.0%	100.0%	100.0%	100.0%	100.0%
Never married	30.9	99.1	83.9	50.8	29.5	21.5	14.2	6.3	4.3	3.3
Ever married	69.1	0.9	16.1	49.2	70.5	78.5	85.8	93.7	95.7	96.7
Married once	53.4	0.9	16.0	46.3	60.8	66.2	65.1	62.6	67.5	75.5
Still married	43.7	0.6	14.3	39.6	52.3	53.0	53.1	49.5	58.0	58.1
Married twice	12.5	0.0	0.1	2.8	8.7	10.9	17.1	23.2	21.3	16.5
Still married	9.9	0.0	0.1	2.6	7.4	9.1	13.8	17.6	17.0	12.2
Married three or more times	3.2	0.0	0.0	0.1	1.1	1.4	3.6	8.0	6.8	4.7
Still married	2.4	0.0	0.0	0.1	0.8	1.2	2.9	5.7	5.1	3.5
Ever divorced	21.0	0.1	1.0	7.5	15.4	22.9	29.5	40.8	30.9	18.6
Currently divorced	8.8	0.0	0.8	4.7	7.0	12.5	12.5	16.9	9.7	5.5
Ever widowed	3.6	0.0	0.0	0.1	0.3	0.5	1.3	2.9	7.6	23.1
Currently widowed	2.4	0.0	0.0	0.1	0.0	0.2	0.8	1.8	4.5	16.8

Source: Bureau of the Census, Number, Timing, and Duration of Marriages and Divorces: 2001, Current Population Reports, P70–97, 2005; Internet site http://www.census.gov/population/www/socdemo/marr-div.html

Table 6.18   Marriages Reaching Specified Anniversary by Year of Marriage, 1955–59 to 1990–94

(percent of marriages reaching specified anniversary by year of marriage, marriage order, and sex, 2001)

	anniversary				
	5-year	10-year	15-year	20-year	25-year
FIRST MARRIAGES					
Men					
1955 to 1959	96.1%	89.5%	82.2%	76.2%	72.3%
1960 to 1964	94.0	81.6	71.1	66.1	62.3
1965 to 1969	93.0	78.3	67.8	62.1	58.0
1970 to 1974	90.4	72.5	61.3	55.8	52.9
1975 to 1979	89.3	72.2	63.4	58.4	–
1980 to 1984	89.8	74.5	66.2	–	–
1985 to 1989	87.6	74.7	–	–	–
1990 to 1994	90.1	–	–	–	–
Women					
1955 to 1959	94.0	86.8	78.6	73.1	67.0
1960 to 1964	93.8	84.0	72.9	66.9	60.9
1965 to 1969	91.3	77.9	65.7	59.2	55.5
1970 to 1974	87.8	70.2	60.3	54.1	49.1
1975 to 1979	84.7	67.7	58.5	52.6	–
1980 to 1984	87.3	71.5	64.2	–	–
1985 to 1989	86.6	74.7	–	–	–
1990 to 1994	86.9	–	–	–	–
SECOND MARRIAGES					
Men					
1975 to 1979	90.8	81.0	57.6	49.0	–
1980 to 1984	90.9	71.8	54.9	–	–
1985 to 1989	90.0	72.2	–	–	–
1990 to 1994	88.8	–	–	–	–
Women					
1975 to 1979	86.3	75.9	55.9	47.2	–
1980 to 1984	89.2	71.0	54.6	–	–
1985 to 1989	86.9	67.8	–	–	–
1990 to 1994	86.8	–	–	–	–

Note: "–" means not applicable.
Source: Bureau of the Census, Number, Timing, and Duration of Marriages and Divorces: 2001, Current Population Reports, P70–97, 2005; Internet site http://www.census.gov/population/www/socdemo/marr-div.html

Marrying Young Often Leads to Divorce

Most women who married before age 18 have seen the marriage end.

Among ever-married women aged 15 to 44, more than one-third—35 percent—have seen their first marriage dissolve. Among their male counterparts, the figure is 31 percent.

The younger the woman at first marriage, the more likely the marriage has ended. Sixty-three percent of women who married for the first time before age 18 have seen their marriage end. Among women who married for the first time at age 23 or older, only 22 percent have ended their marriage. The pattern is the same for men. Fifty-nine percent of men who married for the first time before the age of 20 have seen that marriage end. Among men who first married at age 25 or older, only 19 percent have seen the marriage dissolve.

Educational attainment also has a big impact on marital stability. Among women who did not graduate from high school, 41 percent have dissolved their first marriage. For college graduates, the figure is only 20 percent. Among men, the respective figures are 34 percent for high school dropouts and 17 percent for college graduates.

The number of spouses or cohabiting partners in a lifetime naturally rises with age. Forty-two percent of women and 48 percent of men aged 40 to 44 have had two or more spouses or cohabiting partners. Again, education greatly influences these figures, as does family structure while growing up.

■ Men and women who lived in two-parent families while growing up have had fewer spouses or cohabiting partners in their lifetime than those from single-parent families.

The less educated have more partners

(percent of men aged 15 to 44 with three or more wives or cohabiting partners in lifetime, by education, 2002)

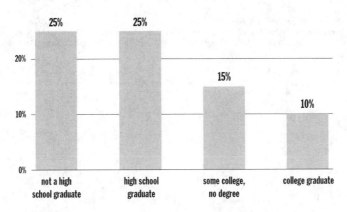

Table 6.19 Cumulative Percentage of Women Whose First Marriage Has Dissolved, 2002

(number of ever-married women aged 15 to 44 and cumulative percentage of those whose first marriage dissolved through separation, annulment, or divorce, by selected characteristics and years since first marriage, 2002; numbers in thousands)

	total		years since first marriage			all marital
	number	percent	one year	five years	ten years	durations
Total ever-married women aged 15 to 44	**35,849**	**100.0%**	**5.5%**	**19.9%**	**29.1%**	**34.7%**
Age at first marriage						
Under age 18	2,983	100.0	6.7	34.2	48.1	62.6
Aged 18 to 19	6,155	100.0	10.4	28.3	39.1	50.1
Aged 20 to 22	10,094	100.0	5.6	21.5	31.9	37.8
Aged 23 or older	16,617	100.0	3.5	13.3	20.2	22.0
First cohabitation relative to first marriage						
Did not cohabit before first marriage	18,572	100.0	5.0	18.4	28.6	35.3
Cohabited with first husband	13,385	100.0	6.1	22.2	30.9	35.9
Cohabited with someone else	3,892	100.0	6.3	19.2	25.2	27.1
Race and Hispanic origin						
Black, non-Hispanic	3,242	100.0	7.7	23.9	37.1	42.8
Hispanic	5,269	100.0	4.7	17.4	25.6	30.0
White, non-Hispanic	24,817	100.0	5.1	19.6	28.9	35.1
Education						
Not a high school graduate	3,816	100.0	7.6	23.5	31.7	40.6
High school graduate or GED	10,691	100.0	7.0	25.0	38.2	45.4
Some college, no degree	10,728	100.0	5.5	21.3	31.3	36.4
Bachelor's degree or more	9,728	100.0	2.9	11.8	17.0	20.3
Family structure at age 14						
Living with both parents	26,839	100.0	5.1	18.0	25.8	31.6
Other	9,009	100.0	6.9	25.6	38.8	43.8

Note: Education categories include only people aged 22 to 44.
Source: National Center for Health Statistics, Fertility, Family Planning, and Reproductive Health of U.S. Women: Data from the 2002 National Survey of Family Growth, Vital and Health Statistics, Series 23, No. 25, 2005; Internet site http://www .cdc.gov/nchs/nsfg.htm

Table 6.20 Cumulative Percentage of Men Whose First Marriage Has Dissolved, 2002

(number of ever-married men aged 15 to 44 and cumulative percentage of those whose first marriage dissolved through separation, annulment, or divorce, by selected characteristics and years since first marriage, 2002; numbers in thousands)

| | total | | years since first marriage | | | all marital |
	number	percent	one year	five years	ten years	durations
Total ever-married men aged 15 to 44	**30,972**	**100.0%**	**5.8%**	**19.3%**	**26.7%**	**30.6%**
Age at first marriage						
Under age 20	3,854	100.0	15.8	42.6	50.2	58.6
Aged 20 to 22	7,249	100.0	6.3	20.8	30.1	35.5
Aged 23 to 25	8,101	100.0	5.0	19.3	27.2	29.8
Aged 25 or older	11,767	100.0	2.7	10.8	16.7	18.9
First cohabitation relative to first marriage						
Did not cohabit before first marriage	13,649	100.0	5.9	18.8	25.5	29.8
Cohabited with first husband	12,734	100.0	5.4	20.7	28.0	31.8
Cohabited with someone else	4,566	100.0	5.8	16.8	26.5	29.2
Race and Hispanic origin						
Black, non-Hispanic	2,894	100.0	5.6	22.8	34.8	39.2
Hispanic	5,064	100.0	5.2	15.3	19.7	22.3
White, non-Hispanic	20,611	100.0	5.5	19.8	27.7	31.8
Education						
Not a high school graduate	4,037	100.0	9.7	26.2	32.0	34.4
High school graduate or GED	10,793	100.0	6.1	23.0	33.9	39.9
Some college, no degree	7,695	100.0	5.6	19.7	27.6	30.5
Bachelor's degree or more	8,131	100.0	3.3	10.8	14.2	17.0
Family structure at age 14						
Living with both parents	23,270	100.0	5.5	17.9	24.5	29.0
Other	7,702	100.0	6.5	23.7	33.5	35.5

Note: Education categories include only people aged 22 to 44.
Source: National Center for Health Statistics, Fertility, Contraception, and Fatherhood: Data on Men and Women from Cycle 6 of the 2002 National Survey of Family Growth, Vital and Health Statistics, Series 23, No. 26, 2006; Internet site http://www.cdc .gov/nchs/nsfg.htm

Table 6.21 Number of Husbands and Cohabiting Partners in Lifetime among Women, 2002

(total number of women aged 15 to 44 and percent distribution by number of husbands or cohabiting partners in lifetime, by selected characteristics, 2002; numbers in thousands)

	total		never married	number of husbands or cohabiting partners in lifetime		
	number	percent	or cohabited	one	two	three or more
Total women aged 15 to 44	**61,561**	**100.0%**	**27.2%**	**48.4%**	**16.4%**	**8.0%**
Aged 15 to 24	19,674	100.0	66.4	28.1	4.3	1.2
Aged 25 to 29	9,249	100.0	16.0	62.3	17.0	4.8
Aged 30 to 34	10,272	100.0	9.1	59.2	21.0	10.7
Aged 35 to 39	10,853	100.0	6.6	58.1	23.2	11.2
Aged 40 to 44	11,512	100.0	5.1	53.2	25.9	15.8
Race and Hispanic origin						
Black, non-Hispanic	8,250	100.0	37.3	41.5	16.2	5.1
Hispanic	9,107	100.0	24.4	55.4	15.1	5.2
White, non-Hispanic	39,498	100.0	25.5	48.3	16.9	9.3
Education						
Not a high school graduate	5,627	100.0	8.9	55.6	22.9	12.7
High school grad. or GED	14,264	100.0	7.8	51.3	25.3	15.6
Some college, no degree	14,279	100.0	12.1	57.4	21.7	8.8
Bachelor's degree or more	13,551	100.0	18.3	63.8	13.0	4.9
Family structure at age 14						
Living with both parents	43,921	100.0	27.2	51.1	15.3	6.4
Other	17,640	100.0	27.4	41.6	19.0	12.1

Note: Education categories include only people aged 22 to 44.
Source: National Center for Health Statistics, Fertility, Family Planning, and Reproductive Health of U.S. Women: Data from the 2002 National Survey of Family Growth, Vital and Health Statistics, Series 23, No. 25, 2005; Internet site http://www.cdc.gov/nchs/nsfg.htm

Table 6.22   Number of Wives and Cohabiting Partners in Lifetime among Men, 2002

(total number of men aged 15 to 44 and percent distribution by number of wives or cohabiting partners in lifetime, by selected characteristics, 2002; numbers in thousands)

| | total | | never married or cohabited | number of wives or cohabiting partners in lifetime | | |
	number	percent		one	two	three or more
Total men aged 15 to 44	**61,147**	**100.0%**	**32.8%**	**37.2%**	**15.6%**	**14.4%**
Aged 15 to 24	20,091	100.0	75.3	14.2	7.5	3.1
Aged 25 to 29	9,226	100.0	20.4	48.3	18.5	12.8
Aged 30 to 34	10,138	100.0	12.4	51.8	19.0	16.8
Aged 35 to 39	10,557	100.0	9.0	49.4	20.2	21.5
Aged 40 to 44	11,135	100.0	7.8	44.8	20.6	26.9
Race and Hispanic origin						
Black, non-Hispanic	6,940	100.0	36.6	28.0	16.5	18.9
Hispanic	10,188	100.0	30.2	41.5	17.1	11.3
White, non-Hispanic	38,738	100.0	32.2	38.1	15.3	14.5
Education						
Not a high school graduate	6,355	100.0	11.6	41.8	21.5	25.1
High school grad. or GED	15,659	100.0	11.8	42.2	21.6	24.5
Some college, no degree	13,104	100.0	22.1	43.8	19.0	15.2
Bachelor's degree or more	11,901	100.0	18.2	56.9	15.2	9.7
Family structure at age 14						
Living with both parents	45,166	100.0	33.3	39.5	15.4	11.8
Other	15,981	100.0	31.5	30.8	16.2	21.6

Note: Education categories include only people aged 22 to 44.
Source: National Center for Health Statistics, Fertility, Contraception, and Fatherhood: Data on Men and Women from Cycle 6 of the 2002 National Survey of Family Growth, Vital and Health Statistics, Series 23, No. 26, 2006; Internet site http://www.cdc .gov/nchs/nsfg.htm

Men Place Greater Importance on Marriage than Women

Attitudes toward divorce are mixed.

Contrary to stereotype, men think it is more important to get married than women. Two-thirds of men aged 15 to 44 agree with the statement, "It is better to get married than to go through life being single." Only 51 percent of their female counterparts agree.

The majority of men think it is important to get married, regardless of demographic characteristic. Among men, those most likely to place great importance on marriage are Hispanics (77 percent), the least educated (75 percent), and those for whom religion is very important (74 percent). Among women, those most likely to think marriage is important are Hispanics (62 percent), the least educated (60 percent), and fundamentalist Protestants (59 percent).

Despite the fact that divorce has become commonplace, fewer than half of men and women aged 15 to 44 think divorce is the best solution when a couple cannot work out their marriage problems. There is little variation in this attitude by demographic characteristic. The groups most likely to think divorce is OK are men and women aged 40 to 44, the formerly married, Hispanics, the least educated, and those with no religion.

■ Women's growing financial independence from men has affected their attitudes toward marriage.

Women do not place as much importance on marriage as men

(percent of people aged 15 to 44 who agree with the statement,
"It is better to get married than go through life being single," by sex, 2002)

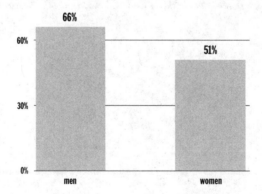

Table 6.23 Attitude toward Marriage by Sex, 2002

"It is better to get married than to go through life being single."

(percent of people aged 15 to 44 agreeing with statement, by selected characteristics and sex, 2002)

	percent agreeing	
	men	women
Total aged 15 to 44	**66.0%**	**50.6%**
Aged 15 to 19	69.1	54.5
Aged 20 to 24	64.3	51.4
Aged 25 to 29	63.7	49.2
Aged 30 to 34	64.4	49.0
Aged 35 to 39	67.7	51.7
Aged 40 to 44	66.3	48.3
Marital status		
Currently married	73.0	55.7
Currently cohabiting	53.9	45.0
Never married, not cohabiting	61.9	48.4
Formerly married, not cohabiting	63.9	40.3
Race and Hispanic origin		
Black, non-Hispanic	64.6	52.9
Hispanic	77.2	62.1
White, non-Hispanic	63.5	47.3
Education		
Not a high school graduate	75.4	59.6
High school graduate or GED	63.5	50.7
Some college, no degree	63.2	45.8
Bachelor's degree or more	64.9	50.0
Current religion		
No religion	55.9	38.5
Fundamentalist Protestant	68.4	59.3
Other Protestant	68.4	51.7
Catholic	69.7	53.4
Other religion	63.2	49.2
Importance of religion		
Very important	73.6	57.0
Somewhat important	65.1	47.5
Not important	56.9	38.7

Source: National Center for Health Statistics, Fertility, Contraception, and Fatherhood: Data on Men and Women from Cycle 6 of the 2002 National Survey of Family Growth, Vital and Health Statistics, Series 23, No. 26, 2006; Internet site http://www.cdc.gov/nchs/nsfg.htm

Table 6.24 Attitude toward Divorce by Sex, 2002

"Divorce is usually the best solution when a couple can't seem to work out their marriage problems."

(percent of people aged 15 to 44 who agree with statement, by selected characteristics and sex, 2002)

	percent agreeing	
	men	women
Total aged 15 to 44	**44.2%**	**46.6%**
Aged 15 to 19	41.7	48.0
Aged 20 to 24	42.6	39.9
Aged 25 to 29	40.2	45.1
Aged 30 to 34	38.8	47.1
Aged 35 to 39	47.8	48.0
Aged 40 to 44	53.1	50.8
Marital status		
Currently married	42.4	43.7
Currently cohabiting	48.3	53.2
Never married, not cohabiting	43.4	46.0
Formerly married, not cohabiting	54.8	56.8
Race and Hispanic origin		
Black, non-Hispanic	44.0	42.8
Hispanic	55.5	61.0
White, non-Hispanic	43.3	44.3
Education		
Not a high school graduate	52.4	64.7
High school graduate or GED	48.9	48.6
Some college, no degree	38.4	43.0
Bachelor's degree or more	42.7	43.1
Current religion		
No religion	52.2	55.6
Fundamentalist Protestant	33.6	33.0
Other Protestant	37.1	41.4
Catholic	50.9	53.2
Other religion	43.1	48.0
Importance of religion		
Very important	34.9	39.6
Somewhat important	49.2	52.4
Not important	51.2	55.6

Source: National Center for Health Statistics, Fertility, Contraception, and Fatherhood: Data on Men and Women from Cycle 6 of the 2002 National Survey of Family Growth, Vital and Health Statistics, Series 23, No. 26, 2006; Internet site http://www.cdc .gov/nchs/nsfg.htm

7

Fertility and Infertility

■ Many Americans seek help for fertility problems. Delayed childbearing has become much more common as American women have made college and career the norm. One consequence is a growing number of men and women seeking help to have children.

■ Nearly one in five women aged 40 to 44 is childless. Childlessness falls with age from 93 percent of women aged 15 to 19 to below 50 percent in the 25-to-29 age group.

■ Twelve percent of women aged 15 to 44 have impaired fecundity. Sixty-five percent of women in the age group are fecund, meaning they are able to have children. Another 22 percent are contraceptively sterile.

■ The childless often seek help for their fertility problems. Older women without children are most likely to have received infertility services. Among women aged 40 to 44 without children, 29 percent have ever received infertility services—most commonly advice and tests.

■ Childlessness does not bother most men and women a "great deal." When childless men and women are asked whether they would be bothered if they never would have any children, only 30 percent of men and 42 percent of women say it would bother them a great deal.

Childlessness Has Grown Slightly Since 1990

Asians are much more likely than Hispanics to be childless.

Among women aged 15 to 44, nearly 45 percent were childless in 2004—up 3 percentage points since 1990. Most will not remain childless because they just have not yet had children. Childlessness falls with age from 93 percent among women aged 15 to 19 to less than 50 percent in the 25-to-29 age group. Among women aged 40 to 44, just 19 percent are childless.

Hispanics are less likely to be childless than women of other racial or ethnic groups. Only 37 percent of Hispanics aged 15 to 44 were childless in 2004 compared with 41 percent of blacks and 47 percent of Asians and non-Hispanic whites. Asians delay childbearing much longer than other women. Among Asian women aged 30 to 34, fully 40 percent are childless compared to just 19 percent of blacks and Hispanics and 31 percent of non-Hispanic whites. By the 40-to-44 age group, however, Asian women are less likely to be childless than blacks or non-Hispanic whites.

■ Few women remain childless voluntarily. Among all women aged 15 to 44, only 6 percent will remain childless by choice.

Women are less likely to be childless than men

(percent of people aged 15 to 44 who are childless, by sex, 2002)

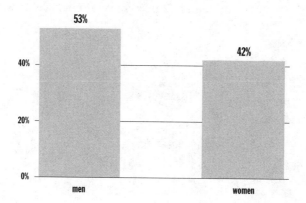

Table 7.1 Childlessness among Women by Age, 1990 to 2004

(percentage of women aged 15 to 44 who are childless by age, 1990 to 2004; percentage point change, 1990–2004)

	2004	2000	1990	percentage point change, 1990–2004
Total women aged 15 to 44	**44.6%**	**42.8%**	**41.6%**	**3.0**
Aged 15 to 19	93.3	90.5	91.9	1.4
Aged 20 to 24	68.9	63.6	64.6	4.3
Aged 25 to 29	44.2	44.2	42.1	2.1
Aged 30 to 34	27.6	28.1	25.7	1.9
Aged 35 to 39	19.6	20.1	17.7	1.9
Aged 40 to 44	19.3	19.0	16.0	3.3

Source: Bureau of the Census, Fertility of American Women, Historical Time Series Tables, Internet site http://www.census.gov/population/www/socdemo/fertility.html#hist; calculations by New Strategist

Table 7.2 Childlessness among Women by Age, Race, and Hispanic Origin, 2004

(percentage of women aged 15 to 44 who are childless by age, race, and Hispanic origin, 2004)

	total	Asian	black	Hispanic	non-Hispanic white
Total women aged 15 to 44	**44.6%**	**47.2%**	**40.5%**	**37.1%**	**47.0%**
Aged 15 to 19	93.3	94.7	90.4	87.9	95.5
Aged 20 to 24	68.9	80.8	57.0	52.8	75.4
Aged 25 to 29	44.2	50.4	33.3	31.5	49.6
Aged 30 to 34	27.6	40.0	18.9	18.6	30.9
Aged 35 to 39	19.6	19.0	17.0	15.1	21.3
Aged 40 to 44	19.3	17.8	21.3	13.8	20.0

Source: Bureau of the Census, Fertility of American Women: June 2004, Current Population Reports, P20–555, 2005; Internet site http://www.census.gov/population/www/socdemo/fertility.html

Table 7.3 Childlessness among Men and Women by Age, Race, and Hispanic Origin, 2002

(percentage of people aged 15 to 44 who are childless by age, race, Hispanic origin, and sex, 2002)

	men	women
Total aged 15 to 44	**53.3%**	**41.6%**
Aged 15 to 19	98.1	92.2
Aged 20 to 24	82.6	67.1
Aged 25 to 29	55.0	39.5
Aged 30 to 34	37.1	26.8
Aged 35 to 39	29.2	16.9
Aged 40 to 44	22.4	14.9
Black, non-Hispanic	50.4	36.7
Hispanic	44.5	32.4
White, non-Hispanic	56.1	44.2

Source: National Center for Health Statistics, Fertility, Contraception, and Fatherhood: Data on Men and Women from Cycle 6 of the 2002 National Survey of Family Growth, Vital and Health Statistics, Series 23, No. 26, 2006; Internet site http://www.cdc.gov/nchs/nsfg.htm

Table 7.4 Voluntary Childlessness among Women, 2002

(total number of women aged 15 to 44 and percent distribution by childlessness status, 2002; numbers in thousands)

	number	percent distribution
Total women aged 15 to 44	**61,561**	**100.0%**
One or more births	35,952	58.4
No births	25,622	41.6
Expect one or more births	20,293	33.0
Expect no births	5,329	8.7
Voluntarily childless	3,830	6.2
Nonvoluntarily childless	1,509	2.5

Note: Voluntarily childless are women who are physically able to have a birth (fecund) and expect to have no children in their lifetime or they are surgically sterile for contraceptive reasons. Nonvoluntarily childless are those who expect to have no children in their lifetime and have either impaired fecundity or are surgically sterile for reasons other than contraception.
Source: National Center for Health Statistics, Fertility, Family Planning, and Reproductive Health of U.S. Women: Data from the 2002 National Survey of Family Growth, Vital and Health Statistics, Series 23, No. 25, 2005; Internet site http://www.cdc.gov/nchs/products/pubs/pubd/series/sr23/pre-1/sr23_25.htm

Twelve Percent of Women Aged 15 to 44 Have Impaired Fecundity

Fertility problems increase with age.

Sixty-five percent of women aged 15 to 44 are fecund, meaning they are able to have children. Another 22 percent are contraceptively sterile, and a substantial 12 percent have impaired fecundity. Impaired fecundity grows with age. Among women aged 40 to 44, 18 percent report impaired fecundity.

Not surprisingly, women who have never had children are much more likely to report impaired fecundity than others. Among childless women aged 40 to 44, 37 percent have impaired fecundity. This compares with 15 percent of women in the age group who have had one or more children.

Men are much less likely to have fertility problems than women. Among all men aged 15 to 44, only 1 percent report a fertility problem. The proportion reaches 2 percent among men aged 35 or older.

■ Women with fertility problems are greatly outnumbered by those who have chosen to become contraceptively sterile.

More than one-third of childless women aged 40 to 44 have impaired fecundity

(percent of childless women aged 15 to 44 with impaired fecundity, by age, 2002)

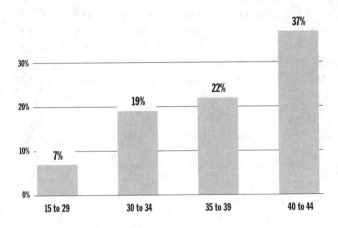

Table 7.5 Fecundity Status of Women by Age, 2002

(total number of women aged 15 to 44 and percent distribution by age and fecundity status, 2002; numbers in thousands)

	total		fecund	surgically sterile		impaired fecundity
	number	percent		contraceptive	noncontraceptive	
Total women aged 15 to 44	**61,561**	**100.0%**	**64.8%**	**22.0%**	**1.5%**	**11.8%**
Aged 15 to 29	28,923	100.0	86.4	5.0	0.1	8.4
Aged 30 to 34	10,272	100.0	60.8	24.2	0.9	14.1
Aged 35 to 39	10,853	100.0	47.1	38.7	2.1	12.1
Aged 40 to 44	11,512	100.0	30.4	46.8	4.9	17.9

Source: National Center for Health Statistics, Fertility, Family Planning, and Reproductive Health of U.S. Women: Data from the 2002 National Survey of Family Growth, Vital and Health Statistics, Series 23, No. 25, 2005; Internet site http://www.cdc .gov/nchs/products/pubs/pubd/series/sr23/pre-1/sr23_25.htm

Table 7.6 Fecundity Status of Women by Marital Status, 2002

(total number of women aged 15 to 44 and percent distribution by marital and fecundity status, 2002; numbers in thousands)

	total		fecund	surgically sterile		impaired fecundity
	number	percent		contraceptive	noncontraceptive	
Total women aged 15 to 44	**61,561**	**100.0%**	**64.8%**	**22.0%**	**1.5%**	**11.8%**
Currently married	28,237	100.0	50.1	32.7	2.1	15.1
First marriage	23,082	100.0	54.6	28.9	1.7	14.7
Second marriage	5,245	100.0	30.1	49.4	3.7	16.7
Currently cohabiting	5,570	100.0	65.3	20.8	1.3	12.6
Never married, not cohabiting	21,568	100.0	88.2	4.4	0.4	7.1
Formerly married, not cohabiting	6,096	100.0	49.4	35.2	3.0	12.3

Source: National Center for Health Statistics, Fertility, Family Planning, and Reproductive Health of U.S. Women: Data from the 2002 National Survey of Family Growth, Vital and Health Statistics, Series 23, No. 25, 2005; Internet site http://www.cdc .gov/nchs/products/pubs/pubd/series/sr23/pre-1/sr23_25.htm

Table 7.7 Fecundity Status of Women by Number of Births and Age, 2002

(total number of women aged 15 to 44 and percent distribution by number of births, age, and fecundity status, 2002; numbers in thousands)

| | total | | fecund | surgically sterile | | impaired fecundity |
	number	percent		contraceptive	noncontraceptive	
Total women aged 15 to 44	**61,561**	**100.0%**	**64.8%**	**22.0%**	**1.5%**	**11.8%**
No births	**25,622**	**100.0**	**85.4**	**2.1**	**0.9**	**11.7**
Aged 15 to 29	19,313	100.0	92.3	0.3	0.0	7.4
Aged 30 to 34	2,752	100.0	78.2	1.8	1.0	19.0
Aged 35 to 39	1,837	100.0	60.8	13.2	3.7	22.3
Aged 40 to 44	1,721	100.0	45.3	10.3	7.6	36.8
One or more births	**35,938**	**100.0**	**50.1**	**36.2**	**1.9**	**11.9**
Aged 15 to 29	9,611	100.0	74.7	14.4	0.3	10.6
Aged 30 to 34	7,521	100.0	54.5	32.4	0.9	12.3
Aged 35 to 39	9,016	100.0	44.3	43.9	1.8	10.4
Aged 40 to 44	9,791	100.0	27.8	53.3	4.4	14.6

Source: National Center for Health Statistics, Fertility, Family Planning, and Reproductive Health of U.S. Women: Data from the 2002 National Survey of Family Growth, Vital and Health Statistics, Series 23, No. 25, 2005; Internet site http://www.cdc .gov/nchs/products/pubd/series/sr23/pre-1/sr23_25.htm

Table 7.8 Fecundity Status of Women by Race and Hispanic Origin, 2002

(total number of women aged 15 to 44 and percent distribution by race, Hispanic origin, and fecundity status, 2002; numbers in thousands)

| | total | | fecund | surgically sterile | | impaired fecundity |
	number	percent		contraceptive	noncontraceptive	
Total women aged 15 to 44	**61,561**	**100.0%**	**64.8%**	**22.0%**	**1.5%**	**11.8%**
Black, non-Hispanic	8,250	100.0	64.3	23.7	1.6	10.5
Hispanic	9,107	100.0	65.9	22.4	0.9	10.7
White, non-Hispanic	39,498	100.0	63.6	22.4	1.6	12.4

Source: National Center for Health Statistics, Fertility, Family Planning, and Reproductive Health of U.S. Women: Data from the 2002 National Survey of Family Growth, Vital and Health Statistics, Series 23, No. 25, 2005; Internet site http://www.cdc .gov/nchs/products/pubd/series/sr23/pre-1/sr23_25.htm

Table 7.9 Fecundity Status of Women by Education, 2002

(total number of women aged 15 to 44 and percent distribution by education and fecundity status, 2002; numbers in thousands)

	total			surgically sterile		impaired fecundity
	number	percent	fecund	contraceptive	noncontraceptive	
Total women aged 15 to 44	**61,561**	**100.0%**	**64.8%**	**22.0%**	**1.5%**	**11.8%**
Not a high school graduate	5,627	100.0	43.6	39.9	2.7	13.8
High school grad. or GED	14,264	100.0	48.3	35.7	1.8	14.2
Some college, no degree	14,279	100.0	55.9	28.1	2.4	13.7
Bachelor's degree or more	13,551	100.0	70.4	15.8	1.3	12.6

Note: Educational categories include only people aged 22 to 44.
Source: National Center for Health Statistics, Fertility, Family Planning, and Reproductive Health of U.S. Women: Data from the 2002 National Survey of Family Growth, Vital and Health Statistics, Series 23, No. 25, 2005; Internet site http://www.cdc .gov/nchs/products/pubs/pubd/series/sr23/pre-1/sr23_25.htm

Table 7.10 Men with Infertility Problems, 2002

(total number of men aged 15 to 44 and percent with an infertility problem by selected characteristics, 2002; numbers in thousands)

| | total | with fertility problem | | |
		any	semen problem	varicocele
Total men aged 15 to 44	**61,147**	**1.2%**	**0.9%**	**0.4%**
Aged 15 to 29	29,317	0.4	–	–
Aged 30 to 34	10,138	1.7	1.6	–
Aged 35 to 39	10,557	2.1	1.3	–
Aged 40 to 44	11,135	2.0	1.8	–
Marital status				
Married	25,808	2.4	1.9	0.9
Unmarried	35,340	0.3	1.9	–
Number of biological children				
None	32,593	0.9	0.7	–
One or more	28,554	1.5	1.1	–
Race and Hispanic origin				
Black, non-Hispanic	6,940	–	–	–
Hispanic	10,188	0.6	0.6	–
White, non-Hispanic	38,738	1.6	1.1	0.6
Education				
Less than bachelor's degree	35,118	0.8	0.6	–
Bachelor's degree or more	11,901	3.7	2.8	1.8

Note: "–" means zero or sample is too small to make a reliable estimate.
Source: National Center for Health Statistics, Fertility, Contraception, and Fatherhood: Data on Men and Women from Cycle 6 of the 2002 National Survey of Family Growth, Vital and Health Statistics, Series 23, No. 26, 2006; Internet site http://www.cdc .gov/nchs/nsfg.htm

A Large Proportion of Women Take Advantage of Infertility Services

Many men seek services as well.

Infertility services offered by clinics and doctor's offices are popular among young and middle-aged adults. Twelve percent of women aged 15 to 44 have received infertility services at some point in their lives, as have 8 percent of their male counterparts.

Older women without children are most likely to have received infertility services. Among women aged 15 to 44 without children, 29 percent have ever received infertility services—most commonly advice and tests. Six percent have received artificial insemination.

Two percent of women aged 15 to 44 have sought medical help to become pregnant in the past year, with the figure peaking at 4 percent among women aged 30 to 34. Among childless women aged 30 to 34, 9 percent have sought medical help to become pregnant in the past year.

■ Educated men and women are much more likely to use infertility services than those with less education.

Artificial insemination is uncommon, even among older childless women

(percent of childless women aged 15 to 44 who have ever received artificial insemination, by age, 2002)

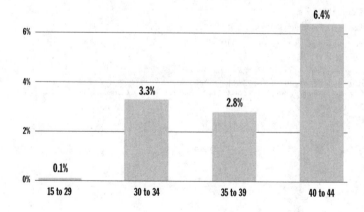

Table 7.11 Women Receiving Infertility Services by Age, 2002

(total number of women aged 15 to 44 and percent ever having received infertility services by type of service and age, 2002; numbers in thousands)

	total	15 to 29	30 to 34	35 to 39	40 to 44
Total women, number	**61,561**	**28,923**	**10,272**	**10,853**	**11,512**
Total women, percent	**100.0%**	**100.0%**	**100.0%**	**100.0%**	**100.0%**
Any infertility service	11.9	4.9	17.7	17.3	19.2
Advice	6.1	2.1	9.9	9.5	9.7
Tests on woman or man	4.8	1.4	6.4	6.7	10.0
Ovulation drugs	3.8	1.0	5.3	4.6	8.4
Medical help to prevent miscarriage	5.5	2.7	7.5	7.7	8.7
Surgery or treatment of blocked tubes	0.7	0.1	1.0	1.3	1.5
Artificial insemination	1.1	0.2	1.8	1.4	2.6
Assisted reproductive technology	0.3	0.0	0.4	0.3	0.7

Source: National Center for Health Statistics, Fertility, Family Planning, and Reproductive Health of U.S. Women: Data from the 2002 National Survey of Family Growth, Vital and Health Statistics, Series 23, No. 25, 2005; Internet site http://www.cdc .gov/nchs/products/pubs/pubd/series/sr23/pre-1/sr23_25.htm

Table 7.12 Men Receiving Infertility Services by Age, 2002

(total number of men aged 15 to 44 and percent ever having received infertility services by type of service and age, 2002; numbers in thousands)

	total	15 to 29	30 to 34	35 to 39	40 to 44
Total men, number	**61,147**	**29,317**	**10,138**	**10,557**	**11,135**
Total men, percent	**100.0%**	**100.0%**	**100.0%**	**100.0%**	**100.0%**
Any infertility service	7.6	3.7	8.5	13.2	9.1
Advice	4.6	2.2	5.1	9.9	5.6
Tests on man or woman	3.2	0.7	4.6	7.6	4.6
Ovulation drugs	2.1	0.8	2.7	4.5	2.8
Surgery for blocked tubes	0.8	–	–	1.8	1.9
Artificial insemination	0.6	–	–	1.9	1.0
Treatment for varicocele	0.4	–	–	–	–

Note: "–" means zero or sample is too small to make a reliable estimate.
Source: National Center for Health Statistics, Fertility, Contraception, and Fatherhood: Data on Men and Women from Cycle 6 of the 2002 National Survey of Family Growth, Vital and Health Statistics, Series 23, No. 26, 2006; Internet site http://www.cdc .gov/nchs/nsfg.htm

Table 7.13 Women Receiving Infertility Services by Number of Births and Age, 2002

(total number of women aged 15 to 44 and percent ever having received infertility services by type of service, number of births, and age, 2002; numbers in thousands)

			no births		
	total	15 to 29	30 to 34	35 to 39	40 to 44
Total women, number	**25,622**	**19,313**	**2,752**	**1,837**	**1,721**
Total women, percent	**100.0%**	**100.0%**	**100.0%**	**100.0%**	**100.0%**
Any infertility service	7.1	2.9	17.3	15.2	29.1
Advice	4.5	1.3	13.5	9.9	19.6
Tests on woman or man	3.8	1.1	9.6	8.5	19.6
Ovulation drugs	2.6	0.8	6.7	6.5	12.0
Medical help to prevent miscarriage	2.3	1.5	4.3	4.0	6.9
Surgery or treatment of blocked tubes	0.5	0.1	0.6	1.6	4.4
Artificial insemination	1.1	0.1	3.3	2.8	6.4
Assisted reproductive technology	0.3	0.0	1.0	1.0	1.8

			one or more births		
	total	15 to 29	30 to 34	35 to 39	40 to 44
Total women, number	**35,938**	**9,610**	**7,521**	**9,016**	**9,791**
Total women, percent	**100.0%**	**100.0%**	**100.0%**	**100.0%**	**100.0%**
Any infertility service	15.3	9.0	17.8	17.7	17.5
Advice	7.3	3.6	8.6	9.5	8.0
Tests on woman or man	5.5	2.0	5.2	6.3	8.3
Ovulation drugs	4.6	1.5	4.8	4.2	7.8
Medical help to prevent miscarriage	7.7	5.1	8.7	8.4	9.0
Surgery or treatment of blocked tubes	0.9	0.1	1.1	1.3	1.0
Artificial insemination	1.2	0.3	1.3	1.2	1.9
Assisted reproductive technology	0.2	0.0	0.1	0.2	0.6

Source: National Center for Health Statistics, Fertility, Family Planning, and Reproductive Health of U.S. Women: Data from the 2002 National Survey of Family Growth, Vital and Health Statistics, Series 23, No. 25, 2005; Internet site http://www.cdc .gov/nchs/products/pubs/pubd/series/sr23/pre-1/sr23_25.htm

Table 7.14 Men Receiving Infertility Services by Number of Biological Children and Age, 2002

(total number of men aged 15 to 44 and percent ever having received infertility services by type of service, number of biological children, and age, 2002; numbers in thousands)

	no biological children			
	total	15 to 29	30 to 34	35 to 44
Total men, number	**32,593**	**23,254**	**3,765**	**5,575**
Total men, percent	**100.0%**	**100.0%**	**100.0%**	**100.0%**
Any infertility service	4.8	2.7	4.6	11.5
Advice	3.1	1.7	3.6	8.5
Tests on man or woman	1.8	0.6	2.1	6.6
Ovulation drugs	1.0	–	–	3.1
Surgery for blocked tubes	0.5	–	–	2.4
Artificial insemination	0.5	–	–	2.3
Treatment for varicocele	0.1	–	–	–

	one or more biological children			
	total	15 to 29	30 to 34	35 to 39
Total men, number	**28,554**	**6,064**	**6,373**	**16,117**
Total men, percent	**100.0%**	**100.0%**	**100.0%**	**100.0%**
Any infertility service	9.9	6.4	10.6	11.0
Advice	6.4	4.3	6.0	7.4
Tests on man or woman	4.9	1.0	6.0	5.9
Ovulation drugs	3.4	2.2	3.5	3.8
Surgery for blocked tubes	1.0	–	–	1.6
Artificial insemination	0.6	–	–	1.1
Treatment for varicocele	0.8	–	–	–

Note: "–" means zero or sample is too small to make a reliable estimate.
Source: National Center for Health Statistics, Fertility, Contraception, and Fatherhood: Data on Men and Women from Cycle 6 of the 2002 National Survey of Family Growth, Vital and Health Statistics, Series 23, No. 26, 2006; Internet site http://www.cdc .gov/nchs/nsfg.htm

Table 7.15 Women Receiving Infertility Services by Number of Births and Marital Status, 2002

(total number of women aged 15 to 44 and percent ever having received infertility services by type of service, number of births, and marital status, 2002; numbers in thousands)

	no births			
	total	married	cohabiting	neither
Total women aged 15 to 44, number	25,622	5,142	2,287	18,194
Total women aged 15 to 44, percent	100.0%	100.0%	100.0%	100.0%
Any infertility service	7.1	23.8	5.8	2.5
Advice	4.5	17.7	3.0	0.9
Tests on woman or man	3.8	15.4	1.6	0.7
Ovulation drugs	2.6	10.8	1.4	0.4
Medical help to prevent miscarriage	2.3	6.0	2.1	1.3
Surgery or treatment of blocked tubes	0.5	2.2	0.0	0.1
Artificial insemination	1.1	4.3	0.0	0.3
Assisted reproductive technology	0.3	1.4	0.0	0.0

	one or more births			
	total	married	cohabiting	neither
Total women aged 15 to 44, number	35,938	23,185	3,283	9,471
Total women aged 15 to 44, percent	100.0%	100.0%	100.0%	100.0%
Any infertility service	15.3	18.4	10.5	9.5
Advice	7.3	9.6	2.6	3.3
Tests on woman or man	5.5	7.9	0.4	1.3
Ovulation drugs	4.6	6.5	0.3	1.2
Medical help to prevent miscarriage	7.7	8.9	6.2	5.4
Surgery or treatment of blocked tubes	0.9	1.2	0.0	0.2
Artificial insemination	1.2	1.5	1.3	0.4
Assisted reproductive technology	0.2	0.3	0.0	0.1

Source: National Center for Health Statistics, Fertility, Family Planning, and Reproductive Health of U.S. Women: Data from the 2002 National Survey of Family Growth, Vital and Health Statistics, Series 23, No. 25, 2005; Internet site http://www.cdc .gov/nchs/products/pubs/pubd/series/sr23/pre-1/sr23_25.htm

Table 7.16   Men Receiving Infertility Services by Number of Biological Children and Marital Status, 2002

(total number of men aged 15 to 44 and percent ever having received infertility services by type of service, number of biological children, and marital status, 2002; numbers in thousands)

	total	no biological children		one or more biological children	
		married	unmarried	married	unmarried
Total men aged 15 to 44, number	**61,147**	**5,491**	**27,102**	**20,316**	**8,238**
Total men aged 15 to 44, percent	**100.0%**	**100.0%**	**100.0%**	**100.0%**	**100.0%**
Any infertility service	7.6	18.3	0.9	12.0	4.9
Advice	4.6	15.5	0.5	8.0	2.6
Tests on man or woman	3.2	9.0	0.3	5.9	2.6
Ovulation drugs	2.1	5.3	–	4.3	1.0
Surgery for blocked tubes	0.8	2.6	–	1.4	–
Artificial insemination	0.6	2.9	–	0.9	–
Treatment for varicocele	0.4	–	–	1.0	–

Note: "–" means zero or sample is too small to make a reliable estimate.
Source: National Center for Health Statistics, Fertility, Contraception, and Fatherhood: Data on Men and Women from Cycle 6 of the 2002 National Survey of Family Growth, Vital and Health Statistics, Series 23, No. 26, 2006; Internet site http://www.cdc .gov/nchs/nsfg.htm

Table 7.17 Women Receiving Infertility Services by Race and Hispanic Origin, 2002

(total number of women aged 15 to 44 and percent ever having received infertility services by type of service, race, and Hispanic origin, 2002; numbers in thousands)

	total	non-Hispanic black	Hispanic	non-Hispanic white
Total women aged 15 to 44, number	61,561	8,250	9,107	39,498
Total women aged 15 to 44, percent	100.0%	100.0%	100.0%	100.0%
Any infertility service	11.9	8.4	8.2	13.8
Advice	6.1	2.8	3.2	7.7
Tests on woman or man	4.8	1.6	2.2	6.3
Ovulation drugs	3.8	1.3	1.9	4.9
Medical help to prevent miscarriage	5.5	4.8	3.8	6.2
Surgery or treatment of blocked tubes	0.7	0.6	0.4	0.9
Artificial insemination	1.1	0.2	0.4	1.5
Assisted reproductive technology	0.3	0.1	0.1	0.4

Source: National Center for Health Statistics, Fertility, Family Planning, and Reproductive Health of U.S. Women: Data from the 2002 National Survey of Family Growth, Vital and Health Statistics, Series 23, No. 25, 2005; Internet site http://www.cdc .gov/nchs/products/pubs/pubd/series/sr23/pre-1/sr23_25.htm

Table 7.18 Men Receiving Infertility Services by Race and Hispanic Origin, 2002

(total number of men aged 15 to 44 and percent ever having received infertility services by type of service, race, and Hispanic origin, 2002; numbers in thousands)

	total	non-Hispanic black	Hispanic	non-Hispanic white
Total men aged 15 to 44, number	61,147	6,940	10,188	38,738
Total men aged 15 to 44, percent	100.0%	100.0%	100.0%	100.0%
Any infertility service	7.6	6.3	5.2	8.7
Advice	4.6	3.8	3.5	5.2
Tests on man or woman	3.2	2.3	1.3	4.2
Ovulation drugs	2.1	1.1	0.8	2.8
Surgery for blocked tubes	0.8	0.5	–	1.1
Artificial insemination	0.6	–	–	0.8
Treatment for varicocele	0.4	–	–	0.6

Note: "–" means zero or sample is too small to make a reliable estimate.
Source: National Center for Health Statistics, Fertility, Contraception, and Fatherhood: Data on Men and Women from Cycle 6 of the 2002 National Survey of Family Growth, Vital and Health Statistics, Series 23, No. 26, 2006; Internet site http://www.cdc .gov/nchs/nsfg.htm

Table 7.19 Women Receiving Infertility Services by Education, 2002

(number of women aged 22 to 44 and percent ever having received infertility services by type of service and education, 2002; numbers in thousands)

	not a high school graduate	high school graduate or GED	some college, no degree	bachelor's degree or more
Total women aged 22 to 44, number	**5,627**	**14,264**	**14,279**	**13,551**
Total women aged 22 to 44, percent	**100.0%**	**100.0%**	**100.0%**	**100.0%**
Any infertility service	9.7	12.1	17.0	17.6
Advice	3.0	6.5	8.6	10.4
Tests on woman or man	3.1	4.9	6.2	8.4
Ovulation drugs	1.3	3.4	4.7	7.8
Medical help to prevent miscarriage	5.4	5.4	8.3	6.8
Surgery or treatment of blocked tubes	0.4	0.6	1.1	1.2
Artificial insemination	0.3	1.1	1.4	2.4
Assisted reproductive technology	0.0	0.1	0.4	0.6

Source: National Center for Health Statistics, Fertility, Family Planning, and Reproductive Health of U.S. Women: Data from the 2002 National Survey of Family Growth, Vital and Health Statistics, Series 23, No. 25, 2005; Internet site http://www.cdc .gov/nchs/products/pubs/pubd/series/sr23/pre-1/sr23_25.htm

Table 7.20 Men Receiving Infertility Services by Education, 2002

(number of men aged 22 to 44 and percent ever having received infertility services by type of service and education, 2002; numbers in thousands)

	less than a bachelor's degree	bachelor's degree or more
Total men aged 22 to 44, number	**35,118**	**11,901**
Total men aged 22 to 44, percent	**100.0%**	**100.0%**
Any infertility service	6.4	16.1
Advice	4.1	11.6
Tests on man or woman	2.2	10.2
Ovulation drugs	1.6	6.1
Surgery for blocked tubes	0.6	2.1
Artificial insemination	0.5	1.5
Treatment for varicocele	–	1.4

Note: "–" means zero or sample is too small to make a reliable estimate.
Source: National Center for Health Statistics, Fertility, Contraception, and Fatherhood: Data on Men and Women from Cycle 6 of the 2002 National Survey of Family Growth, Vital and Health Statistics, Series 23, No. 26, 2006; Internet site http://www.cdc .gov/nchs/nsfg.htm

Table 7.21 Women Receiving Medical Help to Become Pregnant in the Past Year by Age, 2002

(total number of women aged 15 to 44 and percent distribution by infertility services ever received and medical help to become pregnant sought in past 12 months, by age, 2002; numbers in thousands)

	total		never had an infertility visit	medical help only to prevent miscarriage	any medical help to become pregnant		
	number	total			total	no visits in past year	one+ visits in past year
Total women aged 15 to 44	**61,561**	**100.0%**	**88.1%**	**3.6%**	**8.3%**	**6.4%**	**1.9%**
Aged 15 to 29	28,923	100.0	95.1	2.2	2.7	1.4	1.3
Aged 30 to 34	10,272	100.0	82.3	5.2	12.5	8.6	3.9
Aged 35 to 39	10,853	100.0	82.7	4.9	12.4	10.1	2.3
Aged 40 to 44	11,512	100.0	80.8	4.5	14.8	13.6	1.2

Source: National Center for Health Statistics, Fertility, Family Planning, and Reproductive Health of U.S. Women: Data from the 2002 National Survey of Family Growth, Vital and Health Statistics, Series 23, No. 25, 2005; Internet site http://www.cdc .gov/nchs/products/pubd/series/sr23/pre-1/sr23_25.htm

Table 7.22 Women Receiving Medical Help to Become Pregnant in the Past Year by Number of Births and Age, 2002

(total number of women aged 15 to 44 and percent distribution by infertility services ever received and medical help to become pregnant sought in past 12 months, by number of births and age, 2002; numbers in thousands)

	total		never had an infertility visit	medical help only to prevent miscarriage	any medical help to become pregnant		
	number	percent			total	no visits in past year	one+ visits in past year
Total women aged 15 to 44	**61,561**	**100.0%**	**88.1%**	**3.6%**	**8.3%**	**6.4%**	**1.9%**
No births	**25,622**	**100.0**	**92.9**	**1.4**	**5.7**	**3.1**	**2.6**
Aged 15 to 29	19,313	100.0	97.1	1.2	1.7	0.5	1.2
Aged 30 to 34	2,752	100.0	82.7	1.6	15.7	6.7	9.0
Aged 35 to 39	1,837	100.0	84.8	0.3	14.9	10.5	4.4
Aged 40 to 44	1,721	100.0	70.9	4.9	24.2	18.9	5.3
One or more births	**35,938**	**100.0**	**84.7**	**5.2**	**10.2**	**8.8**	**1.4**
Aged 15 to 29	9,610	100.0	91.0	4.3	4.7	3.4	1.4
Aged 30 to 34	7,521	100.0	82.2	6.6	11.3	9.2	2.0
Aged 35 to 39	9,016	100.0	82.3	5.8	11.9	10.0	1.9
Aged 40 to 44	9,791	100.0	82.5	4.4	13.1	12.7	0.5

Source: National Center for Health Statistics, Fertility, Family Planning, and Reproductive Health of U.S. Women: Data from the 2002 National Survey of Family Growth, Vital and Health Statistics, Series 23, No. 25, 2005; Internet site http://www.cdc .gov/nchs/products/pubd/series/sr23/pre-1/sr23_25.htm

Table 7.23 Women Receiving Medical Help to Become Pregnant in the Past Year by Number of Births and Marital Status, 2002

(total number of women aged 15 to 44 and percent distribution by infertility services ever received and medical help to become pregnant sought in past 12 months, by number of births and marital status, 2002; numbers in thousands)

	total		never had an infertility visit	medical help only to prevent miscarriage	any medical help to become pregnant		
	number	percent			total	no visits in past year	one+ visits in past year
Total women aged 15 to 44	**61,561**	**100.0%**	**88.1%**	**3.6%**	**8.3%**	**6.4%**	**1.9%**
No births	**25,622**	**100.0**	**92.9**	**1.4**	**5.7**	**3.1**	**2.6**
Married	5,142	100.0	76.2	1.8	22.0	10.4	11.6
Cohabiting	2,287	100.0	94.2	2.1	3.7	2.6	1.2
Neither	18,194	100.0	97.5	1.2	1.3	1.1	0.2
One or more births	**35,938**	**100.0**	**84.7**	**5.2**	**10.2**	**8.8**	**1.4**
Married	23,185	100.0	81.6	5.2	13.2	11.5	1.8
Cohabiting	3,283	100.0	89.5	6.0	4.5	4.3	0.3
Neither	9,471	100.0	90.5	4.8	4.7	3.8	0.9

Source: National Center for Health Statistics, Fertility, Family Planning, and Reproductive Health of U.S. Women: Data from the 2002 National Survey of Family Growth, Vital and Health Statistics, Series 23, No. 25, 2005; Internet site http://www.cdc .gov/nchs/products/pubs/pubd/series/sr23/pre-1/sr23_25.htm

Table 7.24 Women Receiving Medical Help to Become Pregnant in the Past Year by Race and Hispanic Origin, 2002

(total number of women aged 15 to 44 and percent distribution by infertility services ever received and medical help to become pregnant sought in past 12 months, by race and Hispanic origin, 2002; numbers in thousands)

	total		never had an infertility visit	medical help only to prevent miscarriage	any medical help to become pregnant		
	number	percent			total	no visits in past year	one+ visits in past year
Total women aged 15 to 44	**61,561**	**100.0%**	**88.1%**	**3.6%**	**8.3%**	**6.4%**	**1.9%**
Black, non-Hispanic	8,250	100.0	91.6	4.1	4.3	3.4	0.9
Hispanic	9,107	100.0	91.9	3.0	5.2	3.0	2.1
White, non-Hispanic	39,498	100.0	86.2	3.8	10.1	8.0	2.1

Source: National Center for Health Statistics, Fertility, Family Planning, and Reproductive Health of U.S. Women: Data from the 2002 National Survey of Family Growth, Vital and Health Statistics, Series 23, No. 25, 2005; Internet site http://www.cdc .gov/nchs/products/pubs/pubd/series/sr23/pre-1/sr23_25.htm

Table 7.25 Women Receiving Medical Help to Become Pregnant in the Past Year by Education, 2002

(total number of women aged 15 to 44 and percent distribution by infertility services ever received and medical help to become pregnant sought in past 12 months, by education, 2002; numbers in thousands)

	total		never had an infertility visit	medical help only to prevent miscarriage	any medical help to become pregnant		
	number	percent			total	no visits in past year	one+ visits in past year
Total women aged 15 to 44	**61,561**	**100.0%**	**88.1%**	**3.6%**	**8.3%**	**6.4%**	**1.9%**
Not a high school graduate	5,627	100.0	90.3	5.0	4.7	3.1	1.6
High school grad. or GED	14,264	100.0	87.9	3.9	8.3	7.0	1.3
Some college, no degree	14,279	100.0	83.0	4.8	12.3	9.5	2.8
Bachelor's degree or more	13,551	100.0	82.4	3.9	13.7	10.4	3.4

Note: Education categories include only people aged 22 to 44.
Source: National Center for Health Statistics, Fertility, Family Planning, and Reproductive Health of U.S. Women: Data from the 2002 National Survey of Family Growth, Vital and Health Statistics, Series 23, No. 25, 2005; Internet site http://www.cdc .gov/nchs/products/pubs/pubd/series/sr23/pre-1/sr23_25.htm

Men Are Less Troubled by Childlessness than Women

Among both men and women, fewer than half say they would be bothered "a great deal" if they did not have children.

When childless men and women are asked whether they would be bothered if they never would have any children, only 30 percent of men and 42 percent of women say it would bother them a "great deal." Twenty-two percent of men and 15 percent of women say it would not bother them at all.

The percentage of people bothered a great deal by childlessness does not vary much by demographic characteristic. Among both men and women, those most bothered by the idea of childlessness are 15-to-24-year-olds (35 percent of men and 49 percent of women). Those aged 30 or older are much less bothered, in part because they have had more time to get used to the idea. Among childless 30-to-44-year-olds, 29 percent of women and 35 percent of men say the idea of childlessness does not bother them at all.

■ By religion, Catholic women are most bothered by the idea of childlessness. Forty-seven percent say it would bother them a great deal.

The older the woman, the less bothered she is by childlessness

(percent of childless women aged 15 to 44 who say they would be bothered "a great deal" if they did not have children, by age, 2002)

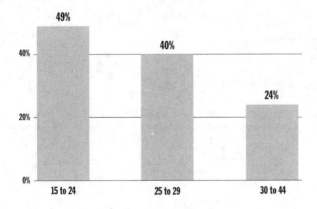

Table 7.26 Women's Attitude toward Childlessness, 2002

"If it turns out that you do not have any children, would that bother you?"

(percent distribution of childless women aged 15 to 44 by response, by selected characteristics, 2002)

	total	a great deal	some or a little	not at all
Total childless women aged 15 to 44	**100.0%**	**42.0%**	**43.0%**	**15.0%**
Aged 15 to 24	100.0	49.2	40.3	10.5
Aged 25 to 29	100.0	40.3	48.2	11.6
Aged 30 to 44	100.0	23.9	46.9	29.2
Race and Hispanic origin				
Black, non-Hispanic	100.0	39.8	42.7	17.5
Hispanic	100.0	42.6	40.3	17.2
White, non-Hispanic	100.0	42.4	43.4	14.2
Education				
Not a high school graduate	100.0	34.2	38.3	27.5
High school graduate or GED	100.0	25.8	46.8	27.3
Some college, no degree	100.0	35.8	45.7	18.6
Bachelor's degree or more	100.0	38.9	46.7	14.4
Religion				
None	100.0	31.2	43.7	25.2
Fundamentalist Protestant	100.0	32.1	51.3	16.7
Other Protestant	100.0	43.4	43.7	12.9
Catholic	100.0	47.3	39.0	13.7
Other religion	100.0	46.8	45.2	8.1
Importance of religion				
Very important	100.0	44.8	42.8	12.4
Somewhat important	100.0	46.3	41.4	12.3
Not important	100.0	31.3	45.3	23.5

Source: National Center for Health Statistics, Fertility, Contraception, and Fatherhood: Data on Men and Women from Cycle 6 of the 2002 National Survey of Family Growth, Vital and Health Statistics, Series 23, No. 26, 2006; Internet site http://www.cdc.gov/nchs/nsfg.htm

Table 7.27 Men's Attitude toward Childlessness, 2002

"If it turns out that you do not have any children, would that bother you?"

(percent distribution of childless men aged 15 to 44 by response, by selected characteristics, 2002)

	total	a great deal	some or a little	not at all
Total childless men aged 15 to 44	**100.0%**	**29.5%**	**48.3%**	**22.2%**
Aged 15 to 24	100.0	34.6	46.7	18.7
Aged 25 to 29	100.0	32.1	55.9	12.1
Aged 30 to 44	100.0	18.1	47.5	34.5
Race and Hispanic origin				
Black, non-Hispanic	100.0	33.2	38.8	28.0
Hispanic	100.0	35.4	41.1	23.5
White, non-Hispanic	100.0	28.2	51.8	20.0
Education				
Not a high school graduate	100.0	21.9	46.1	31.9
High school graduate or GED	100.0	19.3	49.2	31.6
Some college, no degree	100.0	31.7	49.2	19.1
Bachelor's degree or more	100.0	25.6	54.4	20.0
Religion				
None	100.0	22.7	47.9	29.3
Fundamentalist Protestant	100.0	35.1	44.1	20.8
Other Protestant	100.0	32.1	48.7	19.2
Catholic	100.0	31.7	48.1	20.2
Other religion	100.0	27.5	49.6	22.9
Importance of religion				
Very important	100.0	34.2	46.0	19.7
Somewhat important	100.0	31.4	51.2	17.3
Not important	100.0	23.0	47.4	29.7

Source: National Center for Health Statistics, Fertility, Contraception, and Fatherhood: Data on Men and Women from Cycle 6 of the 2002 National Survey of Family Growth, Vital and Health Statistics, Series 23, No. 26, 2006; Internet site http://www.cdc .gov/nchs/nsfg.htm

8

Contraception

■ Young and middle-aged Americans use contraception almost universally. Consequently, the nation's doctor's offices and clinics are full of men and women looking for ways to prevent unwanted pregnancy and control family size.

■ Most women use contraception. Sixty-two percent of women aged 15 to 44 were using contraception in 2002. The pill is the most popular method, used by 19 percent.

■ Religion has little influence on contraceptive use. The majority of women aged 15 to 44 use contraception regardless of religious practice. Even among Catholics, the 60 percent majority are contraceptive users.

■ The type of birth control a woman uses varies by age. The youngest women are most likely to be on the pill. Older women are more likely to be contraceptively sterile.

■ Most men use contraception. Among men aged 15 to 44 who had sexual intercourse in the past 12 months, 71 percent used some method of birth control. Condoms were the most popular method.

■ Condoms have become increasingly popular. The percentage of men who report having used a condom the first time they had sex climbed from 22 percent in 1980 to 73 percent in 1999–2002.

■ Many doctor visits are for birth control. Thirty-four percent of women aged 15 to 44 have visited a medical care provider for birth control in the past 12 months.

More Women Are Using Contraception

Only 7 percent of women are taking their chances.

Sixty-two percent of women aged 15 to 44 were using contraception in 2002, according to the National Center for Health Statistics—up from 56 percent in 1982. Only 7 percent of women are sexually active but not using contraception, pregnant, or trying to get pregnant—in other words, risking an unwanted pregnancy.

The pill is the most popular method of contraception, used by 19 percent of all women aged 15 to 44 and by 31 percent of contraceptive users in the age group. Female sterilization ranks second in popularity, used by 17 percent of all women aged 15 to 44 and by 27 percent of contraceptive users. Condoms, ranked third, are the contraceptive method of choice for 11 percent of women aged 15 to 44 (and 18 percent of contraceptive users).

Nearly 90 percent of sexually active women aged 15 to 44 have used a condom at some point in their lives, making it the most widely used method of contraception. The pill has been used by 82 percent of sexually active women.

■ The HIV threat has boosted condom use during the past 20 years.

Condom use has increased since 1982

(percent of women aged 15 to 44 currently using condoms as their contraceptive method, 1982 and 2002)

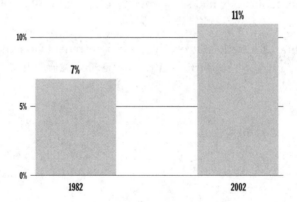

Table 8.1 Current Contraceptive Status of Women, 1982 and 2002

(total number of women aged 15 to 44 and percent distribution by current contraceptive status and method, 1982 and 2002; numbers in thousands)

	2002	1982
Total women agd 15 to 44, number	**61,561**	**54,099**
Total women aged 15 to 44, percent	**100.0%**	**100.0%**
Using contraception	**61.9**	**55.7**
Pill	18.9	15.6
Female sterilization	16.7	12.9
Condom	11.1	6.7
Male sterilization	5.7	6.1
Three-month injectable	3.3	–
Withdrawal	2.5	1.1
Intrauterine device (IUD)	1.3	4.0
Implant, Lunelle, or Patch	0.8	–
Periodic abstinence—calendar rhythm method	0.7	1.8
Diaphragm	0.2	4.5
Periodic abstinence—natural family planning	0.2	0.3
Other methods	0.6	2.7
Not using contraception	**38.1**	**44.3**
Never had intercourse or no intercourse in past three months	18.1	19.5
Pregnant or postpartum	5.3	5.0
Seeking pregnancy	4.2	4.2
Nonsurgically sterile, male or female	1.6	1.2
Surgically sterile, female (noncontraceptive)	1.5	6.3
All other	7.4	8.1

Note: Other methods includes Today® Sponge, cervical cap, female condom, and other methods. "–" means method not available in that year.
Source: National Center for Health Statistics, Use of Contraception and Use of Family Planning Services in the United States: 1982–2002, Advance Data, No. 350, 2004; Internet site http://www.cdc.gov/nchs/nsfg.htm

Table 8.2 Current Contraceptive Method Used by Women Using Contraception, 1982 and 2002

(number of women aged 15 to 44 using contraception and percent distribution by current contraceptive method, 1982 and 2002; numbers in thousands)

	2002	1982
Women aged 15 to 44 using contraception, number	**38,109**	**30,142**
Women 15 to 44 using contraception, percent	**100.0%**	**100.0%**
Pill	30.6	28.0
Female sterilization	27.0	23.2
Condom	18.0	12.0
Male sterilization	9.2	10.9
Three-month injectable	5.3	–
Withdrawal	4.0	2.0
Intrauterine device (IUD)	2.0	7.1
Implant, Lunelle, or Patch	1.2	–
Periodic abstinence—calendar rhythm method	1.2	3.3
Diaphragm	0.3	8.1
Periodic abstinence—natural family planning	0.4	0.6
Other methods	0.9	1.3

Note: Other methods includes Today® Sponge, cervical cap, female condom, and other methods. "–" means method not available in that year.
Source: National Center for Health Statistics, Use of Contraception and Use of Family Planning Services in the United States: 1982–2002, Advance Data, No. 350, 2004; Internet site http://www.cdc.gov/nchs/nsfg.htm

Table 8.3 Contraceptive Methods Ever Used by Women by Age, 2002

(number of women aged 15 to 44 who have had sexual intercourse and percent who have ever used contraceptive method, by age, 2002; numbers in thousands)

	total	15 to 19	20 to 24	25 to 29	30 to 34	35 to 39	40 to 44
Women who have had sexual intercourse, number	**54,190**	**4,598**	**8,530**	**8,939**	**10,077**	**10,686**	**11,360**
Women who have had sexual intercourse, percent	**100.0%**	**100.0%**	**100.0%**	**100.0%**	**100.0%**	**100.0%**	**100.0%**
Any method	98.2	97.7	98.5	99.0	98.4	98.1	97.5
Condom	89.7	93.7	93.1	91.9	91.7	88.2	83.3
Pill	82.3	61.4	77.9	83.9	87.2	87.0	83.9
Withdrawal	56.1	55.0	60.1	62.3	59.8	54.4	46.8
Female sterilization	20.7	0.0	2.6	11.0	20.4	31.9	40.1
Three-month injectable	16.8	20.7	24.4	26.7	18.3	10.9	5.8
Periodic abstinence—calendar rhythm method	16.2	10.8	10.2	10.5	17.8	22.0	20.4
Male sterilization	13.0	0.0	2.1	6.4	10.6	20.0	27.0
Foam alone	12.1	3.1	5.3	9.2	12.9	14.9	19.8
Diaphragm	8.5	0.6	1.4	2.9	6.6	11.6	20.4
Suppository or insert	7.5	3.3	4.4	5.3	9.4	9.2	9.9
Today® Sponge	7.3	0.1	0.2	2.4	9.7	13.7	11.2
Jelly or cream alone	7.3	3.1	5.7	5.6	8.6	8.3	9.4
Intrauterine device (IUD)	5.8	0.2	2.0	4.6	5.2	5.8	12.4
Emergency contraception	4.2	8.1	9.1	5.2	3.5	1.5	1.1
Periodic abstinence—natural family planning	3.5	0.3	1.1	3.5	3.5	5.2	5.1
Implant	2.1	0.1	0.7	4.5	4.0	1.4	0.9
Female condom	1.9	1.7	2.4	1.9	2.1	1.5	1.8
One-month injectable (Lunelle)	0.9	1.0	1.0	1.4	1.0	0.6	0.7
Contraceptive patch	0.9	1.5	1.8	1.4	0.9	0.5	0.0
Other methods	1.0	0.3	0.8	0.9	0.7	0.9	1.7

Source: National Center for Health Statistics, Fertility, Family Planning, and Reproductive Health of U.S. Women: Data from the 2002 National Survey of Family Growth, Vital and Health Statistics, Series 23, No. 25, 2005; Internet site http://www.cdc .gov/nchs/products/pubs/pubd/series/sr23/pre-1/sr23_25.htm

Sixty Percent of Catholics Use Contraception

Seventy-three percent of married women use contraception.

American women are surprisingly uniform in their contraceptive use. By age, from 61 to 71 percent of women ranging in age from 20 to 44 use contraception. Among women aged 15 to 19, only 32 percent are contraceptive users—but that is because many are not sexually active.

More than 70 percent of women who are married or living with a partner use contraception compared with only 44 percent of never-married women. By race and Hispanic origin, non-Hispanic whites are slightly more likely to use contraception (65 percent) than blacks (57 percent) or Hispanics (59 percent).

Interestingly, even religion has little influence on contraceptive use. The majority of women aged 15 to 44 use contraception regardless of their religious practice. Even among Catholics, the 60 percent majority are contraceptive users.

■ Contraceptive use is the norm because it allows families to control their growth and well-being.

The influence of religion on contraceptive use is surprisingly small

(percent of women aged 15 to 44 using contraception, by current religion, 2002)

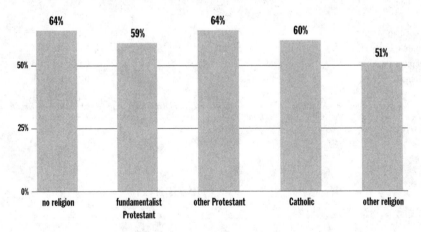

Table 8.4 Contraceptive Status among Women by Age, 2002

(total number of women aged 15 to 44 and percent distribution by contraceptive status and age, 2002; numbers in thousands)

	total		using contraception	not using contraception
	number	percent		
Total women aged 15 to 44	**61,561**	**100.0%**	**61.9%**	**38.1%**
Aged 15 to 19	9,834	100.0	31.5	68.5
Aged 20 to 24	9,840	100.0	60.7	39.3
Aged 25 to 29	9,249	100.0	68.0	32.0
Aged 30 to 34	10,272	100.0	69.2	30.8
Aged 35 to 39	10,853	100.0	70.8	29.2
Aged 40 to 44	11,512	100.0	69.1	30.9

Source: National Center for Health Statistics, Use of Contraception and Use of Family Planning Services in the United States: 1982–2002, Advance Data, No. 350, 2004; Internet site http://www.cdc.gov/nchs/nsfg.htm

Table 8.5 Contraceptive Status among Women by Marital Status, 2002

(total number of women aged 15 to 44 and percent distribution by contraceptive status and marital status, 2002; numbers in thousands)

	total		using contraception	not using contraception
	number	percent		
Total women aged 15 to 44	**61,561**	**100.0%**	**61.9%**	**38.1%**
Currently married	28,327	100.0	72.9	27.1
Currently cohabiting	5,570	100.0	72.5	27.5
Never married	21,568	100.0	44.0	56.0
Formerly married	6,096	100.0	64.4	35.6

Source: National Center for Health Statistics, Use of Contraception and Use of Family Planning Services in the United States: 1982–2002, Advance Data, No. 350, 2004; Internet site http://www.cdc.gov/nchs/nsfg.htm

Table 8.6 Contraceptive Status among Women by Race and Hispanic Origin, 2002

(total number of women aged 15 to 44 and percent distribution by contraceptive status, race, and Hispanic origin, 2002; numbers in thousands)

	total		using contraception	not using contraception
	number	percent		
Total women aged 15 to 44	**61,561**	**100.0%**	**61.9%**	**38.1%**
Black, non-Hispanic	8,587	100.0	57.4	42.6
Hispanic	9,107	100.0	59.0	41.0
White, non-Hispanic	40,420	100.0	64.5	35.5

Source: National Center for Health Statistics, Use of Contraception and Use of Family Planning Services in the United States: 1982–2002, Advance Data, No. 350, 2004; Internet site http://www.cdc.gov/nchs/nsfg.htm

Table 8.7 Contraceptive Status among Women by Current Religion, 2002

(total number of women aged 15 to 44 and percent distribution by contraceptive status and current religion, 2002; numbers in thousands)

	total		using contraception	not using contraception
	number	percent		
Total women aged 15 to 44	**61,561**	**100.0%**	**61.9%**	**38.1%**
No religion	8,692	100.0	63.7	36.3
Fundamentalist Protestant	3,714	100.0	58.9	41.1
Other Protestant	27,877	100.0	64.0	36.0
Catholic	17,653	100.0	60.1	39.9
Other religion	3,624	100.0	50.6	49.4

Source: National Center for Health Statistics, Fertility, Family Planning, and Reproductive Health of U.S. Women: Data from the 2002 National Survey of Family Growth, Vital and Health Statistics, Series 23, No. 25, 2005; Internet site Internet site http://www.cdc.gov/nchs/nsfg.htm

Most Young Women Who Use Contraception Are on the Pill

Condoms rank second in popularity among women under age 30.

The type of contraceptive a woman uses varies depending on her age, marital status, and other characteristics. The youngest women are most likely to be on the pill. Among women under age 25 who use contraception, 52 to 53 percent are on the pill. Another 23 to 27 percent use condoms. Pill and condom use decline with age. Just 11 percent of women aged 40 to 44 are on the pill, and 12 percent use condoms.

Among contraceptive users, never-married women are more likely to be on the pill than married ones, 49 versus 24 percent. Non-Hispanic whites are more likely to be on the pill (34 percent) than blacks (23 percent) or Hispanics (22 percent). Black and Hispanic women are more likely than non-Hispanic white women to use three-month injectable contraceptives.

College graduates are far more likely to use the pill than those with less education. Forty-two percent of college-educated women who use contraceptives are on the pill compared with only 19 percent of women who went no further than high school. Condom use is also higher among college graduates, while female sterilization is greater among the less educated.

■ As women complete their families with age, they opt for more permanent methods of contraception such as female sterilization.

The use of the birth control pill declines with age

(percent of women aged 15 to 44 using contraception who use the birth control pill, by age, 2002)

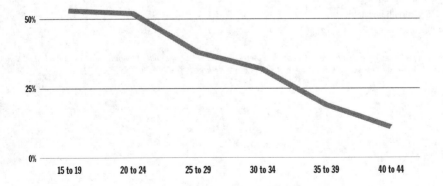

Table 8.8 Current Method of Contraception among Women by Age, 2002

(percent distribution of women aged 15 to 44 using contraception by type of contraceptive used and age, 2002; numbers in thousands)

	total	15 to 19	20 to 24	25 to 29	30 to 34	35 to 39	40 to 44
Women aged 15 to 44 using contraception	**100.0%**	**100.0%**	**100.0%**	**100.0%**	**100.0%**	**100.0%**	**100.0%**
Pill	30.6	52.8	52.3	37.6	31.5	18.6	10.9
Female sterilization	27.0	0.0	3.6	15.1	27.5	41.2	50.3
Condom	18.0	27.0	23.1	20.5	17.1	15.7	11.5
Male sterilization	9.2	0.0	0.8	4.2	9.2	14.2	18.4
Three-month injectable	5.3	13.9	10.1	6.5	4.2	2.1	1.6
Other methods	9.9	6.3	10.1	16.2	10.7	8.2	7.3

Source: National Center for Health Statistics, Use of Contraception and Use of Family Planning Services in the United States: 1982–2002, Advance Data, No. 350, 2004; Internet site http://www.cdc.gov/nchs/nsfg.htm

Table 8.9 Current Method of Contraception among Women by Marital Status, 2002

(percent distribution of women aged 15 to 44 using contraception by type of contraceptive used and marital status, 2002; numbers in thousands)

	total	currently married	currently cohabiting	never married	formerly married
Women aged 15 to 44 using contraception	**100.0%**	**100.0%**	**100.0%**	**100.0%**	**100.0%**
Pill	30.6	23.6	33.2	49.4	19.1
Female sterilization	27.0	29.8	25.4	10.0	54.9
Condom	18.0	16.4	18.1	23.4	12.5
Male sterilization	9.2	15.4	3.1	0.9	3.3
Three-month injectable	5.3	3.1	9.3	9.6	2.7
Other methods	9.9	11.7	11.0	6.7	7.5

Source: National Center for Health Statistics, Use of Contraception and Use of Family Planning Services in the United States: 1982–2002, Advance Data, No. 350, 2004; Internet site http://www.cdc.gov/nchs/nsfg.htm

Table 8.10 Current Method of Contraception among Women by Race and Hispanic Origin, 2002

(percent distribution of women aged 15 to 44 using contraception by type of contraceptive used, race, and Hispanic origin, 2002; numbers in thousands)

	total	black, non-Hispanic	Hispanic	white, non-Hispanic
Women aged 15 to 44 using contraception	**100.0%**	**100.0%**	**100.0%**	**100.0%**
Pill	30.6	22.5	22.0	34.4
Female sterilization	27.0	38.9	33.8	24.0
Condom	18.0	20.0	18.5	16.6
Male sterilization	9.2	2.4	4.4	11.6
Three-month injectable	5.3	9.8	7.3	4.3
Other methods	9.9	6.5	14.1	9.2

Source: National Center for Health Statistics, Use of Contraception and Use of Family Planning Services in the United States: 1982–2002, Advance Data, No. 350, 2004; Internet site http://www.cdc.gov/nchs/nsfg.htm

Table 8.11 Current Method of Contraception among Women by Education, 2002

(percent distribution of women aged 15 to 44 using contraception by type of contraceptive used and education, 2002; numbers in thousands)

	total	not a high school graduate	high school graduate or GED	some college, no degree	bachelor's degree or more
Women aged 15 to 44 using contraception	**100.0%**	**100.0%**	**100.0%**	**100.0%**	**100.0%**
Pill	30.6	10.6	19.0	27.6	41.8
Female sterilization	27.0	55.3	41.5	28.7	12.8
Condom	18.0	13.2	13.1	17.9	20.8
Male sterilization	9.2	2.8	10.8	12.1	12.8
Three-month injectable	5.3	7.4	4.9	3.2	1.9
Other methods	9.9	10.7	10.8	10.4	10.0

Note: Education categories include only people aged 22 to 44.
Source: National Center for Health Statistics, Use of Contraception and Use of Family Planning Services in the United States: 1982–2002, Advance Data, No. 350, 2004; Internet site http://www.cdc.gov/nchs/nsfg.htm

Most Men Used Contraception the Last Time They Had Sex

Condoms are the most popular birth control method among men.

Among men aged 15 to 44 who had sexual intercourse in the past 12 months, 71 percent used a method of birth control. Condoms were the most popular method, used by 30 percent. A slightly smaller 26 percent depended on the birth control pill. Never-married men are much more likely than married men to have used a condom at last sexual intercourse (63 versus 13 percent).

Condoms are the most popular contraceptive regardless of race and Hispanic origin. Among unmarried black men, 59 percent used a condom at last sexual intercourse. The figure was a smaller 44 percent among Hispanics and 45 percent among non-Hispanic whites. The pill is more popular among unmarried non-Hispanic white men (41 percent) than blacks (21 percent) or Hispanics (23 percent).

Condom use rises sharply with men's educational attainment. Fifty-one percent of unmarried men with a bachelor's degree used a condom at last sexual intercourse compared with only 27 percent of unmarried men who did not graduate from high school.

■ Many men depend on their partner's use of the birth control pill to prevent unwanted pregnancy.

Thirty percent of men say they used a condom the last time they had sexual intercourse

(percent distribution of men aged 15 to 44 who had sex in the past 12 months, by type of birth control used at last sexual intercourse, 2002)

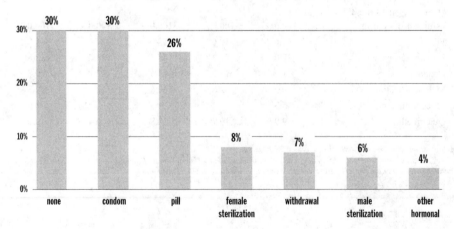

Table 8.12 Contraceptive Use at Last Sexual Intercourse among Men by Age, 2002

(number of total and unmarried men aged 15 to 44 who had sex in the past 12 months and percent distribution by contraceptive used at last sexual intercourse, by age and type of contraceptive, 2002; numbers in thousands)

	total			method used at last sexual intercourse							
	number	percent	no method used	any	pill	other hormonal	condom	withdrawal	female sterilization	male sterilization	other
Total men aged 15 to 44 who have had sexual intercourse in past year	**48,249**	**100.0%**	**29.5%**	**70.5%**	**25.6%**	**3.5%**	**29.5%**	**7.1%**	**8.1%**	**5.7%**	**7.8%**
Aged 15 to 19	4,058	100.0	10.5	89.5	31.9	5.2	72.0	14.7	0.1	0.0	8.4
Aged 20 to 24	7,936	100.0	18.3	81.7	42.8	5.5	47.3	9.7	0.5	0.0	7.5
Aged 25 to 29	8,053	100.0	28.6	71.4	31.7	4.3	31.4	8.7	4.5	1.4	7.2
Aged 30 to 34	9,190	100.0	33.9	66.1	24.4	4.1	20.4	6.1	8.7	4.6	7.1
Aged 35 to 39	9,391	100.0	35.3	64.7	20.2	1.4	14.9	4.9	15.0	8.1	9.2
Aged 40 to 44	9,622	100.0	37.9	62.1	10.3	1.7	18.0	3.5	13.4	15.1	7.5
Unmarried men aged 15 to 44 who have had sexual intercourse in past year	**22,912**	**100.0**	**19.2**	**80.8**	**33.8**	**3.9**	**47.8**	**9.2**	**5.0**	**1.0**	**8.1**
Aged 15 to 19	4,016	100.0	9.7	90.3	32.1	5.3	72.5	14.7	0.1	0.0	8.3
Aged 20 to 24	6,423	100.0	14.0	86.0	45.5	4.3	54.5	11.1	0.3	0.0	8.0
Aged 25 to 29	3,887	100.0	19.3	80.7	38.1	3.8	44.2	9.9	4.0	1.0	5.1
Aged 30 to 34	3,067	100.0	24.7	75.3	30.5	5.4	36.3	6.4	7.2	0.4	9.5
Aged 35 to 39	2,536	100.0	23.3	76.7	25.5	1.5	28.9	5.6	14.1	3.3	8.3
Aged 40 to 44	2,983	100.0	33.9	66.1	15.6	1.3	32.9	2.5	12.8	3.2	10.2

Note: Numbers may not add to total because more than one type of contraceptive may have been used. "Other" methods include spermicidal foam, jelly, cream, rhythm, and so on.
Source: National Center for Health Statistics, Fertility, Contraception, and Fatherhood: Data on Men and Women from Cycle 6 of the 2002 National Survey of Family Growth, Vital and Health Statistics, Series 23, No. 26, 2006; Internet site http://www.cdc .gov/nchs/nsfg.htm

Table 8.13 Contraceptive Use at Last Sexual Intercourse among Men by Marital Status, 2002

(total number of men aged 15 to 44 who had sex in the past 12 months and percent distribution by contraceptive used at last sexual intercourse, by marital status and type of contraceptive, 2002; numbers in thousands)

	total			method used at last sexual intercourse							
	number	percent	no method used	any	pill	other hormonal	condom	withdrawal	female sterilization	male sterilization	other
Total men aged 15 to 44 who have had sexual intercourse in past year	**48,249**	**100.0%**	**29.5%**	**70.5%**	**25.6%**	**3.5%**	**29.5%**	**7.1%**	**8.1%**	**5.7%**	**7.8%**
Currently married	25,337	100.0	38.9	61.1	18.3	3.1	12.9	5.2	10.9	9.9	7.5
Currently cohabiting	5,559	100.0	31.1	68.9	31.5	7.0	17.8	7.5	12.5	1.0	8.6
Never married, not cohabiting	13,955	100.0	12.3	87.7	37.2	2.9	63.2	11.2	1.0	0.1	7.8
Formerly married, not cohabiting	3,397	100.0	28.3	71.7	23.7	2.7	33.7	3.5	8.9	4.8	8.3

Note: Numbers may not add to total because more than one type of contraceptive may have been used. "Other" methods include spermicidal foam, jelly, cream, rhythm, and so on.
Source: National Center for Health Statistics, Fertility, Contraception, and Fatherhood: Data on Men and Women from Cycle 6 of the 2002 National Survey of Family Growth, Vital and Health Statistics, Series 23, No. 26, 2006; Internet site http://www.cdc.gov/nchs/nsfg.htm

---

Table 8.14 Contraceptive Use at Last Sexual Intercourse among Unmarried Men by Number of Biological Children and Number of Sex Partners, 2002

(number of unmarried men aged 15 to 44 who had sex in the past 12 months and percent distribution by contraceptive used at last sexual intercourse, by number of biological children, number of sex partners in past 12 months, and type of contraceptive, 2002; numbers in thousands)

	total			method used at last sexual intercourse							
	number	percent	no method used	any	pill	other hormonal	condom	withdrawal	female sterilization	male sterilization	other
Unmarried men aged 15 to 44 who have had sexual intercourse in past year	**22,912**	**100.0%**	**19.2%**	**80.8%**	**33.8%**	**3.9%**	**47.8%**	**9.2%**	**5.0%**	**1.0%**	**8.1%**
Number of biological children											
No children	15,759	100.0	13.8	86.2	38.7	3.2	57.2	10.5	1.3	0.3	8.7
One or more	7,153	100.0	31.1	68.9	23.0	5.3	27.2	6.3	13.1	2.5	6.9
Number of female partners in past 12 months											
One	13,985	100.0	22.8	77.2	32.9	4.2	40.9	9.1	6.2	1.0	8.9
Two or more	8,927	100.0	13.5	86.5	35.2	3.3	58.7	9.3	3.0	0.9	6.9

Note: Numbers may not add to total because more than one type of contraceptive may have been used. "Other" methods include spermicidal foam, jelly, cream, rhythm, and so on.
Source: National Center for Health Statistics, Fertility, Contraception, and Fatherhood: Data on Men and Women from Cycle 6 of the 2002 National Survey of Family Growth, Vital and Health Statistics, Series 23, No. 26, 2006; Internet site http://www.cdc.gov/nchs/nsfg.htm

Table 8.15 Contraceptive Use at Last Sexual Intercourse among Unmarried Men by Race and Hispanic Origin, 2002

(number of unmarried men aged 15 to 44 who had sex in the past 12 months and percent distribution by contraceptive used at last sexual intercourse, by race, Hispanic origin, and type of contraceptive, 2002; numbers in thousands)

	total			method used at last sexual intercourse							
	number	percent	no method used	any	pill	other hormonal	condom	withdrawal	female sterilization	male sterilization	other
Unmarried men aged 15 to 44 who have had sexual intercourse in past year	**22,912**	**100.0%**	**19.2%**	**80.8%**	**33.8%**	**3.9%**	**47.8%**	**9.2%**	**5.0%**	**1.0%**	**8.1%**
Black, non-Hispanic	3,611	100.0	25.0	75.0	21.4	3.4	58.9	4.0	4.6	0.5	5.9
Hispanic	4,175	100.0	26.4	73.6	22.8	6.1	43.9	10.6	5.1	0.0	7.9
White, non-Hispanic	13,477	100.0	15.5	84.5	41.4	3.5	45.4	10.2	4.1	1.6	9.2

Note: Numbers may not add to total because more than one type of contraceptive may have been used. "Other" methods include spermicidal foam, jelly, cream, rhythm, and so on.
Source: National Center for Health Statistics, Fertility, Contraception, and Fatherhood: Data on Men and Women from Cycle 6 of the 2002 National Survey of Family Growth, Vital and Health Statistics, Series 23, No. 26, 2006; Internet site http://www.cdc.gov/nchs/nsfg.htm

Table 8.16 Contraceptive Use at Last Sexual Intercourse among Unmarried Men by Education, 2002

(number of unmarried men aged 15 to 44 who had sex in the past 12 months and percent distribution by contraceptive used at last sexual intercourse, by education and type of contraceptive, 2002; numbers in thousands)

	total			method used at last sexual intercourse							
	number	percent	no method used	any	pill	other hormonal	condom	withdrawal	female sterilization	male sterilization	other
Unmarried men aged 15 to 44 who have had sexual intercourse in past year	**22,912**	**100.0%**	**19.2%**	**80.8%**	**33.8%**	**3.9%**	**47.8%**	**9.2%**	**5.0%**	**1.0%**	**8.1%**
Not a high school grad.	2,305	100.0	38.6	61.4	18.4	8.1	26.5	8.1	10.1	0.0	4.2
High school graduate or GED	5,622	100.0	29.0	71.0	26.4	4.4	33.5	6.7	9.8	2.0	7.1
Some college, no degree	5,170	100.0	17.3	82.7	41.2	1.6	42.7	6.9	4.9	1.3	8.6
Bachelor's degree or higher	2,919	100.0	9.4	90.6	39.1	1.0	50.5	8.6	3.0	1.6	11.0

Note: Education categories include only people aged 22 to 44. Numbers may not add to total because more than one type of contraceptive may have been used. "Other" methods include spermicidal foam, jelly, cream, rhythm, and so on.
Source: National Center for Health Statistics, Fertility, Contraception, and Fatherhood: Data on Men and Women from Cycle 6 of the 2002 National Survey of Family Growth, Vital and Health Statistics, Series 23, No. 26, 2006; Internet site http://www.cdc.gov/nchs/nsfg.htm

Among Women Who Do Not Use Birth Control, 11 Percent Are Trying to Become Pregnant

A larger number of women have no reason for not using birth control.

Among women aged 15 to 44 who are not using contraception, nearly half had no sexual intercourse for the past three months. Twenty-five percent are pregnant, postpartum, or trying to get pregnant. Eight percent are sterile for noncontraceptive reasons. That leaves 19 percent who have no reason for not using birth control.

The percentage of sexually active women without a reason for not using contraceptives is highest among cohabiting women, at 30 percent. The percentage of women who do not use contraceptives because they are trying to become pregnant is highest among 30-to-34-year-olds and currently married women, at 23 and 26 percent, respectively.

Some women stop using birth control because of side effects. Overall, 29 percent of women aged 15 to 44 who have ever used the birth control pill have discontinued its use. Sixty-five percent of those who discontinued the pill said side effects were the reason. Twelve percent of women have discontinued the use of condoms, with the biggest reason being a decrease in sexual pleasure for their partner or themselves.

■ Although few sexually active women do not use birth control, problems with birth control methods still result in many unwanted pregnancies.

Most women have a reason for not using birth control

(percent distribution of women aged 15 to 44 who are not currently using contraception, by reason, 2002)

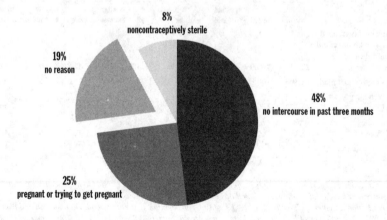

8%
noncontraceptively sterile

19%
no reason

48%
no intercourse in past three months

25%
pregnant or trying to get pregnant

Table 8.17 Reason for Not Using Contraceptives among Women by Age, 2002

(percent distribution of women aged 15 to 44 not using contraception by reason and age, 2002; numbers in thousands)

	total	15 to 19	20 to 24	25 to 29	30 to 34	35 to 39	40 to 44
Women aged 15 to 44 not using contraception	100.0%	100.0%	100.0%	100.0%	100.0%	100.0%	100.0%
Never had intercourse or no intercourse in past three months	47.5	82.0	45.5	27.8	24.7	31.2	35.0
No reason for not using contraception	19.4	10.1	21.4	25.0	22.7	26.4	21.7
Pregnant or postpartum	13.9	5.1	24.2	26.3	22.4	13.0	2.6
Seeking pregnancy	11.0	1.8	7.1	17.2	22.7	17.5	10.7
Nonsurgically sterile, male or female	4.2	1.0	1.8	2.8	4.5	4.1	14.2
Surgically sterile, female (noncontraceptive)	3.9	0.0	0.0	1.3	2.9	7.2	15.9

Source: National Center for Health Statistics, Use of Contraception and Use of Family Planning Services in the United States: 1982–2002, Advance Data, No. 350, 2004; Internet site http://www.cdc.gov/nchs/nsfg.htm

Table 8.18 Reason for Not Using Contraceptives among Women by Marital Status, 2002

(percent distribution of women aged 15 to 44 not using contraception by reason and marital status, 2002; numbers in thousands)

	total	currently married	currently cohabiting	never married	formerly married
Women aged 15 to 44 not using contraception	100.0%	100.0%	100.0%	100.0%	100.0%
Never had intercourse or no intercourse in past three months	47.5	8.5	8.7	76.6	49.7
No reason for not using contraception	19.4	23.2	30.2	15.2	23.3
Pregnant or postpartum	13.9	27.7	31.6	4.1	6.2
Seeking pregnancy	11.0	25.5	19.3	1.4	5.6
Nonsurgically sterile, male or female	4.2	7.4	5.1	1.8	7.0
Surgically sterile, female (noncontraceptive)	3.9	7.7	4.7	0.7	8.4

Source: National Center for Health Statistics, Use of Contraception and Use of Family Planning Services in the United States: 1982–2002, Advance Data, No. 350, 2004; Internet site http://www.cdc.gov/nchs/nsfg.htm

Table 8.19 Reason for Not Using Contraceptives among Women by Race and Hispanic Origin, 2002

(percent distribution of women aged 15 to 44 not using contraception by reason, race, and Hispanic origin, 2002; numbers in thousands)

	total	black, non-Hispanic	Hispanic	white, non-Hispanic
Women aged 15 to 44 not using contraception	**100.0%**	**100.0%**	**100.0%**	**100.0%**
Never had intercourse or no intercourse in past three months	47.5	45.5	45.6	47.9
No reason for not using contraception	19.4	23.9	18.8	18.9
Pregnant or postpartum	13.9	13.8	16.8	13.0
Seeking pregnancy	11.0	9.9	12.7	11.0
Nonsurgically sterile, male or female	4.2	3.5	4.1	4.8
Surgically sterile, female (noncontraceptive)	3.9	3.5	2.2	4.8

Source: National Center for Health Statistics, Use of Contraception and Use of Family Planning Services in the United States: 1982–2002, Advance Data, No. 350, 2004; Internet site http://www.cdc.gov/nchs/nsfg.htm

Table 8.20 Discontinuation of Contraceptive Method among Woman by Type and Reason, 2002

(number of women aged 15 to 44 who ever used contraceptive type, percent who discontinued type, and percent distribution by reason for discontinuation, 2002; numbers in thousands)

	pill	condom	Depo-ProveraTM	NorplantTM
Total women aged 15 to 44 ever having used contraceptive	**45,616**	**48,642**	**9,226**	**1,150**
Percent discontinuing contraceptive	**29.2%**	**11.9%**	**42.3%**	**41.6%**
Reason for discontinuation				
Side effects	64.6	17.9	72.3	70.6
Worried about side effects	13.1	2.0	4.2	–
Did not like changes to menstrual cycle	12.7	1.5	33.7	19.3
Method failed, user became pregnant	10.4	7.5	5.7	8.3
Doctor's orders	8.5	2.5	5.7	9.2
Too difficult to use	5.2	8.6	0.7	–
Decreased sexual pleasure	4.1	37.9	8.2	–
Too expensive	3.2	2.2	2.1	–
Worried method might not work	3.0	13.2	2.2	0.0
Partner disliked it	2.8	38.6	2.6	–
Method did not protect against disease	2.1	1.1	1.3	0.0
Too difficult to obtain	1.8	1.5	2.0	0.0
Too messy	1.2	9.5	–	0.0
Other	10.6	15.4	8.1	10.2

Note: Figures will not sum to 100 because more than one reason may have been cited. "–" means sample is too small to make a reliable estimate.
Source: National Center for Health Statistics, Fertility, Family Planning, and Reproductive Health of U.S. Women: Data from the 2002 National Survey of Family Growth, Vital and Health Statistics, Series 23, No. 25, 2005; Internet site Internet site http://www.cdc.gov/nchs/nsfg.htm

Condom Use at First Sexual Intercourse Has Greatly Increased

Most sexually active singles used a condom during the past year.

The fear of AIDS and other sexually transmitted diseases has made condoms increasingly popular. The percentage of men and women aged 15 to 44 who report having used a condom the first time they had sex climbed from 22 percent for those who first had sex before 1980 to 67 to 73 percent for those first having sex in 1999–2002.

Fifty-six percent of unmarried women who have had sexual intercourse in the past year used a condom at least once. Among men the figure is an even greater 67 percent. Nearly two out of three men say they use condoms for both pregnancy and disease prevention.

Most young men say they would not be embarrassed to discuss condom use with a new partner. Most also say there is at least a "good chance" that a new partner would appreciate the use of a condom. But most young men also admit condom use means they will feel less physical pleasure.

■ The advantages of the condom far outweigh the disadvantages, according to most sexually active men and women.

Most men use condoms to prevent both pregnancy and disease

(percent distribution of men aged 15 to 44 who had sexual intercourse in the past year and who used a condom at last sexual intercourse, by reason for condom use, 2002)

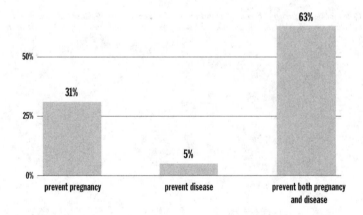

Table 8.21 Condom Use at First Sexual Intercourse by Year of First Sexual Intercourse, 2002

(percent of people aged 15 to 44 who have ever had premarital sexual intercourse who used a condom at first intercourse, by year of first intercourse and sex, 2002)

	percent using condom	
	men	women
Percent of people aged 15 to 44 who ever had premarital sex and who used a condom at first sexual intercourse	**48.7%**	**45.0%**
First intercourse in 1999–2002	73.0	67.2
First intercourse in 1995–1998	70.9	61.7
First intercourse in 1990–1994	58.6	58.0
First intercourse in 1980–1989	44.3	38.1
First intercourse before 1980	21.7	21.7

Source: National Center for Health Statistics, Teenagers in the United States: Sexual Activity, Contraceptive Use, and Childbearing, 2002, Vital and Health Statistics, Series 23, No. 24, 2004; Internet site http://www.cdc.gov/nchs/nsfg.htm

Table 8.22 Condom Use in Past Year Reported by Women, 2002

(number of total and unmarried women aged 15 to 44 who ever used a condom and who had sex in the past 12 months, and percent using a condom in the past 12 months by selected characteristics and consistency of condom use, 2002; numbers in thousands)

	number	condom used in past 12 months		
		any use	some of the time	every time
Total women aged 15 to 44 ever using a condom and having sex in past year	**50,247**	**38.4%**	**25.5%**	**12.9%**
Marital status				
Currently married	27,963	24.6	16.3	8.3
Currently cohabiting	5,433	37.9	29.8	8.1
Never married, not cohabiting	12,152	70.6	44.2	26.4
Formerly married, not cohabiting	4,700	37.9	26.5	11.4
Unmarried women aged 15 to 44 ever using a condom and having sex in past year	**22,284**	**55.6**	**36.9**	**18.7**
Age				
Aged 15 to 19	4,061	82.3	54.8	27.5
Aged 20 to 24	5,891	67.7	45.2	22.5
Aged 25 to 29	3,724	50.2	35.6	14.6
Aged 30 to 44	8,609	37.2	23.4	13.8
Currently cohabiting				
Yes	5,433	37.9	29.8	8.1
No	16,852	61.5	39.3	22.2
Children ever borne				
None	11,354	69.0	44.7	24.3
One or more	10,930	41.9	28.9	13.0
Race and Hispanic origin				
Black, non-Hispanic	4,589	60.5	37.9	22.6
Hispanic	3,374	50.7	35.9	14.8
White, non-Hispanic	12,657	55.0	35.8	19.2
Education				
Not a high school graduate	2,493	34.7	19.7	15.0
High school graduate or GED	5,191	42.0	31.4	10.6
Some college, no degree	4,594	48.3	33.5	14.8
Bachelor's degree or higher	3,461	58.6	37.6	21.0

Note: Education categories include only people aged 22 to 44.
Source: National Center for Health Statistics, Fertility, Family Planning, and Reproductive Health of U.S. Women: Data from the 2002 National Survey of Family Growth, Vital and Health Statistics, Series 23, No. 25, 2005; Internet site http://www.cdc .gov/nchs/products/pubs/pubd/series/sr23/pre-1/sr23_25.htm

Table 8.23 Condom Use in Past Year Reported by Men, 2002

(number of total and unmarried men aged 15 to 44 who had sex in the past 12 months and percent distribution by how often a condom was used, by selected characteristics and consistency of condom use, 2002; numbers in thousands)

	number	condom used in past 12 months		
		any use	some of the time	every time
Total men aged 15 to 44 ever using a condom and having sex in past year	**48,249**	**45.3%**	**29.1%**	**16.2%**
Marital status				
Currently married	25,337	27.0	19.5	7.5
Currently cohabiting	5,559	39.7	33.1	6.6
Never married, not cohabiting	13,955	84.0	46.6	37.4
Formerly married, not cohabiting	3,397	48.3	29.6	18.7
Unmarried men aged 15 to 44 ever using a condom and having sex in past year	**22,912**	**67.1**	**40.5**	**26.6**
Age				
Aged 15 to 19	4,016	89.3	42.4	47.0
Aged 20 to 24	6,423	79.4	51.3	28.2
Aged 25 to 29	3,887	67.7	49.8	17.9
Aged 30 to 34	3,067	53.0	31.7	21.4
Aged 35 to 39	2,536	48.5	29.4	19.1
Aged 40 to 44	2,983	42.2	21.3	20.9
Number of biological children				
None	15,759	76.9	44.1	32.8
One or more	7,153	46.6	33.1	13.6
Number of female partners in past 12 months				
One	13,985	56.2	30.6	25.6
Two or more	8,927	83.6	55.6	28.0
Race and Hispanic origin				
Black, non-Hispanic	3,611	72.1	37.0	35.1
Hispanic	4,175	67.1	41.1	26.0
White, non-Hispanic	13,477	65.1	40.0	25.1
Education				
Not a high school graduate	2,305	45.9	28.3	17.7
High school graduate or GED	5,622	52.8	34.6	18.2
Some college, no degree	5,170	62.5	39.1	23.4
Bachelor's degree or higher	2,919	73.0	51.0	22.1

Note: Education categories include only people aged 22 to 44.
Source: National Center for Health Statistics, Fertility, Contraception, and Fatherhood: Data on Men and Women from Cycle 6 of the 2002 National Survey of Family Growth, Vital and Health Statistics, Series 23, No. 26, 2006; Internet site http://www.cdc .gov/nchs/nsfg.htm

Table 8.24 Reason for Condom Use Reported by Men, 2002

(number of unmarried men aged 15 to 44 who had sexual intercourse in the past 12 months and who used a condom at last sexual intercourse, by selected characteristics and reason for condom use, 2002; numbers in thousands)

	total		reason for condom use at last sexual intercourse		
	number	percent	prevent pregnancy	prevent disease	both pregnancy and disease prevention
Unmarried men aged 15 to 44 who had sexual intercourse in the past year and used a condom at last sexual intercourse	**10,240**	**100.0%**	**30.9%**	**4.9%**	**62.6%**
Number of female partners in past year					
One partner	5,374	100.0	37.6	4.1	57.0
Two or more partners	4,866	100.0	23.6	5.8	68.7
Race and Hispanic origin					
Black, non-Hispanic	2,087	100.0	31.5	8.7	58.6
Hispanic	1,853	100.0	31.2	5.4	61.3
White, non-Hispanic	5,529	100.0	30.2	3.3	64.7
Education					
Not a high school graduate	604	100.0	36.9	16.0	41.6
High school graduate or GED	1,806	100.0	27.9	7.2	62.7
Some college, no degree	2,146	100.0	24.5	3.6	69.8
Bachelor's degree or higher	1,343	100.0	38.1	4.0	57.4

Note: Education categories include only people aged 22 to 44. Numbers may not sum to 100 because "other reason" is not shown.
Source: National Center for Health Statistics, Fertility, Contraception, and Fatherhood: Data on Men and Women from Cycle 6 of the 2002 National Survey of Family Growth, Vital and Health Statistics, Series 23, No. 26, 2006; Internet site http://www.cdc.gov/nchs/nsfg.htm

Table 8.25 Attitude toward Condom Use among Men Aged 15 to 24, 2002: Embarrassment

"What is the chance that it would be embarrassing for you
and a new partner to discuss using a condom?"

(percent distribution of men aged 15 to 24 by selected characteristics and response toward statement, 2002)

	total	no chance	a little chance	50/50 chance	a good chance	almost certain
Total men aged 15 to 24	**100.0%**	**54.5%**	**21.8%**	**12.3%**	**6.3%**	**5.2%**
Ever had sexual intercourse						
No	100.0	34.4	30.0	19.4	10.0	6.2
Yes	100.0	64.3	17.8	8.9	4.4	4.7
Age at first sexual intercourse						
Under age 15	100.0	71.0	13.2	6.4	4.1	5.3
Age 15 to 17	100.0	63.7	19.5	8.8	4.3	3.7
Age 18 to 19	100.0	68.0	17.3	8.9	4.3	–
Aged 20 or older	100.0	43.6	19.8	15.4	6.5	–

Note: "–" means sample is too small to make a reliable estimate.
Source: National Center for Health Statistics, Fertility, Contraception, and Fatherhood: Data on Men and Women from Cycle 6 of the 2002 National Survey of Family Growth, Vital and Health Statistics, Series 23, No. 26, 2006; Internet site http://www.cdc .gov/nchs/nsfg.htm

Table 8.26 Attitude toward Condom Use among Men Aged 15 to 24, 2002: Appreciation

"What is the chance that if you used a condom, a new partner would appreciate it?"

(percent distribution of men aged 15 to 24 by selected characteristics and response toward statement, 2002)

	total	no chance	a little chance	50/50 chance	a good chance	almost certain
Total men aged 15 to 24	**100.0%**	**2.1%**	**3.0%**	**12.4%**	**39.2%**	**43.4%**
Ever had sexual intercourse						
No	100.0	3.2	4.1	12.1	40.4	40.3
Yes	100.0	1.5	2.5	12.5	38.6	44.9
Age at first sexual intercourse						
Under age 15	100.0	0.9	3.0	13.0	38.3	44.8
Age 15 to 17	100.0	1.9	2.2	13.1	40.9	42.0
Age 18 to 19	100.0	–	3.2	8.5	34.1	53.3
Aged 20 or older	100.0	–	–	15.3	32.2	48.2

Note: "–" means sample is too small to make a reliable estimate.
Source: National Center for Health Statistics, Fertility, Contraception, and Fatherhood: Data on Men and Women from Cycle 6 of the 2002 National Survey of Family Growth, Vital and Health Statistics, Series 23, No. 26, 2006; Internet site http://www.cdc.gov/nchs/nsfg.htm

Table 8.27 Attitude toward Condom Use among Men Aged 15 to 24, 2002: Physical Pleasure

"What is the chance that if you used a condom during sex, you would feel less physical pleasure?"

(percent distribution of men aged 15 to 24 by selected characteristics and response toward statement, 2002)

	total	no chance	a little chance	50/50 chance	a good chance	almost certain
Total men aged 15 to 24	**100.0%**	**13.6%**	**27.0%**	**28.3%**	**19.4%**	**11.7%**
Ever had sexual intercourse						
No	100.0	13.6	30.8	38.0	12.5	5.1
Yes	100.0	13.6	25.2	23.8	22.7	14.8
Age at first sexual intercourse						
Under age 15	100.0	13.6	20.7	24.2	21.2	20.3
Age 15 to 17	100.0	13.1	25.3	23.5	24.8	13.4
Age 18 to 19	100.0	10.7	31.5	26.0	19.6	12.3
Aged 20 or older	100.0	22.5	25.1	20.7	18.7	13.1

Source: National Center for Health Statistics, Fertility, Contraception, and Fatherhood: Data on Men and Women from Cycle 6 of the 2002 National Survey of Family Growth, Vital and Health Statistics, Series 23, No. 26, 2006; Internet site http://www.cdc .gov/nchs/nsfg.htm

Contraceptive Sterilization Is Popular with Increasing Age

Tubal sterilization is the most common operation.

Among women aged 15 to 44, a substantial 22 percent are contraceptively sterile. Female sterilization is more common than male sterilization, and the likelihood of being sterilized rises sharply with age. Among women aged 40 to 44, fully 47 are contraceptively sterile or their partners have been sterilized.

The most popular type of sterilization is tubal, with 16 percent of women aged 15 to 44 having had the operation. Among women aged 40 to 44, fully 34 percent have had a tubal sterilization. Six percent of men aged 15 to 44 have had a vasectomy, the proportion peaking at 28 percent among married men aged 40 to 44.

■ Contraceptive sterilization is a permanent solution to the problems of birth control use.

Twenty-eight percent of married men aged 40 to 44 have had a vasectomy

(percent of married men aged 25 to 44 who have had a vasectomy, by age, 2002)

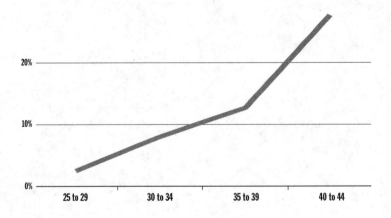

Table 8.28 Contraceptive Sterilization, 2002

(total number of women aged 15 to 44 and percent contraceptively sterile or with a partner who is contraceptively sterile, by selected characteristics, 2002; numbers in thousands)

| | number | contraceptively sterile | | |
		total	female sterilization	male sterilization
Total women aged 15 to 44	**61,561**	**22.4%**	**16.7%**	**5.7%**
Age				
Aged 15 to 19	9,834	0.0	0.0	0.0
Aged 20 to 24	9,840	2.7	2.2	0.5
Aged 25 to 29	9,249	13.1	10.3	2.8
Aged 30 to 34	10,272	25.4	19.0	6.4
Aged 35 to 39	10,853	39.2	29.2	10.0
Aged 40 to 44	11,512	47.4	34.7	12.7
Marital status				
Currently married	28,327	32.9	21.7	11.2
Currently cohabiting	5,570	20.6	18.4	2.2
Never married, not cohabiting	21,568	4.8	4.4	0.4
Formerly married, not cohabiting	6,096	37.5	35.3	2.2
Race and Hispanic origin				
Black, non-Hispanic	8,587	23.7	22.3	1.4
Hispanic	9,107	22.5	19.9	2.6
White, non-Hispanic	40,420	23.0	15.5	7.5

National Center for Health Statistics, Use of Contraception and Use of Family Planning Services in the United States: 1982–2002, Advance Data, No. 350, 2004; Internet site http://www.cdc.gov/nchs/nsfg.htm

Table 8.29 Reason for Contraceptive Sterilization Operation Reported by Women, 2002

(total number of women aged 15 to 44 who had a sterilization operation or whose current husband or cohabiting partner had a vasectomy in 1997 or later, percent citing reason for operation, and percent distribution by main reason, 2002; numbers in thousands)

	tubal sterilization	hysterectomy	vasectomy
REASON FOR OPERATION			
Women aged 15 to 44 with operation since 1997, number	**3,768**	**1,445**	**2,073**
Women aged 15 to 44 with operation since 1997, percent	**100.0%**	**100.0%**	**100.0%**
Woman had all the children she wanted	90.6	75.3	89.7
Husband or cohabiting partner had all the children he wanted	77.7	64.5	93.6
Any medical reason	28.0	99.1	13.0
Medical problems with female organs	11.3	86.3	–
Pregnancy would be dangerous to woman's health	13.1	12.0	8.2
Would probably lose a pregnancy	4.9	7.4	2.4
Would probably have an unhealthy child	1.8	3.8	0.5
Husband or cohabiting partner had health problem	–	–	0.0
Other medical reason	6.0	15.0	3.4
Any problems with birth control methods	15.1	1.2	16.2
Any health-related problems with birth control methods	7.4	1.1	5.2
MAIN REASON FOR OPERATION			
Women aged 15 to 44 with operation since 1997, number	**3,768**	**1,445**	**2,073**
Women aged 15 to 44 with operation since 1997, percent	**100.0%**	**100.0%**	**100.0%**
Woman had all the children she wanted	65.2	9.2	47.0
Husband or cohabiting partner had all the children he wanted	7.2	0.0	36.4
Medical reasons	18.3	89.5	5.0
Problems with other methods of birth control	2.4	0.0	0.5
Other reason	6.9	1.3	11.1

Note: "Reason for operation" may not sum to 100 because more than one reason may have been cited. "–" means not applicable.
Source: National Center for Health Statistics, Fertility, Family Planning, and Reproductive Health of U.S. Women: Data from the 2002 National Survey of Family Growth, Vital and Health Statistics, Series 23, No. 25, 2005; Internet site http://www.cdc.gov/nchs/nsfg.htm

Table 8.30 Contraceptive Sterilization Operation Reported by Women, 2002

(total number of women aged 15 to 44 and percent having had a sterilization operation or whose current husband or cohabiting partner has had a vasectomy, by selected characteristics, 2002; numbers in thousands)

		sterilizing operation				
	total	any	tubal sterilization	vasectomy	hysterectomy	other
Total women aged 15 to 44	**61,561**	**23.6%**	**16.2%**	**6.2%**	**4.1%**	**2.5%**
Age						
Aged 15 to 24	19,674	1.3	1.1	0.3	0.0	0.1
Aged 25 to 29	9,249	13.3	10.2	2.9	0.5	1.0
Aged 30 to 34	10,272	25.2	18.8	5.4	3.1	1.6
Aged 35 to 39	10,853	41.2	28.1	11.6	7.0	3.7
Aged 40 to 44	11,512	52.0	33.6	14.5	12.3	7.4
Marital status						
Currently married	28,327	35.1	21.3	12.8	5.3	3.1
First marriage	23,082	30.9	17.9	12.0	4.0	2.1
Second or later marriage	5,245	53.6	36.2	16.6	11.3	7.7
Currently cohabiting	5,570	22.1	18.4	3.0	4.2	2.7
Never married, not cohabiting	21,568	4.8	4.0	–	0.9	0.6
Formerly married, not cohabiting	6,096	38.5	34.2	–	9.9	0.6
Children ever borne						
None	25,622	3.0	1.0	1.3	1.0	0.9
One	11,173	12.1	7.2	3.1	3.3	2.1
Two	13,402	43.5	28.7	13.2	8.2	4.3
Three or more	11,343	58.1	45.0	11.9	7.2	4.0
Race and Hispanic origin						
Black, non-Hispanic	8,250	25.3	21.6	1.3	4.8	2.7
Hispanic	9,107	23.4	19.8	2.8	2.1	2.3
White, non-Hispanic	39,498	24.2	14.9	8.2	4.6	2.5
Education						
Not a high school graduate	5,627	42.8	37.8	2.1	6.0	4.4
High school graduate or GED	14,264	37.8	27.8	8.2	7.3	4.0
Some college, no degree	14,279	30.5	19.8	9.2	5.8	3.4
Bachelor's degree or higher	13,551	17.4	7.9	8.7	2.5	1.5
Region						
Northeast	9,704	19.7	13.8	5.1	2.3	1.2
Midwest	14,100	25.1	16.3	7.9	4.2	2.5
South	22,939	26.5	19.4	5.2	5.6	3.2
West	14,818	20.4	13.0	6.6	3.1	2.0
Religion raised						
None	4,773	18.0	11.5	7.0	2.6	2.2
Fundamentalist Protestant	3,620	30.0	24.6	3.8	7.1	3.8
Other Protestant	28,120	26.1	17.8	6.8	5.3	2.9
Catholic	21,517	22.1	14.8	6.2	2.7	1.9
Other religion	3,324	13.3	10.0	2.9	2.0	0.9

Note: Numbers may not add to total because some women reported more than one type of sterilizing operation. Education categories include only people aged 22 to 44. "–" means not applicable.
Source: National Center for Health Statistics, Use of Contraception and Use of Family Planning Services in the United States: 1982–2002, Advance Data, No. 350, 2004; Internet site http://www.cdc.gov/nchs/nsfg.htm

Table 8.31 Contraceptive Sterilization Operation Reported by Men, 2002

(total number of men aged 15 to 44 and percent having had a vasectomy or whose current wife or cohabiting partner has had a sterilizing operation, by selected characteristics and type of operation, 2002; numbers in thousands)

| | | sterilizing operation | | | |
| | | | wife or partner | | |
	total	any	vasectomy	tubal sterilization	hysterectomy
Total men aged 15 to 44	**61,147**	**14.5%**	**6.2%**	**7.6%**	**1.9%**
Age					
Aged 15 to 24	20,091	0.7	–	0.4	0.0
Aged 25 to 29	9,226	5.6	1.6	4.4	–
Aged 30 to 34	10,138	14.9	5.3	8.3	1.3
Aged 35 to 39	10,557	28.2	9.3	14.5	5.9
Aged 40 to 44	11,135	33.7	18.8	15.9	3.1
Marital status					
Currently married	25,808	28.6	13.3	14.4	3.9
Currently cohabiting	5,653	19.1	0.7	16.2	2.5
Never married, not cohabiting	25,412	0.4	–	–	–
Formerly married, not cohabiting	4,274	7.2	6.8	–	–
Number of biological children					
None	32,593	2.9	0.7	1.3	1.2
One	10,457	13.6	6.1	6.4	1.9
Two	9,829	27.6	15.1	12.3	3.3
Three or more	8,269	45.7	17.6	28.1	3.0
Race and Hispanic origin					
Black, non-Hispanic	6,940	10.4	1.9	6.8	2.3
Hispanic	10,188	11.0	2.3	8.2	0.8
White, non-Hispanic	38,738	15.2	8.0	6.2	2.3
Education					
Not a high school graduate	6,355	20.9	6.6	12.8	2.3
High school graduate or GED	15,659	23.8	8.0	14.1	4.5
Some college, no degree	13,104	17.8	9.8	7.8	1.4
Bachelor's degree or higher	11,901	12.4	7.1	4.9	0.9
Region					
Northeast	8,361	11.7	6.3	5.2	–
Midwest	12,766	16.0	8.2	6.8	2.0
South	24,543	15.5	5.6	9.2	2.8
West	15,477	13.3	5.6	6.8	1.1
Religion raised					
None	4,981	12.6	10.2	3.2	–
Fundamentalist Protestant	2,747	9.5	3.1	5.2	–
Other Protestant	27,152	16.9	7.1	8.7	3.2
Catholic	21,821	13.0	5.3	6.9	0.9
Other religion	4,263	13.0	2.6	9.8	–

Note: Numbers may not add to total because some women reported more than one type of sterilizing operation. Education categories include only people aged 22 to 44. "–" means sample is too small to make a reliable estimate or not applicable.
Source: National Center for Health Statistics, Fertility, Contraception, and Fatherhood: Data on Men and Women from Cycle 6 of the 2002 National Survey of Family Growth, Vital and Health Statistics, Series 23, No. 26, 2006; Internet site http://www.cdc.gov/nchs/nsfg.htm

Table 8.32 Vasectomies among Married Men, 2002

(percent of married men aged 15 to 44 who have had a vasectomy, by selected characteristics, 2002; numbers in thousands)

	percent having had a vasectomy
Married men aged 15 to 44	**13.3%**
Age	
Aged 15 to 24	–
Aged 25 to 29	2.5
Aged 30 to 34	8.0
Aged 35 to 39	12.7
Aged 40 to 44	27.7
Number of biological children	
None	3.2
One	8.5
Two	17.4
Three or more	22.0
Race and Hispanic origin	
Black, non-Hispanic	5.1
Hispanic	4.4
White, non-Hispanic	16.2
Education	
Not a high school graduate	11.8
High school graduate or GED	12.8
Some college, no degree	18.4
Bachelor's degree or higher	10.6
Region	
Northeast	15.3
Midwest	17.0
South	11.8
West	11.8

Note: "–" means sample is too small to make a reliable estimate.
Source: National Center for Health Statistics, Fertility, Contraception, and Fatherhood: Data on Men and Women from Cycle 6 of the 2002 National Survey of Family Growth, Vital and Health Statistics, Series 23, No. 26, 2006; Internet site http://www.cdc.gov/nchs/nsfg.htm

Table 8.33 Use of Contraceptive Sterilization by Birth Control Users, 2002

(total number of women aged 15 to 44 using contraception and percent using female and male sterilization by selected characteristics, 2002; numbers in thousands)

		contraceptively sterile		
	number	total	female	male
Women aged 15 to 44 using contraception	**38,109**	**36.2%**	**27.0%**	**9.2%**
Age				
Aged 15 to 19	3,096	0.0	0.0	0.0
Aged 20 to 24	5,975	4.4	3.6	0.8
Aged 25 to 29	6,291	19.3	15.1	4.2
Aged 30 to 34	7,105	36.7	27.5	9.2
Aged 35 to 39	7,688	55.4	41.2	14.2
Aged 40 to 44	7,955	68.7	50.3	18.4
Marital status				
Currently married	20,655	45.2	29.8	15.4
Currently cohabiting	4,039	28.5	25.4	3.1
Never married, not cohabiting	9,491	10.9	10.0	0.9
Formerly married, not cohabiting	3,924	58.2	54.9	3.3
Children ever borne				
None	11,786	5.2	2.0	3.2
One	6,702	17.7	13.0	4.7
Two	10,415	53.7	38.2	15.5
Three or more	9,205	69.6	56.4	13.2
Race and Hispanic origin				
Black, non-Hispanic	4,925	41.3	38.9	2.4
Hispanic	5,371	38.2	33.8	4.4
White, non-Hispanic	26,062	35.6	24.0	11.6
Education				
Not a high school graduate	3,887	58.1	55.3	2.8
High school graduate or GED	9,996	52.3	41.5	10.8
Some college, no degree	9,954	40.8	28.7	12.1
Bachelor's degree or higher	8,741	25.6	12.8	12.8

Note: Education categories include only people aged 22 to 44.
Source: National Center for Health Statistics, Use of Contraception and Use of Family Planning Services in the United States: 1982–2002, Advance Data, No. 350, 2004; Internet site http://www.cdc.gov/nchs/nsfg.htm

Many Women Use Family Planning Services

More than 40 percent of women aged 15 to 44 have received family planning services from a medical care provider in the past year.

American women are frequent visitors to the doctor's office or clinic for birth control and other family planning services. Forty-two percent of women aged 15 to 44 have visited a medical care provider for family planning services in the past 12 months, and 34 percent have received a birth control method. The proportion of women who receive birth control peaks at 54 percent among women aged 20 to 24.

Men are not strangers to the doctor's office either. Eleven percent of men aged 15 to 44 have received birth control counseling from a medical care provider in the past 12 months. Sixteen percent of men aged 15 to 24 have visited a family planning clinic in the past year themselves, and another 8 percent have visited with a partner.

■ Ready access to birth control is important to young and middle-aged men and women.

Most women aged 20 to 24 have received birth control from a medical care provider in the past year

*(percent of women aged 15 to 44 who have received birth control
from a medical care provider in the past year, by age, 2002)*

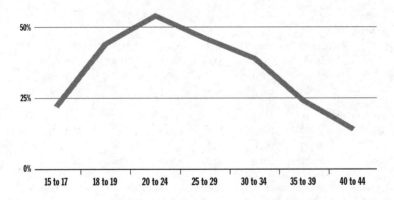

Table 8.34 Women's Use of Family Planning Services, 2002

(total number of women aged 15 to 44 and percent having received at least one family planning service from a medical care provider in the past 12 months, by selected characteristics and type of service, 2002; numbers in thousands)

	total		family planning service received in past year					
	number	percent	any	birth control method	birth control counseling	birth control checkup or test	sterilization counseling	sterilization operation
Total women aged 15 to 44	**61,561**	**100.0%**	**41.7%**	**33.9%**	**18.6%**	**23.6%**	**4.4%**	**1.9%**
Age								
Aged 15 to 19	9,834	100.0	39.9	31.1	22.1	22.0	1.1	0.0
Aged 15 to 17	5,819	100.0	31.8	22.2	19.0	15.8	0.9	0.0
Aged 18 to 19	4,016	100.0	51.6	43.9	26.5	31.0	1.4	0.0
Aged 20 to 24	9,840	100.0	63.3	54.0	30.6	35.7	3.6	1.2
Aged 25 to 29	9,249	100.0	55.4	46.3	23.8	30.2	7.1	2.2
Aged 30 to 34	10,272	100.0	47.0	39.1	18.3	27.2	6.6	2.6
Aged 35 to 39	10,853	100.0	30.5	23.9	12.7	18.6	5.2	3.0
Aged 40 to 44	11,512	100.0	19.5	14.0	7.0	10.8	3.0	2.0
Marital status								
Currently married	28,327	100.0	39.5	31.5	16.0	21.3	5.8	2.5
Currently cohabiting	5,570	100.0	50.4	43.2	21.5	30.2	4.6	1.8
Never married, not cohabiting	21,568	100.0	44.4	36.4	22.5	25.4	2.4	0.7
Formerly married, not cohabiting	6,096	100.0	34.5	28.0	14.3	22.0	4.7	3.1
Children ever borne								
None	25,622	100.0	45.3	38.8	20.8	27.1	1.3	0.3
One	11,193	100.0	51.0	43.0	22.9	27.6	4.5	1.4
Two	13,402	100.0	38.1	29.3	16.5	21.4	6.3	3.7
Three or more	11,343	100.0	28.6	19.5	11.8	14.5	9.2	3.8
Race and Hispanic origin								
Black, non-Hispanic	8,587	100.0	39.6	30.6	20.7	21.5	5.0	2.2
Hispanic	9,107	100.0	39.7	28.9	22.6	20.6	7.0	2.3
White, non-Hispanic	40,420	100.0	43.2	36.4	17.4	25.4	3.7	1.7

Source: National Center for Health Statistics, Use of Contraception and Use of Family Planning Services in the United States: 1982–2002, Advance Data, No. 350, 2004; Internet site http://www.cdc.gov/nchs/nsfg.htm

Table 8.35 Men's Use of Family Planning Services, 2002

(total number of men aged 15 to 44 and percent having received family planning services from a medical care provider in the past 12 months, by selected characteristics and type of service, 2002; numbers in thousands)

		percent receiving	
	number	birth control counseling	advice about sterilization
Total men aged 15 to 44	**61,147**	**10.6%**	**2.2%**
Age			
Aged 15 to 19	10,208	17.5	1.1
Aged 20 to 24	9,883	16.9	1.1
Aged 25 to 29	9,226	12.4	2.2
Aged 30 to 44	31,830	5.9	2.8
Marital status			
Currently married	25,808	6.0	3.2
Currently cohabiting	5,653	8.5	3.1
Never married, not cohabiting	25,412	16.1	1.0
Formerly married, not cohabiting	4,274	8.4	1.0
Number of biological children			
None	32,593	13.2	1.1
One	10,457	9.5	3.0
Two	9,829	8.5	4.4
Three or more	8,269	4.5	2.7
Race and Hispanic origin			
Black, non-Hispanic	6,940	20.3	3.5
Hispanic	10,188	14.9	2.3
White, non-Hispanic	38,738	7.9	1.9

Source: National Center for Health Statistics, Fertility, Contraception, and Fatherhood: Data on Men and Women from Cycle 6 of the 2002 National Survey of Family Growth, Vital and Health Statistics, Series 23, No. 26, 2006; Internet site http://www.cdc.gov/nchs/nsfg.htm

Table 8.36 Visits by Men Aged 15 to 24 to Family Planning Clinics, 2002

(number of men aged 15 to 24 and percent having visited a family planning clinic in the past 12 months by himself or with a female partner, by selected characteristics and type of service, 2002; numbers in thousands)

		percent visiting	
	number	by himself	with female partner
Total men aged 15 to 24	**20,091**	**15.9%**	**7.5%**
Age			
Aged 15 to 19	10,208	17.9	4.7
Aged 20 to 24	9,883	13.8	10.4
Marital status			
Currently married	1,559	14.8	13.7
Currently cohabiting	1,517	12.9	21.9
Not currently married or cohabiting	17,016	16.2	5.6
Number of biological children			
None	18,181	15.9	6.3
One or more	1,910	15.4	19.0
Race and Hispanic origin			
Black, non-Hispanic	2,550	15.9	8.7
Hispanic	3,579	18.3	9.0
White, non-Hispanic	12,311	15.7	6.6

Source: National Center for Health Statistics, Fertility, Contraception, and Fatherhood: Data on Men and Women from Cycle 6 of the 2002 National Survey of Family Growth, Vital and Health Statistics, Series 23, No. 26, 2006; Internet site http://www.cdc.gov/nchs/nsfg.htm

9

Pregnancy

■ Pregnancy is an almost universal experience among women, more welcome to some than to others. The likelihood of a pregnancy ending in a live birth, abortion, or fetal loss differs by demographic characteristic.

■ Most women have experienced a pregnancy by their mid-twenties. The percentage of women who have been pregnant surpasses 50 percent in the 25-to-29 age group and peaks at 91 percent among women aged 40 to 44.

■ Some pregnancies are unwanted. Overall, 64 percent of pregnancies are intended, 22 percent are mistimed, and 14 percent are unwanted.

■ Many pregnancies do not result in births. Of the 6.4 million pregnancies in 2000, more than 4 million (63 percent) ended in a live birth. Another 1.3 million ended in an abortion, and just over 1 million ended in a spontaneous fetal loss (or miscarriage).

■ The abortion rate fell from 27.4 abortions per 1,000 women in 1990 to 21.3 in 2000. The rate fell in every age group but one.

■ Prenatal care is commonplace. Fully 91 percent of pregnancies receive prenatal care in the first three months.

■ Many women smoke during pregnancy. Thirteen percent of women smoked during their pregnancy, another 11 percent smoked only before the pregnancy, and 75 percent never smoked.

Two-Thirds of Women Aged 15 to 44 Have Had at Least One Pregnancy

A smaller 47 percent of their male counterparts have fathered a pregnancy.

Most women aged 15 to 44 have been pregnant at least once in their lives, the proportion naturally rising with age. Only 14 percent of teen girls aged 15 to 19 have had a pregnancy, as have 42 percent of women aged 20 to 24. The proportion surpasses 50 percent in the 25-to-29 age group.

Black and Hispanic women are more likely to have had a pregnancy than non-Hispanic white women. Seventy-two to 73 percent of black and Hispanic women have had at least one pregnancy versus 63 percent of non-Hispanic white women. Perhaps the biggest difference is by education. Fully 94 percent of women who did not graduate from high school have experienced at least one pregnancy compared with just 64 percent of women with a college degree.

■ Women who were raised without a religion are less likely than fundamentalist Protestants to have had a pregnancy, 58 versus 68 percent.

More than 90 percent of women aged 40 to 44 have had at least one pregnancy

(percent of women aged 15 to 44 who have had at least one pregnancy in their lifetime, by age, 2002)

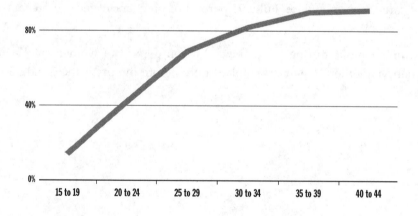

Table 9.1 Number of Pregnancies in Lifetime by Age, 2002

(total number of women aged 15 to 44 and percent distribution by number of pregnancies in lifetime, by age, 2002; numbers in thousands)

| | total | | | pregnancies in lifetime | | | | |
| | | | | | one or more | | | |
	number	percent	none	total	one	two	three	four or more
Total women aged 15 to 44	**61,561**	**100.0%**	**34.3%**	**65.8%**	**15.7%**	**18.4%**	**14.6%**	**17.1%**
Aged 15 to 19	9,834	100.0	85.6	14.2	9.8	3.7	0.7	–
Aged 20 to 24	9,840	100.0	58.0	42.0	19.4	11.9	7.2	3.5
Aged 25 to 29	9,249	100.0	31.4	68.7	20.0	18.7	14.7	15.3
Aged 30 to 34	10,272	100.0	18.0	81.9	17.9	25.9	18.9	19.2
Aged 35 to 39	10,853	100.0	10.3	89.7	14.4	26.4	22.9	26.0
Aged 40 to 44	11,512	100.0	9.4	90.6	13.1	22.0	21.3	34.2

Note: "–" means sample is too small to make a reliable estimate.
Source: National Center for Health Statistics, Fertility, Family Planning, and Reproductive Health of U.S. Women: Data from the 2002 National Survey of Family Growth, Vital and Health Statistics, Series 23, No. 25, 2005; Internet site http://www .cdc.gov/nchs/nsfg.htm

Table 9.2 Number of Pregnancies in Lifetime by Marital Status, 2002

(total number of women aged 15 to 44 and percent distribution by number of pregnancies in lifetime, by marital status, 2002; numbers in thousands)

| | total | | | pregnancies in lifetime | | | | |
| | | | | | one or more | | | |
	number	percent	none	total	one	two	three	four or more
Total women aged 15 to 44	**61,561**	**100.0%**	**34.3%**	**65.8%**	**15.7%**	**18.4%**	**14.6%**	**17.1%**
Married	28,327	100.0	12.1	88.0	16.9	26.5	21.6	23.0
First marriage	23,082	100.0	14.0	86.2	17.9	28.0	20.3	20.0
Second marriage	5,245	100.0	4.0	96.0	12.4	19.9	27.6	36.1
Cohabiting	5,570	100.0	28.0	72.0	20.8	16.3	14.1	20.8
Never married, not cohabiting	21,568	100.0	72.2	27.8	12.1	6.6	4.1	5.0
Formerly married, not cohabiting	6,096	100.0	8.6	91.3	17.8	24.6	19.9	29.0

Source: National Center for Health Statistics, Fertility, Family Planning, and Reproductive Health of U.S. Women: Data from the 2002 National Survey of Family Growth, Vital and Health Statistics, Series 23, No. 25, 2005; Internet site http://www .cdc.gov/nchs/nsfg.htm

Table 9.3 Number of Pregnancies in Lifetime by Race and Hispanic Origin, 2002

(total number of women aged 15 to 44 and percent distribution by number of pregnancies in lifetime, by race and Hispanic origin, 2002; numbers in thousands)

| | total | | | pregnancies in lifetime | | | | |
| | | | | | one or more | | | |
	number	percent	none	total	one	two	three	four or more
Total women aged 15 to 44	**61,561**	**100.0%**	**34.3%**	**65.8%**	**15.7%**	**18.4%**	**14.6%**	**17.1%**
Black, non-Hispanic	8,250	100.0	27.4	72.6	17.2	17.8	15.1	22.5
Hispanic	9,107	100.0	27.8	72.2	15.6	20.0	16.8	19.8
White, non-Hispanic	39,498	100.0	36.8	63.2	15.2	18.1	14.1	15.8

Source: National Center for Health Statistics, Fertility, Family Planning, and Reproductive Health of U.S. Women: Data from the 2002 National Survey of Family Growth, Vital and Health Statistics, Series 23, No. 25, 2005; Internet site http://www .cdc.gov/nchs/nsfg.htm

Table 9.4 Number of Pregnancies in Lifetime by Education, 2002

(total number of women aged 15 to 44 and percent distribution by number of pregnancies in lifetime, by education, 2002; numbers in thousands)

| | total | | | pregnancies in lifetime | | | | |
| | | | | | one or more | | | |
	number	percent	none	total	one	two	three	four or more
Total women aged 15 to 44	**61,561**	**100.0%**	**34.3%**	**65.8%**	**15.7%**	**18.4%**	**14.6%**	**17.1%**
Not a high school graduate	5,627	100.0	6.1	93.9	10.8	21.1	25.8	36.2
High school grad. or GED	14,264	100.0	12.0	88.0	17.5	23.7	21.1	25.7
Some college, no degree	14,279	100.0	21.0	79.1	16.4	24.1	16.5	22.1
Bachelor's degree or more	13,551	100.0	36.1	63.9	18.7	18.9	14.5	11.8

Note: Education categories include only people aged 22 to 44.
Source: National Center for Health Statistics, Fertility, Family Planning, and Reproductive Health of U.S. Women: Data from the 2002 National Survey of Family Growth, Vital and Health Statistics, Series 23, No. 25, 2005; Internet site Internet site http://www .cdc.gov/nchs/nsfg.htm

Table 9.5 Number of Pregnancies in Lifetime by Religion Raised, 2002

(total number of women aged 15 to 44 and percent distribution by number of pregnancies in lifetime, by religion raised, 2002; numbers in thousands)

	total			pregnancies in lifetime				
					one or more			
	number	percent	none	total	one	two	three	four or more
Total women aged 15 to 44	**61,561**	**100.0%**	**34.3%**	**65.8%**	**15.7%**	**18.4%**	**14.6%**	**17.1%**
None	4,773	100.0	42.1	57.8	19.1	16.5	11.4	10.8
Fundamentalist Protestant	3,620	100.0	31.6	68.3	13.5	19.7	19.7	15.4
Other Protestant	28,120	100.0	34.1	66.0	16.2	18.7	13.8	17.3
Catholic	21,517	100.0	32.5	67.6	14.7	18.9	15.2	18.8
Other religion	3,324	100.0	40.0	60.0	14.4	14.6	16.4	14.6

Source: National Center for Health Statistics, Fertility, Family Planning, and Reproductive Health of U.S. Women: Data from the 2002 National Survey of Family Growth, Vital and Health Statistics, Series 23, No. 25, 2005; Internet site Internet site http://www .cdc.gov/nchs/nsfg.htm

Table 9.6 Number of Pregnancies Fathered in Lifetime, 2002

(total number of men aged 15 to 44, average number of pregnancies fathered in lifetime, and percent distribution by number of pregnancies fathered, 2002; numbers in thousands)

	total			pregnancies fathered in lifetime				
					one or more			
	number	percent	none	total	one	two	three or more	average number
Total men aged 15 to 44	**61,147**	**100.0%**	**53.0%**	**47.0%**	**11.0%**	**14.4%**	**21.6%**	**1.3**
Age								
Aged 15 to 24	20,091	100.0	90.3	9.8	5.1	2.2	2.5	0.2
Aged 25 to 29	9,226	100.0	54.9	45.1	12.4	16.7	16.0	1.0
Aged 30 to 34	10,138	100.0	36.6	63.5	16.9	23.0	23.6	1.6
Aged 35 to 39	10,557	100.0	29.0	71.1	13.2	23.0	34.9	2.0
Aged 40 to 44	11,135	100.0	21.8	78.1	12.9	18.6	46.6	2.4
Marital status								
Married	25,808	100.0	21.2	78.8	15.8	25.1	37.9	2.2
Cohabiting	5,653	100.0	45.3	54.7	15.6	12.2	26.9	1.4
Never married, not cohabiting	25,412	100.0	92.3	7.6	3.5	2.4	1.7	0.2
Formerly married, not cohabiting	4,274	100.0	21.3	78.7	20.0	23.7	35.0	2.2

Source: National Center for Health Statistics, Fertility, Contraception, and Fatherhood: Data on Men and Women from Cycle 6 of the 2002 National Survey of Family Growth, Vital and Health Statistics, Series 23, No. 26, 2006; Internet site http://www.cdc. gov/nchs/nsfg.htm

On a Scale of 1 to 10, Women Rate Their Happiness with Pregnancies an 8

One in seven pregnancies is unwanted.

Many pregnancies are unwanted, and women who find themselves with an unwanted pregnancy are not happy about it. Women aged 15 to 44 were asked about their pregnancies in the past three years and to rate how happy they were to be pregnant on a scale of 1 (very unhappy) to 10 (very happy). On average, women rated their happiness at 7.9. If the pregnancy was intended, the happiness rating rose to 9.2. If the pregnancy was mistimed, the rating stood at 6.4. If the pregnancy was unwanted, the rating fell to a lowly 4.2.

The older the woman at the time of pregnancy, the greater the likelihood the pregnancy was intended and the happier the woman was to be pregnant. Non-Hispanic white women are much more likely than black or Hispanic women to report their pregnancy was intended (71 percent versus 45 and 55 percent, respectively), which boosts their happiness rating. Non-Hispanic white women rate their happiness about pregnancy at 8.2 overall, while Hispanics rate their happiness at 8.0, and blacks theirs at 6.6.

■ Overall, 64 percent of pregnancies are intended, 22 percent are mistimed, and 14 percent are unwanted.

Women are not happy with unwanted pregnancies

(on a scale of 1 to 10, with 10 being "very happy," happiness of women aged 15 to 44 with pregnancies by wantedness of birth, for pregnancies ending in live births or fetal losses between 1999 and 2002)

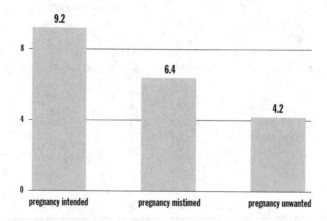

Table 9.7 Happiness with Pregnancy by Wantedness of Birth, 2002

(total number of pregnancies to women aged 15 to 44 since January 1999 including pregnancies current at time of interview, percent distribution by wantedness and by how happy the woman was to be pregnant, and average happiness rating, 2002; numbers in thousands)

	number	percent distribution	happiness scale total	1–3	4–7	8–10	average rating
Total pregnancies	**22,808**	**100.0%**	**100.0%**	**12.6%**	**18.3%**	**69.2%**	**7.9**
Pregnancy intended	14,611	64.1	100.0	2.5	8.8	89.0	9.2
Pregnancy mistimed	4,989	21.9	100.0	18.2	39.4	42.4	6.4
Less than two years too soon	2,047	9.0	100.0	8.1	32.6	59.4	7.5
More than two years too soon	2,743	12.0	100.0	26.3	44.0	29.7	5.5
Pregnancy unwanted	3,170	13.9	100.0	49.8	30.5	19.7	4.2

Note: Happiness scale extends from 1 to 10, with 1 being "very unhappy to be pregnant" and 10 being "very happy to be pregnant." Pregnancies exclude those ending in abortion. Numbers may not add to total because pregnancies with missing wantedness status are not shown.
Source: National Center for Health Statistics, Fertility, Family Planning, and Reproductive Health of U.S. Women: Data from the 2002 National Survey of Family Growth, Vital and Health Statistics, Series 23, No. 25, 2005; Internet site http://www .cdc.gov/nchs/nsfg.htm; calculations by New Strategist

Table 9.8 Happiness with Pregnancy by Wantedness of Birth and Age, 2002

(total number of pregnancies to women aged 15 to 44 since January 1999 including pregnancies current at time of interview, percent distribution by wantedness and by how happy the woman was to be pregnant, and average happiness rating, by age, 2002; numbers in thousands)

	number	percent distribution	happiness scale total	1–3	4–7	8–10	average rating
Total pregnancies	**22,808**	**–**	**100.0%**	**12.6%**	**18.3%**	**69.2%**	**7.9**
Under age 20	**2,373**	**100.0%**	**100.0**	**24.2**	**33.2**	**42.7**	**6.2**
Pregnancy intended	563	23.7	100.0	–	10.3	83.7	8.8
Pregnancy mistimed	1,319	55.6	100.0	24.2	41.2	34.6	5.8
Pregnancy unwanted	491	20.7	100.0	46.9	35.7	11.6	4.1
Aged 20 to 29	**11,589**	**100.0**	**100.0**	**12.7**	**20.5**	**66.9**	**7.8**
Pregnancy intended	7,208	62.2	100.0	3.4	10.5	86.2	9.1
Pregnancy mistimed	2,790	24.1	100.0	16.8	39.4	43.9	6.5
Pregnancy unwanted	1,571	13.6	100.0	47.7	33.1	19.2	4.3
Aged 30 to 44	**8,846**	**100.0**	**100.0**	**9.3**	**11.4**	**79.3**	**8.5**
Pregnancy intended	6,841	77.3	100.0	1.5	6.1	92.4	9.5
Pregnancy mistimed	879	9.9	100.0	13.6	36.9	49.4	6.9
Pregnancy unwanted	1,108	12.5	100.0	54.1	24.6	21.2	4.1

Note: Happiness scale extends from 1 to 10, with 1 being "very unhappy to be pregnant" and 10 being "very happy to be pregnant." Pregnancies exclude those ending in abortion. "–" means not applicable or sample is too small to make a reliable estimate. Numbers may not add to total because pregnancies with missing wantedness status are not shown.
Source: National Center for Health Statistics, Fertility, Family Planning, and Reproductive Health of U.S. Women: Data from the 2002 National Survey of Family Growth, Vital and Health Statistics, Series 23, No. 25, 2005; Internet site http://www .cdc.gov/nchs/nsfg.htm; calculations by New Strategist

Table 9.9   Happiness with Pregnancy by Wantedness of Birth and Marital Status, 2002

(total number of pregnancies to women aged 15 to 44 since January 1999 including pregnancies current at time of interview, percent distribution by wantedness and by how happy the woman was to be pregnant, and average happiness rating, by marital status, 2002; numbers in thousands)

	number	percent distribution	happiness scale total	1–3	4–7	8–10	average rating
Total pregnancies	**22,808**	–	**100.0%**	**12.6%**	**18.3%**	**69.2%**	**7.9**
Married	**14,439**	**100.0%**	**100.0**	**7.1**	**13.1**	**79.9**	**8.7**
Pregnancy intended	11,145	77.2	100.0	1.6	6.2	92.2	9.5
Pregnancy mistimed	2,020	14.0	100.0	13.3	42.8	43.9	6.7
Pregnancy unwanted	1,245	8.6	100.0	46.6	26.8	26.6	4.6
Cohabiting	**3,247**	**100.0**	**100.0**	**18.0**	**25.3**	**56.7**	**7.1**
Pregnancy intended	1,443	44.4	100.0	4.1	11.4	84.5	8.9
Pregnancy mistimed	1,155	35.6	100.0	20.6	36.0	43.5	6.3
Pregnancy unwanted	644	19.8	100.0	44.4	36.8	18.7	4.3
Neither married nor cohabiting	**5,122**	**100.0**	**100.0**	**24.6**	**28.5**	**47.0**	**6.4**
Pregnancy intended	2,023	39.5	100.0	6.7	18.7	74.6	8.2
Pregnancy mistimed	1,813	35.4	100.0	22.3	37.8	40.0	6.1
Pregnancy unwanted	1,281	25.0	100.0	55.6	31.0	13.4	3.8

Note: Happiness scale extends from 1 to 10, with 1 being "very unhappy to be pregnant" and 10 being "very happy to be pregnant." Pregnancies exclude those ending in abortion. "–" means not applicable. Numbers may not add to total because pregnancies with missing wantedness status are not shown.
Source: National Center for Health Statistics, Fertility, Family Planning, and Reproductive Health of U.S. Women: Data from the 2002 National Survey of Family Growth, Vital and Health Statistics, Series 23, No. 25, 2005; Internet site http://www .cdc.gov/nchs/nsfg.htm; calculations by New Strategist

Table 9.10 Happiness with Pregnancy by Wantedness of Birth, Race, and Hispanic Origin, 2002

(total number of pregnancies to women aged 15 to 44 since January 1999 including pregnancies current at time of interview, percent distribution by wantedness and by how happy the woman was to be pregnant, and average happiness rating, by race and Hispanic origin, 2002; numbers in thousands)

	number	percent distribution	happiness scale total	1–3	4–7	8–10	average rating
Total pregnancies	**22,808**	–	**100.0%**	**12.6%**	**18.3%**	**69.2%**	**7.9**
Black, non-Hispanic	**3,125**	**100.0%**	**100.0**	**22.8**	**26.8**	**50.4**	**6.6**
Pregnancy intended	1,407	45.0	100.0	3.9	13.2	82.9	8.8
Pregnancy mistimed	929	29.7	100.0	25.1	40.2	34.6	5.8
Pregnancy unwanted	789	25.2	100.0	54.0	35.2	10.8	3.7
Hispanic	**4,183**	**100.0**	**100.0**	**13.5**	**16.2**	**70.3**	**8.0**
Pregnancy intended	2,292	54.8	100.0	6.1	4.0	89.9	9.2
Pregnancy mistimed	1,137	27.2	100.0	13.1	31.0	55.9	7.3
Pregnancy unwanted	743	17.8	100.0	37.2	30.9	31.9	5.2
White, non-Hispanic	**13,642**	**100.0**	**100.0**	**9.9**	**16.8**	**73.4**	**8.2**
Pregnancy intended	9,632	70.6	100.0	1.1	8.2	90.7	9.4
Pregnancy mistimed	2,572	18.9	100.0	18.5	42.3	39.2	6.1
Pregnancy unwanted	1,414	10.4	100.0	54.2	28.7	17.2	3.9

Note: Happiness scale extends from 1 to 10, with 1 being "very unhappy to be pregnant" and 10 being "very happy to be pregnant." Pregnancies exclude those ending in abortion. "–" means not applicable. Numbers may not add to total because pregnancies with missing wantedness status are not shown.
Source: National Center for Health Statistics, Fertility, Family Planning, and Reproductive Health of U.S. Women: Data from the 2002 National Survey of Family Growth, Vital and Health Statistics, Series 23, No. 25, 2005; Internet site http://www .cdc.gov/nchs/nsfg.htm; calculations by New Strategist

Most Teen Girls Would Be Very Upset If They Became Pregnant

A smaller majority of teen boys would be "very upset."

Not surprisingly, most teenagers would be "very upset" if they or their girlfriend became pregnant. Sixty percent of girls aged 15 to 19 say they would be very upset. Only 5 percent would be "very pleased." Interestingly, a smaller 51 percent of teen boys say they would be very upset if their girlfriend became pregnant.

The older the teen girl, the more likely she would be very upset by a pregnancy. Only 37 percent of girls under age 15 say they would be very upset compared with 57 percent of girls aged 17 to 19. The pattern is the same among teens boys. Eleven percent of boys under age 15 say they would be very pleased if their girlfriend became pregnant.

Non-Hispanic whites would be more upset by a pregnancy than blacks or Hispanics. Among girls, 66 percent of non-Hispanic white teens say they would be very upset if they became pregnant now. This compares with a smaller 51 percent of blacks and 46 percent of Hispanics. Ten percent of Hispanic girls say they would be very pleased by a pregnancy. The pattern is the same for boys, with non-Hispanic whites more upset by a potential pregnancy than blacks or Hispanics.

■ Family structure plays a role in teen attitudes toward pregnancy, and teens from two-parent families would be more upset by a pregnancy than those from other types of families.

Older teens would be more upset by pregnancy

(percent of girls aged 15 to 19 who would be "very upset" if they got pregnant now, by age, 2002)

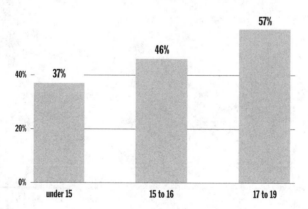

Table 9.11 Attitude of Teenage Girls toward Pregnancy, 2002

"If you got pregnant now, how would you feel?"

(number of never-married females aged 15 to 19 and percent distribution by response to statement, by selected characteristics, 2002; numbers in thousands)

	total		very upset	a little upset	a little pleased	very pleased
	number	percent				
Total never-married women aged 15 to 19	**9,598**	**100.0%**	**60.2%**	**26.7%**	**8.0%**	**4.7%**
Age						
Aged 15 to 17	5,815	100.0	67.5	21.2	8.2	2.8
Aged 18 to 19	3,783	100.0	49.0	35.1	7.8	7.6
Age at first intercourse						
Never had sex	5,236	100.0	72.1	20.3	5.1	2.5
Under age 15	1,248	100.0	36.7	39.9	13.8	7.2
Aged 15 to 16	2,095	100.0	45.8	35.0	10.3	8.9
Aged 17 to 19	1,019	100.0	57.2	26.5	11.1	3.9
Race and Hispanic Origin						
Black, non-Hispanic	1,496	100.0	50.5	32.5	11.7	5.0
Hispanic	1,447	100.0	46.4	29.0	14.9	9.8
White, non-Hispanic	6,099	100.0	65.8	24.2	5.5	3.8
Family structure at age 14						
Living with both parents	6,078	100.0	63.4	27.5	6.1	2.8
Other	3,520	100.0	54.7	25.3	11.3	7.9

Source: National Center for Health Statistics, Teenagers in the United States: Sexual Activity, Contraceptive Use, and Childbearing, 2002, Vital and Health Statistics, Series 23, No. 24, 2004; Internet site http://www.cdc.gov/nchs/nsfg.htm

Table 9.12 Attitude of Teenage Boys toward Pregnancy, 2002

"If you got a female pregnant now, how would you feel?"

(number of never-married males aged 15 to 19 and percent distribution by response to statement, by selected characteristics, 2002; numbers in thousands)

	total number	total percent	very upset	a little upset	a little pleased	very pleased
Total never-married men aged 15 to 19	**10,139**	**100.0%**	**51.4%**	**33.4%**	**11.0%**	**3.7%**
Age						
Aged 15 to 17	5,726	100.0	58.9	29.9	8.1	2.8
Aged 18 to 19	4,413	100.0	41.8	37.8	14.6	4.7
Age at first intercourse						
Never had sex	5,511	100.0	62.1	30.9	4.8	1.8
Under age 15	1,483	100.0	25.7	39.4	23.7	11.0
Aged 15 to 16	1,947	100.0	41.0	41.5	13.0	3.2
Aged 17 to 19	1,199	100.0	51.6	24.0	20.0	3.9
Race and Hispanic Origin						
Black, non-Hispanic	1,468	100.0	35.9	43.1	14.0	6.3
Hispanic	1,603	100.0	38.2	35.1	17.0	9.7
White, non-Hispanic	6,462	100.0	59.0	30.6	8.5	1.3
Family structure at age 14						
Living with both parents	6,974	100.0	54.4	31.9	9.7	3.6
Other	3,165	100.0	45.0	36.5	13.8	3.9

Source: National Center for Health Statistics, Teenagers in the United States: Sexual Activity, Contraceptive Use, and Childbearing, 2002, Vital and Health Statistics, Series 23, No. 24, 2004; Internet site http://www.cdc.gov/nchs/nsfg.htm

The Average Woman Has Three Pregnancies in Her Lifetime

The number of pregnancies per woman has dropped slightly since 1990.

In 2000, the average American woman could expect to have 3.2 pregnancies in her lifetime, according to the National Center for Health Statistics. This figure was slightly lower than the 3.4 pregnancies in 1990. Black women have the most pregnancies in their lifetime—4.5 on average, as measured in 2000. But the figure was a higher 5.2 in 1990. Non-Hispanic white women have the fewest pregnancies, just 2.7.

The average woman has 2.1 live births in her lifetime, a figure that has not changed since 1990. Hispanic women have the largest number of births, an average of 2.7. This is down from 3.0 in 1990. Non-Hispanic white women have the fewest births, just 1.9—although this marks an increase from the 1.8 measured in 1990.

The average woman has 0.7 abortions in her lifetime, down slightly from 0.8 in 1990. Black women have the largest number of lifetime abortions, an average of 1.8. Non-Hispanic white women have the fewest, only 0.4.

■ Black women have more pregnancies and abortions than Hispanic or non-Hispanic white women, which means they have more unwanted pregnancies.

Black and Hispanic women have more than four pregnancies, on average, in their lifetime

(average number of pregnancies in lifetime, by race and Hispanic origin, 2000)

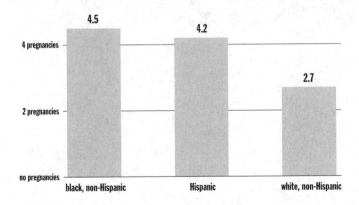

Table 9.13 Lifetime Number of Pregnancies, Births, and Abortions, by Race and Hispanic Origin, 1990 and 2000

(lifetime number of pregnancies, live births, and induced abortions per woman, by race and Hispanic origin, 1990 and 2000)

	2000	1990
NUMBER OF PREGNANCIES		
Average woman	**3.2**	**3.4**
Black, non-Hispanic	4.5	5.2
Hispanic	4.2	4.5
White, non-Hispanic	2.7	2.9
NUMBER OF LIVE BIRTHS		
Average woman	**2.1**	**2.1**
Black, non-Hispanic	2.2	2.5
Hispanic	2.7	3.0
White, non-Hispanic	1.9	1.8
NUMBER OF INDUCED ABORTIONS		
Average woman	**0.7**	**0.8**
Black, non-Hispanic	1.8	1.9
Hispanic	0.9	1.0
White, non-Hispanic	0.4	0.6

Source: National Center for Health Statistics, Estimated Pregnancy Rates for the United States, 1990–2000: An Update, National Vital Statistics Report, Vol. 52, No. 23, 2004; Internet site http://www.cdc.gov/nchs/pressroom/04facts/pregestimates.htm

Pregnancy Rate among Women under Age 30 Has Declined

Rates are lower for blacks, Hispanics, and non-Hispanic whites.

The number of pregnancies per 1,000 women fell by 10 percent between 1990 and 2000. The biggest drop occurred among the youngest women. The number of pregnancies per 1,000 girls under age 15 fell by 40 percent during those years, from 3.5 to 2.1. The pregnancy rate among women aged 30 or older has risen as women who had postponed childbearing make the decision to wait no longer.

As did pregnancy rates, so did birth rates fall between 1990 and 2000. The decline was greatest among the youngest women. Again, women aged 30 or older saw their birth rate rise.

The abortion rate fell from 27.4 abortions per 1,000 women in 1990 to 21.3 in 2000. The rate fell in every age group but one, remaining unchanged among women aged 40 or older. The abortion rate was down 41 percent among non-Hispanic white women during those years and dropped by a smaller 13 to 14 percent among blacks and Hispanics.

■ With pregnancy rates down, fetal loss rates have also fallen.

The abortion rate has fallen

(number of abortions per 1,000 women, 1990 and 2000)

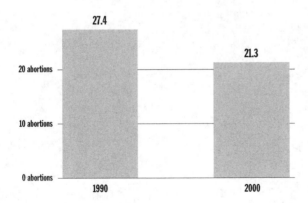

Table 9.14 Pregnancy Rate by Age, Race, and Hispanic Origin, 1990 and 2000

(number of pregnancies per 1,000 women, by age, race, and Hispanic origin, 1990 and 2000)

	2000	1990	percent change 1990–2000
Total women	**104.0**	**115.6**	**−10.0%**
Under age 15	2.1	3.5	−40.0
Aged 15 to 19	84.5	116.3	−27.3
Aged 15 to 17	53.5	80.3	−33.4
Aged 18 to 19	129.9	162.4	−20.0
Aged 20 to 24	178.2	196.7	−9.4
Aged 25 to 29	169.3	179.6	−5.7
Aged 30 to 34	132.2	120.2	10.0
Aged 35 to 39	66.4	56.1	18.4
Aged 40 or older	15.2	11.3	34.5
Black, non-Hispanic	148.7	180.2	−17.5
Hispanic	145.4	163.2	−10.9
White, non-Hispanic	85.2	97.9	−13.0

Source: National Center for Health Statistics, Estimated Pregnancy Rates for the United States, 1990–2000: An Update, National Vital Statistics Report, Vol. 52, No. 23, 2004; Internet site http://www.cdc.gov/nchs/pressroom/04facts/pregestimates.htm; calculations by New Strategist

Table 9.15 Birth Rate by Age, Race, and Hispanic Origin, 1990 and 2000

(number of live births per 1,000 women by age, race, and Hispanic origin, 1990 and 2000)

	2000	1990	percent change 1990–2000
Total women	**65.9**	**70.9**	**–7.1%**
Under age 15	0.9	1.4	–35.7
Aged 15 to 19	47.7	59.9	–20.4
Aged 15 to 17	26.9	37.5	–28.3
Aged 18 to 19	78.1	88.6	–11.9
Aged 20 to 24	109.7	116.5	–5.8
Aged 25 to 29	113.5	120.2	–5.6
Aged 30 to 34	91.2	80.8	12.9
Aged 35 to 39	39.7	31.7	25.2
Aged 40 or older	8.4	5.6	50.0
Black, non-Hispanic	71.4	89.0	–19.8
Hispanic	95.9	107.6	–10.9
White, non-Hispanic	58.5	62.8	–6.8

Source: National Center for Health Statistics, Estimated Pregnancy Rates for the United States, 1990–2000: An Update, National Vital Statistics Report, Vol. 52, No. 23, 2004; Internet site http://www.cdc.gov/nchs/pressroom/04facts/pregestimates.htm; calculations by New Strategist

Table 9.16 Abortion Rate by Age, Race, and Hispanic Origin, 1990 and 2000

(number of induced abortions per 1,000 women by age, race, and Hispanic origin, 1990 and 2000)

	2000	1990	percent change 1990–2000
Total women	**21.3**	**27.4**	**−22.3%**
Under age 15	0.9	1.5	−40.0
Aged 15 to 19	24.0	40.3	−40.4
Aged 15 to 17	14.5	26.5	−45.3
Aged 18 to 19	37.7	57.9	−34.9
Aged 20 to 24	46.3	56.7	−18.3
Aged 25 to 29	31.6	33.9	−6.8
Aged 30 to 34	18.7	19.7	−5.1
Aged 35 to 39	9.7	10.8	−10.2
Aged 40 or older	3.2	3.2	0.0
Black, non-Hispanic	57.4	67.0	−14.3
Hispanic	30.6	35.1	−12.8
White, non-Hispanic	11.7	19.7	−40.6

Source: National Center for Health Statistics, Estimated Pregnancy Rates for the United States, 1990–2000: An Update, National Vital Statistics Report, Vol. 52, No. 23, 2004; Internet site http://www.cdc.gov/nchs/pressroom/04facts/pregestimates.htm; calculations by New Strategist

Table 9.17 Fetal Loss Rate by Age, Race, and Hispanic Origin, 1990 and 2000

(number of fetal losses per 1,000 women by age, race, and Hispanic origin, 1990 and 2000)

	2000	1990	percent change 1990–2000
Total women	**16.7**	**17.2**	**–2.9%**
Under age 15	0.3	0.5	–40.0
Aged 15 to 19	12.8	16.1	–20.5
Aged 15 to 17	12.0	16.2	–25.9
Aged 18 to 19	14.1	15.9	–11.3
Aged 20 to 24	22.2	23.5	–5.5
Aged 25 to 29	24.2	25.5	–5.1
Aged 30 to 34	22.3	19.7	13.2
Aged 35 to 39	17.0	13.6	25.0
Aged 40 or older	3.6	2.4	50.0
Black, non-Hispanic	19.9	24.2	–17.8
Hispanic	18.9	20.5	–7.8
White, non-Hispanic	15.0	15.3	–2.0

Source: National Center for Health Statistics, Estimated Pregnancy Rates for the United States, 1990–2000: An Update, National Vital Statistics Report, Vol. 52, No. 23, 2004; Internet site http://www.cdc.gov/nchs/pressroom/04facts/pregestimates.htm; calculations by New Strategist

Sixty-Three Percent of Pregnancies End in a Live Birth

Twenty-one percent end in abortion, and 16 percent in fetal loss.

Of the 6.4 million pregnancies in 2000, more than 4 million (63 percent) ended in a live birth. Another 1.3 million ended in an abortion, and just over 1 million ended in a spontaneous fetal loss (or miscarriage).

Younger women are more likely to end a pregnancy with an abortion, while older women are more likely to experience a miscarriage. Twenty-three to 26 percent of pregnancies to women aged 35 or older ended in a fetal loss—a much greater share than the 16 percent of all pregnancies that end in that manner.

Black women are least likely to have a pregnancy end in a live birth. Only 48 percent of pregnancies to black women in 2000 ended in a live birth. Fully 39 percent ended in an abortion. Among Hispanics, 21 percent of pregnancies ended in abortion. The figure was just 14 percent among non-Hispanic whites.

■ Sixty percent of abortions are performed on women who have given birth at least once.

Most abortions occur within the first 12 weeks of pregnancy

(percent distribution of abortion by weeks of gestation, 2002)

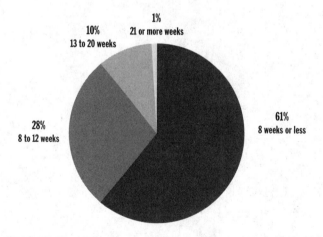

1%
21 or more weeks

10%
13 to 20 weeks

28%
8 to 12 weeks

61%
8 weeks or less

Table 9.18 Pregnancy Outcomes by Age, 2000

(total number of pregnancies and outcome, by age, 2000; numbers in thousands)

	total	live births	induced abortions	fetal losses
Total pregnancies	**6,401**	**4,059**	**1,313**	**1,029**
Under age 15	21	9	9	3
Aged 15 to 19	831	469	235	126
Aged 15 to 17	312	157	85	70
Aged 18 to 19	519	312	151	56
Aged 20 to 24	1,653	1,018	430	206
Aged 25 to 29	1,622	1,088	303	232
Aged 30 to 34	1,347	929	190	228
Aged 35 to 39	756	452	110	194
Aged 40 or older	172	95	37	40
Percent distribution				
Total pregnancies	**100.0%**	**63.4%**	**20.5%**	**16.1%**
Under age 15	100.0	42.9	42.9	14.3
Aged 15 to 19	100.0	56.4	28.3	15.2
Aged 15 to 17	100.0	50.3	27.2	22.4
Aged 18 to 19	100.0	60.1	29.1	10.8
Aged 20 to 24	100.0	61.6	26.0	12.5
Aged 25 to 29	100.0	67.1	18.7	14.3
Aged 30 to 34	100.0	69.0	14.1	16.9
Aged 35 to 39	100.0	59.8	14.6	25.7
Aged 40 or older	100.0	55.2	21.5	23.3

Source: National Center for Health Statistics, Estimated Pregnancy Rates for the United States, 1990–2000: An Update, National Vital Statistics Report, Vol. 52, No. 23, 2004; Internet site http://www.cdc.gov/nchs/pressroom/04facts/pregestimates.htm

Table 9.19 Pregnancy Outcomes by Race and Hispanic Origin, 2000

(total number of pregnancies and outcome, by race and Hispanic origin, 2000; numbers in thousands)

	total	live births	induced abortions	fetal losses
Total pregnancies	**6,401**	**4,059**	**1,313**	**1,029**
Black, non-Hispanic	1,265	607	488	170
Hispanic	1,237	816	261	161
White, non-Hispanic	3,497	2,400	479	618
Percent distribution				
Total pregnancies	**100.0%**	**63.4%**	**20.5%**	**16.1%**
Black, non-Hispanic	100.0	48.0	38.6	13.4
Hispanic	100.0	66.0	21.1	13.0
White, non-Hispanic	100.0	68.6	13.7	17.7

Source: National Center for Health Statistics, Estimated Pregnancy Rates for the United States, 1990–2000: An Update, National Vital Statistics Report, Vol. 52, No. 23, 2004; Internet site http://www.cdc.gov/nchs/pressroom/04facts/pregestimates.htm

Table 9.20 Abortions by Selected Characteristics, 1995 to 2002

(number of legal abortions reported by states and the District of Columbia, and percent distribution by selected characteristics of women, 1995 to 2002)

	2002	2000	1995
Reported abortions, number	**847,622**	**850,293**	**908,243**
Reported abortions, percent	**100.0%**	**100.0%**	**100.0%**
Age			
Under age 20	17.5	18.8	20.1
Aged 20 to 24	33.4	32.8	32.5
Aged 25 or older	49.1	48.4	47.4
Marital status			
Married	18.1	18.7	19.7
Unmarried	81.9	81.3	80.3
Number of births			
None	40.0	40.0	45.2
One	27.3	27.7	26.5
Two	20.2	20.1	18.0
Three or more	12.5	12.2	10.3
Race			
Black	36.6	36.3	35.0
White	55.5	56.6	59.6
Hispanic origin			
Hispanic	18.2	17.2	15.1
Not Hispanic	81.8	82.8	84.9
Weeks of gestation			
8 or less	60.5	58.1	54.0
8 to 12	28.0	30.0	34.0
13 to 20	10.1	10.5	10.6
21 or more	1.4	1.4	1.4
Residence			
In-state	91.2	91.3	91.5
Out-of-state	8.8	8.7	8.5

Note: Not all states provide abortion data. Abortions in Alaska, California, New Hampshire, and Oklahoma are not included in the above figures.
Source: Centers for Disease Control and Prevention, "Abortion Surveillance—United States, 2002," Mortality and Morbidity Weekly Report, Vol. 54/SS07, November 25, 2005; Internet site http://www.cdc.gov/mmwr/preview/mmwrhtml/ss5407a1.htm

Twenty Percent of Women Have Been to a Doctor for a Pregnancy Test in the Past Year

During pregnancy, women gain an average of just over 30 pounds.

Despite the proliferation of over-the-counter pregnancy tests, many women still visit a medical provider for the definitive answer. Among women aged 15 to 44, fully 20 percent have been to a medical provider for a pregnancy test in the past 12 months. The figure peaks at more than 30 percent among women in their twenties. A substantial 11 percent of girls aged 15 to 17 have gone to a medical provider for a pregnancy test in the past year.

Women gained a median of 30.5 pounds during their pregnancy, according to the National Center for Health Statistics. There is little variation in weight gain by race and Hispanic origin.

■ Only 21 percent of married women, but 31 percent of cohabiting women, have gone to a medical provider for a pregnancy test in the past year.

Weight gain during pregnancy does not vary much by race and Hispanic origin

(median weight gain in pounds during pregnancy, by race and Hispanic origin, 2003)

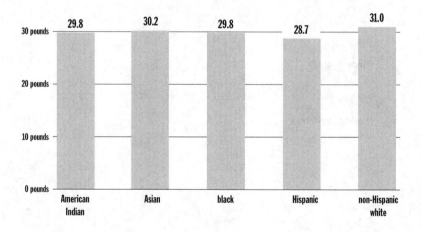

Table 9.21 Pregnancy Test in Past Year, 2002

(total number of women aged 15 to 44 and percent receiving a pregnancy test from a medical care provider in the past 12 months, by selected characteristics, 2002; numbers in thousands)

	number	percent receiving pregnancy test
Total women aged 15 to 44	**61,561**	**19.7%**
Age		
Aged 15 to 19	9,834	18.3
Aged 15 to 17	5,819	11.4
Aged 18 to 19	4,016	28.2
Aged 20 to 24	9,840	31.5
Aged 25 to 29	9,249	30.2
Aged 30 to 34	10,272	22.2
Aged 35 to 39	10,853	13.6
Aged 40 to 44	11,512	5.9
Marital status		
Currently married	28,327	21.1
Currently cohabiting	5,570	31.0
Never married, not cohabiting	21,568	16.5
Formerly married, not cohabiting	6,096	14.1
Children ever borne		
None	25,622	17.4
One	11,193	32.1
Two	13,402	18.8
Three or more	11,343	13.7
Race and Hispanic origin		
Black, non-Hispanic	8,587	23.7
Hispanic	9,107	24.3
White, non-Hispanic	40,420	17.5

Source: National Center for Health Statistics, Use of Contraception and Use of Family Planning Services in the United States: 1982–2002, Advance Data, No. 350, 2004; Internet site http://www.cdc.gov/nchs/nsfg.htm

Table 9.22 Weight Gain during Pregnancy, 2003

(median weight gain in pounds during pregnancy, by race and Hispanic origin, 2003)

	median weight gain
Total pregnancies ending in live births	**30.5**
American Indian	29.8
Asian	30.2
Black	29.8
Hispanic	28.7
White, non-Hispanic	31.0

Source: National Center for Health Statistics, Births: Final Data for 2003, National Vital Statistics Report, Vol. 54, No. 2, 2005; Internet site http://www.cdc.gov/nchs/products/pubs/pubd/nvsr/54/54-pre.htm

More than 90 Percent of Pregnancies Receive Early Prenatal Care

Early prenatal care is least likely among the youngest women.

Most pregnancies come under a doctor's care within the first three months. Fully 91 percent of pregnancies receive prenatal care in the first three months. Another 6 percent are first seen at three to six months, and just 3 percent are not seen at all or only after five or more months of pregnancy.

The pregnancies most likely to receive prenatal care within the first three months are those to older women, non-Hispanic whites, and college graduates. Ninety-three percent of intended pregnancies receive early prenatal care compared with 86 percent of mistimed or unwanted pregnancies.

■ Only 85 to 86 percent of pregnancies to black and Hispanic women receive medical care within the first three months.

Educated women are more likely to get early prenatal care

(percent of pregnancies to women aged 15 to 44 ending in live births in January 1997 to 2002 for which prenatal care began in the first three months, by educational attainment, 2002)

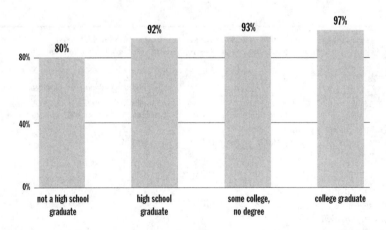

Table 9.23 Prenatal Care by Age, 2002

(total number of pregnancies ending in live births in January 1997 or later to women aged 15 to 44 and percent distribution by months pregnant when prenatal care began, by age at time of birth, 2002; numbers in thousands)

	total		months pregnant when prenatal care began		
	number	percent	less than three months	three to four months	five months or more or no prenatal care
Total pregnancies ending in live births	**23,992**	**100.0%**	**90.7%**	**6.3%**	**3.0%**
Under age 18	1,034	100.0	78.8	13.5	7.8
Aged 18 to 19	1,475	100.0	83.8	11.2	5.0
Aged 20 to 24	6,216	100.0	84.3	10.1	5.6
Aged 25 to 29	6,491	100.0	94.7	4.1	1.3
Aged 30 to 44	8,775	100.0	94.9	3.4	1.6

Note: Numbers may not add to total because pregnancies with missing prenatal care data are not shown.
Source: National Center for Health Statistics, Fertility, Family Planning, and Reproductive Health of U.S. Women: Data from the 2002 National Survey of Family Growth, Vital and Health Statistics, Series 23, No. 25, 2005; Internet site http://www.cdc .gov/nchs/nsfg.htm

Table 9.24 Prenatal Care by Marital Status, 2002

(total number of pregnancies ending in live births in January 1997 or later to women aged 15 to 44 and percent distribution by months pregnant when prenatal care began, by marital status at time of birth, 2002; numbers in thousands)

	total		months pregnant when prenatal care began		
	number	percent	less than three months	three to four months	five months or more or no prenatal care
Total pregnancies ending in live births	**23,992**	**100.0%**	**90.7%**	**6.3%**	**3.0%**
Married	15,636	100.0	94.6	3.8	1.6
Cohabiting	3,320	100.0	82.0	11.8	6.2
Never married, not cohabiting	3,972	100.0	82.2	11.9	5.9
Formerly married, not cohabiting	1,064	100.0	91.9	4.5	3.5

Note: Numbers may not add to total because pregnancies with missing prenatal care data are not shown.
Source: National Center for Health Statistics, Fertility, Family Planning, and Reproductive Health of U.S. Women: Data from the 2002 National Survey of Family Growth, Vital and Health Statistics, Series 23, No. 25, 2005; Internet site http://www.cdc .gov/nchs/nsfg.htm

Table 9.25 Prenatal Care by Wantedness Status at Conception, 2002

(total number of pregnancies ending in live births in January 1997 or later to women aged 15 to 44 and percent distribution by months pregnant when prenatal care began, by wantedness status at conception, 2002; numbers in thousands)

	total		months pregnant when prenatal care began		
	number	percent	less than three months	three to four months	five months or more or no prenatal care
Total pregnancies ending in live births	**23,992**	**100.0%**	**90.7%**	**6.3%**	**3.0%**
Pregnancy intended	15,761	100.0	93.4	4.5	2.1
Pregnancy mistimed	4,883	100.0	85.5	10.3	4.2
Less than two years	1,849	100.0	90.3	6.9	2.8
Two or more years	2,867	100.0	82.5	12.5	5.1
Pregnancy unwanted	3,348	100.0	85.5	8.6	5.9

Note: Numbers may not add to total because pregnancies with missing prenatal care data are not shown.
Source: National Center for Health Statistics, Fertility, Family Planning, and Reproductive Health of U.S. Women: Data from the 2002 National Survey of Family Growth, Vital and Health Statistics, Series 23, No. 25, 2005; Internet site http://www.cdc .gov/nchs/nsfg.htm

Table 9.26 Prenatal Care by Race and Hispanic Origin, 2002

(total number of pregnancies ending in live births in January 1997 or later to women aged 15 to 44 and percent distribution by months pregnant when prenatal care began, by race and Hispanic origin, 2002; numbers in thousands)

	total		months pregnant when prenatal care began		
	number	percent	less than three months	three to four months	five months or more or no prenatal care
Total pregnancies ending in live births	**23,992**	**100.0%**	**90.7%**	**6.3%**	**3.0%**
Black, non-Hispanic	3,184	100.0	84.6	11.1	4.3
Hispanic	4,823	100.0	86.3	6.8	6.9
White, non-Hispanic	14,143	100.0	94.1	4.9	1.0

Note: Numbers may not add to total because pregnancies with missing prenatal care data are not shown.
Source: National Center for Health Statistics, Fertility, Family Planning, and Reproductive Health of U.S. Women: Data from the 2002 National Survey of Family Growth, Vital and Health Statistics, Series 23, No. 25, 2005; Internet site http://www.cdc .gov/nchs/nsfg.htm

Table 9.27 Prenatal Care by Education, 2002

(total number of pregnancies ending in live births in January 1997 or later to women aged 15 to 44 and percent distribution by months pregnant when prenatal care began, by education at time of birth, 2002; numbers in thousands)

	total		months pregnant when prenatal care began		
	number	percent	less than three months	three to four months	five months or more or no prenatal care
Total pregnancies ending in live births	**23,992**	**100.0%**	**90.7%**	**6.3%**	**3.0%**
Not a high school graduate	3,421	100.0	79.8	11.9	8.3
High school graduate or GED	6,959	100.0	92.2	5.7	2.1
Some college, no degree	5,940	100.0	92.5	5.3	2.2
Bachelor's degree or more	5,613	100.0	97.1	2.3	0.6

Note: Numbers may not add to total because pregnancies with missing prenatal care data are not shown. Education categories include only people aged 22 to 44.
Source: National Center for Health Statistics, Fertility, Family Planning, and Reproductive Health of U.S. Women: Data from the 2002 National Survey of Family Growth, Vital and Health Statistics, Series 23, No. 25, 2005; Internet site http://www.cdc.gov/nchs/nsfg.htm

More than One in Ten Women Smoke during Pregnancy

Those with an unwanted pregnancy are more likely to smoke.

Among women aged 15 to 44 who had a pregnancy between January 1997 and 2002, 13 percent smoked during the pregnancy. Another 11 percent smoked only before the pregnancy. Seventy-five percent never smoked.

Some women are more likely to smoke during pregnancy than others. Among those whose pregnancy was intended, 12 percent smoked during the pregnancy. Among those whose pregnancy was unwanted, a much larger 20 percent smoked. Non-Hispanic whites were more likely than blacks or Hispanics to smoke while pregnant (17 percent versus 8 and 5 percent, respectively). Education made the biggest difference in smoking, with only 3 percent of college graduates smoking during pregnancy versus 21 percent of high school dropouts.

■ Among those whose pregnancy ended in fetal loss, 21 percent had smoked during the pregnancy. Among those whose pregnancy ended in a live birth, a smaller 12 percent were smokers.

College graduates are much less likely to smoke during pregnancy

(percent of women aged 15 to 44 with a pregnancy from January 1997 to 2002 who smoked during the pregnancy, by educational attainment, 2002)

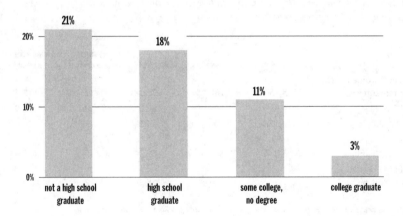

Table 9.28 Smoking during Pregnancy by Age, 2002

(total number of women aged 15 to 44 whose most recent pregnancy ended in a live birth or spontaneous fetal loss in January 1997 or later, and percent distribution by cigarette smoking status during pregnancy, by age, 2002; numbers in thousands)

	total		smoking status		
	number	percent	never smoked	only smoked prior to pregnancy	smoked during pregnancy
Total women with pregnancies	**18,256**	**100.0%**	**75.2%**	**11.4%**	**13.4%**
Under age 18	686	100.0	68.8	13.8	16.5
Aged 18 to 19	812	100.0	64.5	14.6	21.0
Aged 20 to 24	3,969	100.0	65.5	18.8	15.7
Aged 25 to 29	4,712	100.0	74.9	9.6	15.5
Aged 30 to 44	8,077	100.0	81.7	8.4	9.9

Note: Numbers may not add to total because pregnancies with missing smoking status are not shown.
Source: National Center for Health Statistics, Fertility, Family Planning, and Reproductive Health of U.S. Women: Data from the 2002 National Survey of Family Growth, Vital and Health Statistics, Series 23, No. 25, 2005; Internet site http://www.cdc.gov/nchs/nsfg.htm

Table 9.29 Smoking during Pregnancy by Marital Status, 2002

(total number of women aged 15 to 44 whose most recent pregnancy ended in a live birth or spontaneous fetal loss in January 1997 or later, and percent distribution by cigarette smoking status during pregnancy, by marital status at pregnancy outcome, 2002; numbers in thousands)

	total		smoking status		
	number	percent	never smoked	only smoked prior to pregnancy	smoked during pregnancy
Total women with pregnancies	**18,256**	**100.0%**	**75.2%**	**11.4%**	**13.4%**
Married	11,786	100.0	82.0	9.1	8.9
Cohabiting	2,370	100.0	56.7	18.3	25.0
Never married, not cohabiting	3,002	100.0	69.1	15.0	15.9
Formerly married, not cohabiting	1,097	100.0	58.2	12.3	29.5

Note: Numbers may not add to total because pregnancies with missing smoking status are not shown.
Source: National Center for Health Statistics, Fertility, Family Planning, and Reproductive Health of U.S. Women: Data from the 2002 National Survey of Family Growth, Vital and Health Statistics, Series 23, No. 25, 2005; Internet site http://www.cdc.gov/nchs/nsfg.htm

Table 9.30 Smoking during Pregnancy by Wantedness Status, 2002

(total number of women aged 15 to 44 whose most recent pregnancy ended in a live birth or spontaneous fetal loss in January 1997 or later, and percent distribution by cigarette smoking status during pregnancy, by wantedness status at conception, 2002; numbers in thousands)

| | total | | smoking status | | |
	number	percent	never smoked	only smoked prior to pregnancy	smoked during pregnancy
Total women with pregnancies	**18,256**	**100.0%**	**75.2%**	**11.4%**	**13.4%**
Pregnancy intended	11,826	100.0	77.3	10.7	12.0
Pregnancy mistimed	3,580	100.0	74.6	12.4	13.1
Less than two years	1,332	100.0	85.6	7.5	7.0
Two or more years	2,053	100.0	68.9	14.4	16.7
Pregnancy unwanted	2,850	100.0	66.8	13.3	19.9

Note: Numbers may not add to total because pregnancies with missing smoking status are not shown.
Source: National Center for Health Statistics, Fertility, Family Planning, and Reproductive Health of U.S. Women: Data from the 2002 National Survey of Family Growth, Vital and Health Statistics, Series 23, No. 25, 2005; Internet site http://www.cdc .gov/nchs/nsfg.htm

Table 9.31 Smoking during Pregnancy by Pregnancy Outcome, 2002

(total number of women aged 15 to 44 whose most recent pregnancy ended in a live birth or spontaneous fetal loss in January 1997 or later, and percent distribution by cigarette smoking status during pregnancy, by pregnancy outcome, 2002; numbers in thousands)

| | total | | smoking status | | |
	number	percent	never smoked	only smoked prior to pregnancy	smoked during pregnancy
Total women with pregnancies	**18,256**	**100.0%**	**75.2%**	**11.4%**	**13.4%**
Live birth	15,590	100.0	76.4	11.4	12.2
Fetal loss	2,666	100.0	67.7	11.7	20.6

Note: Numbers may not add to total because pregnancies with missing smoking status are not shown.
Source: National Center for Health Statistics, Fertility, Family Planning, and Reproductive Health of U.S. Women: Data from the 2002 National Survey of Family Growth, Vital and Health Statistics, Series 23, No. 25, 2005; Internet site http://www.cdc .gov/nchs/nsfg.htm

Table 9.32 Smoking during Pregnancy by Race and Hispanic Origin, 2002

(total number of women aged 15 to 44 whose most recent pregnancy ended in a live birth or spontaneous fetal loss in January 1997 or later, and percent distribution by cigarette smoking status during pregnancy, by race and Hispanic origin, 2002; numbers in thousands)

	total		smoking status		
	number	percent	never smoked	only smoked prior to pregnancy	smoked during pregnancy
Total women with pregnancies	**18,256**	**100.0%**	**75.2%**	**11.4%**	**13.4%**
Black, non-Hispanic	2,391	100.0	79.5	12.3	8.2
Hispanic	3,566	100.0	88.0	7.0	5.1
White, non-Hispanic	10,978	100.0	70.0	13.0	17.1

Note: Numbers may not add to total because pregnancies with missing smoking status are not shown.
Source: National Center for Health Statistics, Fertility, Family Planning, and Reproductive Health of U.S. Women: Data from the 2002 National Survey of Family Growth, Vital and Health Statistics, Series 23, No. 25, 2005; Internet site http://www.cdc.gov/nchs/nsfg.htm

Table 9.33 Smoking during Pregnancy by Education, 2002

(total number of women aged 15 to 44 whose most recent pregnancy ended in a live birth or spontaneous fetal loss in January 1997 or later, and percent distribution by cigarette smoking status during pregnancy, by education, 2002; numbers in thousands)

	total		smoking status		
	number	percent	never smoked	only smoked prior to pregnancy	smoking during pregnancy
Total women with pregnancies	**18,256**	**100.0%**	**75.2%**	**11.4%**	**13.4%**
Not a high school graduate	2,338	100.0	67.3	11.4	21.4
High school graduate or GED	5,239	100.0	66.9	15.2	17.9
Some college, no degree	4,801	100.0	76.9	12.0	11.2
Bachelor's degree or more	4,161	100.0	90.4	6.2	3.4

Note: Education categories include only people aged 22 to 44.
Source: National Center for Health Statistics, Fertility, Family Planning, and Reproductive Health of U.S. Women: Data from the 2002 National Survey of Family Growth, Vital and Health Statistics, Series 23, No. 25, 2005; Internet site http://www.cdc.gov/nchs/nsfg.htm

10

Births

■ The nation's children and families are becoming increasingly diverse as the Asian, black, and Hispanic populations grow and out-of-wedlock childbearing becomes more common.

■ New mothers are older. The average age at first birth reached 24.9 years in 2000, up from 21.4 years in 1970, as a growing number of women postponed childbearing to go to college.

■ Hispanics account for a growing share of births. Among the 4.1 million babies born in 2004, nearly 1 million were born to Hispanic women—or 23 percent of the total.

■ Most women have had at least one child. Among women aged 15 to 44, the 58 percent majority has had at least one child. Hispanics are most likely to have had children. Non-Hispanic whites are least likely to be parents.

■ The two-child family is the norm. Women aged 15 to 44 have had an average of 1.28 children. They expect to have an additional 0.99 children, for a total of 2.27.

■ Nonmarital childbearing has become commonplace among younger generations. Among women aged 15 to 44 with children, 42 percent have had a child out-of-wedlock.

■ Most births are wanted. But a substantial 31 percent of women aged 15 to 44 have had an unwanted or mistimed birth.

■ Parenting is regarded as a rewarding experience. Ninety-four percent of men and women aged 15 to 44 agree that "the rewards of being a parent are worth it, despite the cost and the work it takes."

Women's Average Age at First Birth Has Increased

American women of Japanese descent are the oldest at first birth, those of Mexican descent the youngest.

Women giving birth to their first child were 21.4 years old, on average, in 1970. Average age at first birth climbed to 24.9 years by 2000 as a growing number of women postponed childbearing because of college. Women's average age at second and higher-order births has also climbed over the years.

There is great variation in age at first birth by race and Hispanic origin. American women of Mexican descent who gave birth to their first child in 2000 were only 22.2 years old, on average. In contrast, American women of Japanese descent were 30.6 years old at first birth.

Because men marry at a slightly older age than women, fathers are older than mothers at their first child's birth. In 2000, men having their first child were 25.1 years old, on average. Among men, average age at first birth is highest for non-Hispanic whites and college graduates.

■ The nation's parents have become older because young adults have postponed childbearing while they attend college.

Average age at first birth rises with education

(average age of men at first child's birth, by education, 2002)

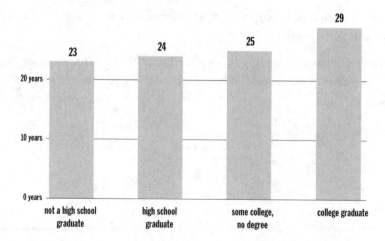

Table 10.1 Average Age of Women When Giving Birth by Birth Order, 1970 and 2000

(average age at which women give birth, by birth order, 1970 and 2000; change in years, 1970–2000)

	average age (years)		
	2000	1970	change
Total women giving birth	**27.2**	**24.6**	**2.6**
First birth	24.9	21.4	3.5
Second birth	27.7	24.1	3.6
Third birth	29.2	26.6	2.6
Fourth birth	30.3	28.7	1.6
Fifth or higher-order birth	32.4	32.0	0.4

National Center for Health Statistics, Mean Age of Mother, National Vital Statistics Report, Vol. 51, No. 1, 2002; Internet site http://www.cdc.gov/nchs/pressroom/02news/ameriwomen.htm

Table 10.2 Average Age of Women at First Child's Birth, 2000

(average age at which women gave birth to their first child, by race and Hispanic Origin, 2000)

	average age at first child's birth
Total women	**24.9 years**
Asian	
Chinese	30.1
Japanese	30.6
Hawaiian	22.6
Filipino	27.3
Black, non-Hispanic	22.3
Hispanic	
Mexican	22.2
Puerto Rican	22.4
Cuban	26.5
Central and South American	24.8
White, non-Hispanic	25.9

National Center for Health Statistics, Mean Age of Mother, National Vital Statistics Report, Vol. 51, No. 1, 2002; Internet site http://www.cdc.gov/nchs/pressroom/02news/ameriwomen.htm; calculations by New Strategist

Table 10.3 Average Age of Men at First Child's Birth, 2002

(average age of men aged 15 to 44 who have fathered at least one biological child at first child's birth, by selected characteristics, 2002)

	average age at first child's birth
Total men aged 15 to 44 with children	**25.1 years**
Marital or cohabiting status	
Currently married	25.7
Currently cohabiting	24.0
Never married, not cohabiting	22.0
Formerly married, not cohabiting	24.1
Race and Hispanic origin	
Black, non-Hispanic	23.5
Hispanic	23.3
White, non-Hispanic	26.1
Education	
Not a high school graduate	22.8
High school graduate or GED	24.0
Some college, no degree	25.4
Bachelor's degree or more	29.4

Source: National Center for Health Statistics, Fertility, Contraception, and Fatherhood: Data on Men and Women from Cycle 6 of the 2002 National Survey of Family Growth, Vital and Health Statistics, Series 23, No. 26, 2006; Internet site http://www.cdc.gov/nchs/nsfg.htm

Birth Rate Has Risen for Women Aged 30 or Older

Teen birth rate has fallen sharply.

The birth rate for women under age 30 has been falling for decades as a growing number of women have gone to college. The birth rate among 15-to-19-year-olds fell 31 percent between 1990 and 2004. The rate for women aged 20 to 24 declined 13 percent during those years, while the rate for women aged 25 to 29 fell 4 percent. Among women aged 30 or older, however, the birth rate has been rising as they play catch-up.

The number of births to girls aged 15 to 19 peaked in 1970 (coinciding with the baby-boom generation passing through the age group) at more than 644,000. Although the number of births to teenagers has fallen, the percentage of babies born to unmarried teens has climbed from just 13 percent in 1950 to more than 81 percent in 2003. Among all babies, the percentage of those born out-of-wedlock has grown from 4 percent in 1950 to 36 percent in 2004.

■ The growing number of children born out-of-wedlock means an increase in the number of single-parent families.

Births to unmarried women have increased

(percent of births to unmarried women, 1950 to 2004)

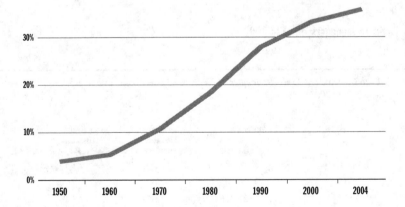

Table 10.4 Birth Rates by Age, 1990 to 2004

(number of live births per 1,000 women aged 15 to 44 and in specified age group, 1990 to 2004; percent change in rate, 1990–2004)

	total	15 to 19	20 to 24	25 to 29	30 to 34	35 to 39	40 to 44	45 to 49
2004	66.3	41.1	101.7	115.5	95.3	45.4	8.9	0.5
2003	66.1	41.6	102.6	115.6	95.1	43.8	8.7	0.5
2002	64.8	43.0	103.6	113.6	91.5	41.4	8.3	0.5
2001	65.3	45.3	106.2	113.4	91.9	40.6	8.1	0.5
2000	65.9	47.7	109.7	113.5	91.2	39.7	8.0	0.5
1999	64.4	48.8	107.9	111.2	87.1	37.8	7.4	0.4
1998	64.3	50.3	108.4	110.2	85.2	36.9	7.4	0.4
1997	63.6	51.3	107.3	108.3	83.0	35.7	7.1	0.4
1996	64.1	53.5	107.8	108.6	82.1	34.9	6.8	0.3
1995	64.6	56.0	107.5	108.8	81.1	34.0	6.6	0.3
1994	65.9	58.2	109.2	111.0	80.4	33.4	6.4	0.3
1993	67.0	59.0	111.3	113.2	79.9	32.7	6.1	0.3
1992	68.4	60.3	113.7	115.7	79.6	32.3	5.9	0.3
1991	69.3	61.8	115.3	117.2	79.2	31.9	5.5	0.2
1990	70.9	59.9	116.5	120.2	80.8	31.7	5.5	0.2
Percent change								
1990 to 2004	–6.5%	–31.4%	–12.7%	–3.9%	17.9%	43.2%	61.8%	150.0%

Source: National Center for Health Statistics, Births: Final Data for 2003, National Vital Statistics Reports, Vol. 54, No. 2, 2005; Internet site http://www.cdc.gov/nchs/births.htm; and Births: Final Data for 2004, Health E-Stats, 2006; Internet site http://www.cdc.gov/nchs/products/pubs/pubd/hestats/finalbirths04/finalbirths04.htm; calculations by New Strategist

Table 10.5 Births to Teenagers, 1950 to 2004

(number of births to women aged 15 to 19, number of births per 1,000 women in age group, and percentage to unmarried women, 1950 to 2004)

	number of births to women aged 15 to 19	births per 1,000 women aged 15 to 19	percent of births to unmarried 15-to-19-year-olds
2004	415,262	41.1	81.3%*
2000	470,506	48.7	78.7
1990	521,826	59.9	67.1
1980	552,161	53.0	47.6
1970	644,708	68.3	29.5
1960	586,966	89.1	14.8
1950	419,535	81.6	13.4

* Figure shown is for 2003.
Source: National Center for Health Statistics, Births to Teenagers in the United States, 1940—2000, National Vital Statistics Report, Vol. 49, No. 10, 2001; Internet site http://www.cdc.gov/nchs/products/pubs/pubd/nvsr/49/49-13.htm and Births: Final Data for 2004, Health E-Stats, 2006; Internet site http://www.cdc.gov/nchs/products/pubs/pubd/hestats/finalbirths04/finalbirths04.htm

Table 10.6 Births to Unmarried Women, 1950 to 2004

(total number of births, and number and percent to unmarried women, 1950 to 2003; births in thousands)

	total births	births to unmarried women	
		number	percent
2004	4,112	1,470	35.8%
2003	4,090	1,416	34.6
2002	4,022	1,366	34.0
2001	4,026	1,349	33.5
2000	4,059	1,347	33.2
1999	3,959	1,305	33.0
1998	3,942	1,294	32.8
1997	3,881	1,257	32.4
1996	3,891	1,260	32.4
1995	3,900	1,254	32.2
1994	3,953	1,290	32.6
1993	4,000	1,240	31.0
1992	4,065	1,225	30.1
1991	4,111	1,214	29.5
1990	4,158	1,165	28.0
1980	3,612	666	18.4
1970	3,731	399	10.7
1960	4,258	224	5.3
1950	3,632	142	3.9

Source: National Center for Health Statistics, Births: Final Data for 2004, Health E-Stats, 2006; Internet site http://www.cdc .gov/nchs/products/pubs/pubd/hestats/finalbirths04/finalbirths04.htm; and earlier reports

Hispanics Have the Highest Birth Rate

More than 8 percent of Hispanic women have given birth in the past year.

Hispanic women have a much higher birth rate than Asians, blacks, or non-Hispanic whites. In 2004, the Hispanic rate was a lofty 97.8 births per 1,000 women, much higher than the 58.4 of non-Hispanic white women. Asian and black women have a birth rate somewhat higher than non-Hispanic whites, at 67.1 and 67.0, respectively. The birth rate varies considerably by age within race and Hispanic origin groups. It peaks among Hispanic women in the 20-to-24 age group at 165.3 births per 1,000 women. The Asian birth rate peaks at 116.9 in the 30-to-34 age group.

Six percent of women aged 15 to 44 have given birth in the past year, the figure peaking at 10 percent among women aged 25 to 29. Among Hispanic women aged 15 to 44, 8.5 percent gave birth in the past year. This compares with only 5.4 percent of non-Hispanic white women.

■ A growing proportion of the nation's children are Hispanic because of their higher birth rate.

Non-Hispanic whites have the lowest birth rate

(number of births per 1,000 women, by race and Hispanic origin, 2004)

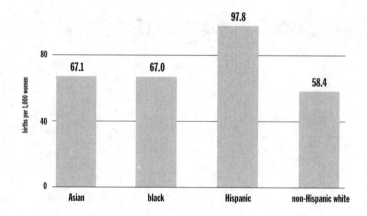

Table 10.7 Birth Rate by Age, Race, and Hispanic Origin, 2004

(number of live births per 1,000 women in age group, by race and Hispanic origin, 2004)

	total	Asian	non-Hispanic black	Hispanic	non-Hispanic white
Total	**66.3**	**67.1**	**67.0**	**97.8**	**58.4**
Under age 15	0.7	0.2	1.6	1.3	0.2
Aged 15 to 17	22.1	8.9	37.1	49.7	12.0
Aged 18 to 19	70.0	29.6	103.9	133.5	48.7
Aged 20 to 24	101.8	59.8	126.9	165.3	81.9
Aged 25 to 29	115.5	108.6	103.0	145.6	110.0
Aged 30 to 34	95.5	116.9	67.4	104.1	97.1
Aged 35 to 39	45.4	62.1	33.7	52.9	44.8
Aged 40 to 44	8.9	13.6	7.8	12.4	8.2
Aged 45 to 54	0.5	1.0	0.5	0.7	0.5

Source: National Center for Health Statistics, Births: Final Data for 2004, Health E-Stats, 2006; Internet site http://www.cdc .gov/nchs/products/pubs/pubd/hestats/finalbirths04/finalbirths04.htm; calculations by New Strategist

Table 10.8 Women Giving Birth in the Past Year, 2004

(total number of women aged 15 to 44, number and percent who gave birth in the past year, and number and percent who had first birth in past year, by age, 2004; numbers in thousands)

	total	gave birth in past year		first birth in past year	
		number	percent	number	percent
Total aged 15 to 44	**61,588**	**3,746**	**6.1%**	**1,474**	**2.4%**
Age					
Aged 15 to 19	9,964	385	3.9	221	2.2
Aged 20 to 24	10,068	882	8.8	433	4.3
Aged 25 to 29	9,498	938	9.9	382	4.0
Aged 30 to 34	10,082	946	9.4	286	2.8
Aged 35 to 39	10,442	443	4.2	120	1.1
Aged 40 to 44	11,535	153	1.3	33	0.3
Race and Hispanic origin					
Asian	3,262	243	7.4	121	3.7
Black	9,065	537	5.9	199	2.2
Hispanic	9,618	817	8.5	269	2.8
Non-Hispanic white	39,120	2,114	5.4	875	2.2
Nativity status					
Native-born	52,107	2,953	5.7	1,181	2.3
Foreign-born	9,481	794	8.4	293	3.1
Region					
Northeast	11,412	656	5.7	254	2.2
Midwest	13,703	898	6.6	339	2.5
South	22,182	1,338	6.0	530	2.4
West	14,291	854	6.0	352	2.5

Source: Bureau of the Census, Fertility of American Women, Current Population Survey—June 2004, Detailed Tables, Internet site http://www.census.gov/population/www/socdemo/fertility/cps2004.html

Forty Percent of Births Are First Births

Among women aged 30 or older, most births are second or higher order.

Of the 4.1 million babies born in 2004, 1.6 million were first births—a substantial 40 percent. The 1.3 million second births accounted for 32 percent of the total. Seventeen percent of babies born in 2004 were third children, and just 11 percent were fourth or higher-order births.

The older the woman, the more likely she is to be having a higher-order birth. The majority of women under age 20 who gave birth in 2004 were having their first child. But among women aged 20 to 24 who gave birth, only 47 percent were having their first child. The 53 percent majority was having a second, third, or higher-order birth. The proportion of mothers having a second or higher-order birth rises with age. Among women aged 30 to 34 who gave birth in 2004, only 29 percent were having their first child and 71 percent were having a second or higher-order birth.

■ Among all first births in 2004, half were born to women under age 25.

Sixty percent of births are second or higher order

(percent distribution of births by birth order, 2004)

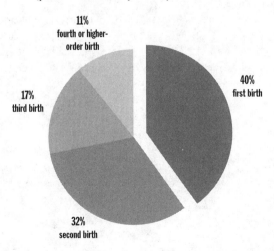

11%
fourth or higher-
order birth

17%
third birth

40%
first birth

32%
second birth

Table 10.9 Births by Age and Birth Order, 2004

(number and percent distribution of births by age and birth order, 2004)

	total	first child	second child	third child	fourth or later child
Total births	**4,115,590**	**1,632,543**	**1,320,853**	**694,584**	**449,049**
Under age 15	6,789	6,642	110	5	0
Aged 15 to 19	415,408	330,238	70,540	11,011	1,508
Aged 20 to 24	1,034,834	483,968	350,739	142,016	53,679
Aged 25 to 29	1,105,297	396,349	370,771	208,216	125,228
Aged 30 to 34	967,008	280,348	342,181	200,365	139,856
Aged 35 to 39	476,123	110,614	155,797	110,077	97,329
Aged 40 or older	110,131	24,385	30,715	22,893	31,449
Percent distribution by birth order					
Total births	**100.0%**	**39.7%**	**32.1%**	**16.9%**	**10.9%**
Under age 15	100.0	97.8	1.6	0.1	0.0
Aged 15 to 19	100.0	79.5	17.0	2.7	0.4
Aged 20 to 24	100.0	46.8	33.9	13.7	5.2
Aged 25 to 29	100.0	35.9	33.5	18.8	11.3
Aged 30 to 34	100.0	29.0	35.4	20.7	14.5
Aged 35 to 39	100.0	23.2	32.7	23.1	20.4
Aged 40 or older	100.0	22.1	27.9	20.8	28.6
Percent distribution by age					
Total births	**100.0%**	**100.0%**	**100.0%**	**100.0%**	**100.0%**
Under age 15	0.2	0.4	0.0	0.0	0.0
Aged 15 to 19	10.1	20.2	5.3	1.6	0.3
Aged 20 to 24	25.1	29.6	26.6	20.4	12.0
Aged 25 to 29	26.9	24.3	28.1	30.0	27.9
Aged 30 to 34	23.5	17.2	25.9	28.8	31.1
Aged 35 to 39	11.6	6.8	11.8	15.8	21.7
Aged 40 or older	2.7	1.5	2.3	3.3	7.0

Note: Numbers will not add to total because "not stated" is not shown.
Source: National Center for Health Statistics, Births: Preliminary Data for 2004, National Vital Statistics Report, Vol. 54, No. 8, 2005; Internet site http://www.cdc.gov/nchs/births.htm; calculations by New Strategist

Hispanics Account for Nearly One in Four Births

Forty-five percent of births to Hispanic women are out-of-wedlock.

The nation's newborns are increasingly diverse. Among the 4.1 million babies born in 2004, nearly 1 million were born to Hispanic women—or 23 percent of the total. Blacks accounted for 14 percent of newborns, and Asians for 6 percent. Non-Hispanic whites accounted for 56 percent of newborns in 2004. The non-Hispanic white share of births rises with age from less than 50 percent for women under age 20 to more than 60 percent for women aged 30 or older.

Out-of-wedlock childbearing is the norm among blacks and American Indians. In 2004, 68 percent of black babies were born to unmarried women. The figure was 61 percent among American Indians. A smaller 45 percent of Hispanic babies were born out-of-wedlock. Among non-Hispanic whites, only 24 percent of babies are born to single mothers, and the proportion bottoms out at 15 percent among Asians.

■ With more than one-third of babies born out-of-wedlock, schools, workplaces, and communities must address the problems of single parents.

More than 40 percent of births are to Asians, blacks, or Hispanics

(percent distribution of births by race and Hispanic origin of mother, 2004)

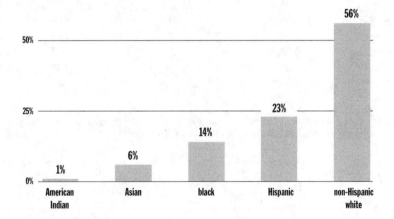

Table 10.10 Births by Age, Race, and Hispanic Origin, 2004

(number and percent distribution of births by age, race, and Hispanic origin of mother, 2004)

	total	American Indian	Asian	non-Hispanic black	Hispanic	non-Hispanic white
Total births	**4,112,052**	**43,927**	**229,123**	**578,772**	**946,349**	**2,296,683**
Under age 15	6,781	139	90	2,729	2,356	1,477
Aged 15 to 19	415,262	7,704	7,632	97,290	133,044	168,795
Aged 20 to 24	1,034,454	15,130	30,662	188,761	279,746	517,148
Aged 25 to 29	1,104,485	10,717	65,040	138,093	254,358	631,726
Aged 30 to 34	965,663	6,488	79,724	92,646	177,762	604,040
Aged 35 to 39	475,606	2,994	37,652	46,945	81,021	304,085
Aged 40 or older	109,801	755	8,323	12,308	18,062	69,412
Percent distribution by age						
Total births	**100.0%**	**100.0%**	**100.0%**	**100.0%**	**100.0%**	**100.0%**
Under age 15	0.2	0.3	0.0	0.5	0.2	0.1
Aged 15 to 19	10.1	17.5	3.3	16.8	14.1	7.3
Aged 20 to 24	25.2	34.4	13.4	32.6	29.6	22.5
Aged 25 to 29	26.9	24.4	28.4	23.9	26.9	27.5
Aged 30 to 34	23.5	14.8	34.8	16.0	18.8	26.3
Aged 35 to 39	11.6	6.8	16.4	8.1	8.6	13.2
Aged 40 or older	2.7	1.7	3.6	2.1	1.9	3.0
Percent distribution by race and Hispanic origin						
Total births	**100.0%**	**1.1%**	**5.6%**	**14.1%**	**23.0%**	**55.9%**
Under age 15	100.0	2.0	1.3	40.2	34.7	21.8
Aged 15 to 19	100.0	1.9	1.8	23.4	32.0	40.6
Aged 20 to 24	100.0	1.5	3.0	18.2	27.0	50.0
Aged 25 to 29	100.0	1.0	5.9	12.5	23.0	57.2
Aged 30 to 34	100.0	0.7	8.3	9.6	18.4	62.6
Aged 35 to 39	100.0	0.6	7.9	9.9	17.0	63.9
Aged 40 or older	100.0	0.7	7.6	11.2	16.4	63.2

Note: Numbers will not add to total because Hispanics may be of any race.
Source: National Center for Health Statistics, Births: Final Data for 2004, Health E-Stats, 2006; Internet site http://www.cdc
.gov/nchs/products/pubs/pubd/hestats/finalbirths04/finalbirths04.htm; calculations by New Strategist

Table 10.11 Births to Unmarried Women by Age, Race, and Hispanic Origin, 2003

(total number of births and number and percent to unmarried women, by age, race, and Hispanic origin of mother, 2003)

	total	American Indian	Asian	black	Hispanic	non-Hispanic white
Total births	**4,089,950**	**43,052**	**221,203**	**599,847**	**912,329**	**2,321,904**
Under age 15	6,661	154	104	2,726	2,356	1,399
Aged 15 to 19	414,580	7,690	7,592	100,951	128,524	172,620
Aged 20 to 24	1,032,305	14,645	30,482	196,268	273,311	522,275
Aged 25 to 29	1,086,366	10,524	64,399	139,947	246,361	627,437
Aged 30 to 34	975,546	6,423	75,692	97,529	169,054	626,315
Aged 35 to 39	467,642	2,906	35,074	49,889	75,801	303,354
Aged 40 or older	106,850	710	7,860	12,537	16,922	68,504
BIRTHS TO UNMARRIED WOMEN						
Total births to unmarried women	**1,415,995**	**26,401**	**33,249**	**409,333**	**410,620**	**546,991**
Under age 15	6,469	152	103	2,715	2,224	1,353
Aged 15 to 19	337,201	6,778	5,544	97,000	97,925	132,482
Aged 20 to 24	549,353	10,002	11,115	160,312	146,729	224,941
Aged 25 to 29	287,205	5,293	7,886	83,421	91,644	101,454
Aged 30 to 34	147,555	2,668	5,238	41,692	46,995	52,167
Aged 35 to 39	69,071	1,193	2,580	19,260	20,158	26,352
Aged 40 or older	19,141	315	783	4,933	4,945	8,242
PERCENT OF BIRTHS TO UNMARRIED WOMEN						
Total births	**34.6%**	**61.3%**	**15.0%**	**68.2%**	**45.0%**	**23.6%**
Under age 15	97.1	98.7	99.0	99.6	94.4	96.7
Aged 15 to 19	81.3	88.1	73.0	96.1	76.2	76.7
Aged 20 to 24	53.2	68.3	36.5	81.7	53.7	43.1
Aged 25 to 29	26.4	50.3	12.2	59.6	37.2	16.2
Aged 30 to 34	15.1	41.5	6.9	42.7	27.8	8.3
Aged 35 to 39	14.8	41.1	7.4	38.6	26.6	8.7
Aged 40 or older	17.9	44.4	10.0	39.3	29.2	12.0

Note: Births by race and Hispanic origin will not add to total because Hispanics may be of any race and "not stated" is not shown.
Source: National Center for Health Statistics, Births: Final Data for 2003, National Vital Statistics Reports, Vol. 54, No. 2, 2005; Internet site http://www.cdc.gov/nchs/births.htm; calculations by New Strategist

Older Mothers Are Better Educated

Many of the youngest mothers did not graduate from high school.

About half the nation's newborns have well-educated mothers. In 2003, fully 47 percent of babies were born to women who had some college experience (21 percent) or who were college graduates (26 percent). Another 51 percent of babies were born to mothers who either had not graduated from high school (21 percent) or had ended their education with a high school diploma (30 percent).

The older the mother, the more likely she is to be a college graduate. Among babies born to women aged 30 or older, an impressive 44 to 47 percent of their mothers are college graduates. Conversely, among babies born to women under age 20, the 59 percent majority of their mothers had not graduated from high school.

■ The economic well-being of babies born to poorly educated women is fragile.

Nearly half of babies are born to women with at least some college experience

(percent distribution of births by educational attainment of mother, 2003)

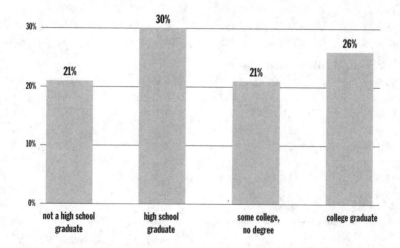

Table 10.12 Births by Age and Educational Attainment, 2003

(number and percent distribution of births in reporting states by age and educational attainment of mother, 2003)

	total	not a high school graduate	high school graduate only	some college	college graduate
Total births	**3,863,502**	**822,123**	**1,162,697**	**811,985**	**1,012,730**
Under age 20	401,260	236,579	137,333	21,114	0
Aged 20 to 24	980,514	268,002	423,305	220,117	56,387
Aged 25 to 29	1,025,666	165,626	299,115	258,304	288,933
Aged 30 to 34	916,840	96,862	190,800	199,543	417,131
Aged 35 to 39	438,771	43,675	90,951	91,675	205,602
Aged 40 or older	100,451	11,379	21,193	21,232	44,677

PERCENT DISTRIBUTION BY EDUCATIONAL ATTAINMENT

	total	not a high school graduate	high school graduate only	some college	college graduate
Total births	**100.0%**	**21.3%**	**30.1%**	**21.0%**	**26.2%**
Under age 20	100.0	59.0	34.2	5.3	0.0
Aged 20 to 24	100.0	27.3	43.2	22.4	5.8
Aged 25 to 29	100.0	16.1	29.2	25.2	28.2
Aged 30 to 34	100.0	10.6	20.8	21.8	45.5
Aged 35 to 39	100.0	10.0	20.7	20.9	46.9
Aged 40 or older	100.0	11.3	21.1	21.1	44.5

PERCENT DISTRIBUTION BY AGE

	total	not a high school graduate	high school graduate only	some college	college graduate
Total births	**100.0%**	**100.0%**	**100.0%**	**100.0%**	**100.0%**
Under age 20	10.4	28.8	11.8	2.6	0.0
Aged 20 to 24	25.4	32.6	36.4	27.1	5.6
Aged 25 to 29	26.5	20.1	25.7	31.8	28.5
Aged 30 to 34	23.7	11.8	16.4	24.6	41.2
Aged 35 to 39	11.4	5.3	7.8	11.3	20.3
Aged 40 or older	2.6	1.4	1.8	2.6	4.4

Note: Data exclude Pennsylvania and Washington. Births by education will not add to total because "not stated" is not shown.
Source: National Center for Health Statistics, Births: Final Data for 2003, National Vital Statistics Reports, Vol. 54, No. 2, 2005;
Internet site http://www.cdc.gov/nchs/births.htm; calculations by New Strategist

More than One in Four Babies Are Born by Caesarean Section

Older women are much more likely to have Caesarean deliveries.

Delayed childbearing can have unanticipated consequences. The older a woman is when she has a child, the greater the likelihood of complications that necessitate Caesarean delivery.

Among babies born in 2003, more than one in four (27 percent) were Caesarean deliveries. Only 23 percent of babies born to women under age 25 were delivered by Caesarean section, but the share stood at 31 percent among women aged 25 to 39, and topped 42 percent among women aged 40 or older.

Perhaps because of the high rate of Caesarean delivery, hospitals are by far the preferred place of delivery and physicians are the attendant of choice at most births. Eighty-seven percent of births in 2003 were attended by a doctor of medicine. Midwives attended only 8 percent of deliveries.

■ As new fertility technologies enable more women to have children later in life, the Caesarean rate is likely to rise further.

Few babies are delivered by midwives

(percent distribution of births by attendant, 2003)

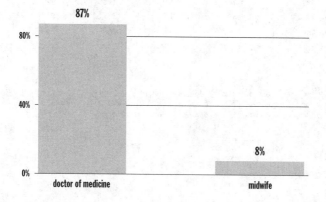

Table 10.13 Births by Age and Method of Delivery, 2003

(number and percent distribution of births by age and method of delivery, 2003)

		vaginal		Caesarean		
	total births	total	after previous Caesarean	total	primary	repeat
Total births	**4,089,950**	**2,949,853**	**51,602**	**1,119,388**	**684,484**	**434,699**
Under age 20	421,241	339,393	1,171	80,182	70,150	10,030
Aged 20 to 24	1,032,305	795,078	9,003	232,579	154,407	78,157
Aged 25 to 29	1,086,366	795,736	14,123	285,231	172,845	112,353
Aged 30 to 34	975,546	665,025	16,004	305,102	170,728	134,296
Aged 35 to 39	467,642	293,643	9,194	171,142	90,685	80,403
Aged 40 or older	106,850	60,978	2,107	45,152	25,669	19,460
PERCENT DISTRIBUTION BY METHOD OF DELIVERY						
Total births	**100.0%**	**72.1%**	**1.3%**	**27.4%**	**16.7%**	**10.6%**
Under age 20	100.0	80.6	0.3	19.0	16.7	2.4
Aged 20 to 24	100.0	77.0	0.9	22.5	15.0	7.6
Aged 25 to 29	100.0	73.2	1.3	26.3	15.9	10.3
Aged 30 to 34	100.0	68.2	1.6	31.3	17.5	13.8
Aged 35 to 39	100.0	62.8	2.0	36.6	19.4	17.2
Aged 40 or older	100.0	57.1	2.0	42.3	24.0	18.2
PERCENT DISTRIBUTION BY AGE						
Total births	**100.0%**	**100.0%**	**100.0%**	**100.0%**	**100.0%**	**100.0%**
Under age 20	10.3	11.5	2.3	7.2	10.2	2.3
Aged 20 to 24	25.2	27.0	17.4	20.8	22.6	18.0
Aged 25 to 29	26.6	27.0	27.4	25.5	25.3	25.8
Aged 30 to 34	23.9	22.5	31.0	27.3	24.9	30.9
Aged 35 to 39	11.4	10.0	17.8	15.3	13.2	18.5
Aged 40 or older	2.6	2.1	4.1	4.0	3.8	4.5

Note: Numbers will not add to total because "not stated" is not shown.
Source: National Center for Health Statistics, Births: Final Data for 2003, National Vital Statistics Reports, Vol. 54, No. 2, 2005;
Internet site http://www.cdc.gov/nchs/births.htm; calculations by New Strategist

Table 10.14 Births by Attendant and Place of Delivery, 2003

(number and percent distribution of births by attendant and place of delivery, 2003)

	total births	physician			midwife			other	unspecified
		total	doctor of medicine	doctor of osteopathy	total	certified nurse midwife	other midwife		
Total births	**4,089,950**	**3,733,750**	**3,554,819**	**178,931**	**328,153**	**310,342**	**17,811**	**20,599**	**7,448**
In hospital	4,053,987	3,730,008	3,551,650	178,358	305,513	300,931	4,582	11,535	6,931
Not in hospital	35,723	3,622	3,049	573	22,588	9,362	13,226	9,015	498
Freestanding birthing center	9,779	923	611	312	8,664	5,828	2,836	185	7
Clinic or doctor's office	397	225	196	29	108	57	51	62	2
Residence	23,221	1,813	1,613	200	13,403	3,272	10,131	7,631	374
Other	2,326	661	629	32	413	205	208	1,137	115
Not specified	240	120	120	0	52	49	3	49	19

PERCENT DISTRIBUTION BY ATTENDANT

	total births	physician			midwife			other	unspecified
Total births	**100.0%**	**91.3%**	**86.9%**	**4.4%**	**8.0%**	**7.6%**	**0.4%**	**0.5%**	**0.2%**
In hospital	100.0	92.0	87.6	4.4	7.5	7.4	0.1	0.3	0.2
Not in hospital	100.0	10.1	8.5	1.6	63.2	26.2	37.0	25.2	1.4
Freestanding birthing center	100.0	9.4	6.2	3.2	88.6	59.6	29.0	1.9	0.1
Clinic or doctor's office	100.0	56.7	49.4	7.3	27.2	14.4	12.8	15.6	0.5
Residence	100.0	7.8	6.9	0.9	57.7	14.1	43.6	32.9	1.6
Other	100.0	28.4	27.0	1.4	17.8	8.8	8.9	48.9	4.9
Not specified	100.0	50.0	50.0	0.0	21.7	20.4	1.3	20.4	7.9

PERCENT DISTRIBUTION BY PLACE OF DELIVERY

	total births	physician			midwife			other	unspecified
Total births	**100.0%**	**100.0%**	**100.0%**	**100.0%**	**100.0%**	**100.0%**	**100.0%**	**100.0%**	**100.0%**
In hospital	99.1	99.9	99.9	99.7	93.1	97.0	25.7	56.0	93.1
Not in hospital	0.9	0.1	0.1	0.3	6.9	3.0	74.3	43.8	6.7
Freestanding birthing center	0.2	0.0	0.0	0.2	2.6	1.9	15.9	0.9	0.1
Clinic or doctor's office	0.0	0.0	0.0	0.0	0.0	0.0	0.3	0.3	0.0
Residence	0.6	0.0	0.0	0.1	4.1	1.1	56.9	37.0	5.0
Other	0.1	0.0	0.0	0.0	0.1	0.1	1.2	5.5	1.5
Not specified	0.0	0.0	0.0	0.0	0.0	0.0	0.0	0.2	0.3

Note: Births in hospital includes births en route to or on arrival at hospital.
Source: National Center for Health Statistics, Births: Final Data for 2003, National Vital Statistics Reports, Vol. 54, No. 2, 2005; Internet site http://www.cdc.gov/nchs/births.htm; calculations by New Strategist

Eight Percent of Babies Have Low Birth Weight

Blacks are most likely to have low birth weight babies.

Among the 4 million babies born in 2003, more than 324,000—or 8 percent—had low birth weight, which is defined as less than 2,500 grams, or 5.5 pounds. Just over 1 percent of births were very low birth weight babies in 2003, weighing less than 3.25 pounds.

Blacks are twice as likely to have a low birth weight than Hispanics or non-Hispanic whites. In 2003, 14 percent of black births were low birth weight babies compared with 7 percent of births to Hispanics and non-Hispanic whites. Low birth weight is also associated with a younger age at giving birth, lower educational levels, late prenatal care, cigarette smoking during pregnancy, and lower income levels.

■ Low birth weight babies are more likely to have developmental problems and to require greater medical care.

Blacks are twice as likely to have a low birth weight baby

(percent of total live births that were low birth weight, by race and Hispanic origin, 2003)

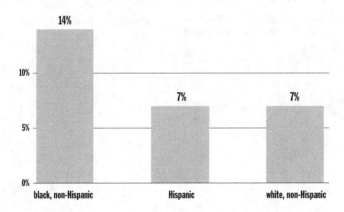

Table 10.15 Births by Birth Weight, 2003

(number and percent distribution of births by birth weight, 2003)

	number	percent distribution
Total births	**4,089,950**	**100.0%**
Less than 500 grams	6,307	0.2
500 to 999 grams	22,980	0.6
1,000 to 1,499 grams	29,930	0.7
1,500 to 1,999 grams	63,791	1.6
2,000 to 2,499 grams	201,056	4.9
2,500 to 2,999 grams	711,003	17.4
3,000 to 3,499 grams	1,557,864	38.1
3,500 to 3,999 grams	1,131,577	27.7
4,000 to 4,499 grams	309,721	7.6
4,500 to 4,999 grams	46,690	1.1
5,000 grams or more	5,431	0.1
Not stated	3,600	0.1
Very low birth weight	59,217	1.4
Low birth weight	324,064	7.9

Note: Very low birth weight is defined as less than 1,500 grams (3.25 pounds). Low birth weight is defined as less than 2,500 grams (5.5 pounds).
Source: National Center for Health Statistics, Births: Final Data for 2003, National Vital Statistics Reports, Vol. 54, No. 2, 2005; Internet site http://www.cdc.gov/nchs/births.htm; calculations by New Strategist

Table 10.16 Low Birth Weight Births by Age, Race, and Hispanic Origin, 2003

(number and percent of babies born weighing 2,500 grams or less, and percent distribution of low birth weight births by by age, race, and Hispanic origin of mother, 2003)

	total	non-Hispanic black	Hispanic	non-Hispanic white
NUMBER				
Total low birth weight births	**324,064**	**77,947**	**60,973**	**163,331**
Under age 15	848	423	244	144
Aged 15 to 19	40,211	13,738	10,120	14,904
Aged 20 to 24	82,494	24,899	17,173	36,764
Aged 25 to 29	76,631	16,668	14,624	39,730
Aged 30 to 34	71,477	12,667	11,122	41,263
Aged 35 to 39	40,550	7,484	5,914	23,634
Aged 40 to 44	10,655	1,933	1,641	6,083
Aged 45 to 54	1,198	135	135	809
PERCENT OF BIRTHS WITH LOW BIRTH WEIGHT				
Total births	**7.9%**	**13.6%**	**6.7%**	**7.0%**
Under age 15	12.7	16.0	10.4	10.3
Aged 15 to 19	9.7	14.1	7.9	8.6
Aged 20 to 24	8.0	13.2	6.3	7.0
Aged 25 to 29	7.1	12.5	5.9	6.3
Aged 30 to 34	7.3	13.6	6.6	6.6
Aged 35 to 39	8.7	15.7	7.8	7.8
Aged 40 to 44	10.6	16.9	10.2	9.4
Aged 45 to 54	20.5	22.0	18.0	20.8
PERCENT DISTRIBUTION BY RACE AND HISPANIC ORIGIN				
Total low birth weight births	**100.0%**	**24.1%**	**18.8%**	**50.4%**
Under age 15	100.0	49.9	28.8	17.0
Aged 15 to 19	100.0	34.2	25.2	37.1
Aged 20 to 24	100.0	30.2	20.8	44.6
Aged 25 to 29	100.0	21.8	19.1	51.8
Aged 30 to 34	100.0	17.7	15.6	57.7
Aged 35 to 39	100.0	18.5	14.6	58.3
Aged 40 to 44	100.0	18.1	15.4	57.1
Aged 45 to 54	100.0	11.3	11.3	67.5

Note: Low birth weight is defined as 2,500 grams (5.5 pounds) or less.
Source: National Center for Health Statistics, Births: Final Data for 2003, National Vital Statistics Reports, Vol. 54, No. 2, 2005; Internet site http://www.cdc.gov/nchs/births.htm; calculations by New Strategist

Table 10.17 Low Birth Weight Births by Selected Characteristics of Mother, 2002

(number of single live births ever born to women aged 15 to 44, and percent that were low birth weight, by selected characteristics, 2002; numbers in thousands)

	total	percent low birth weight
Total live births to women aged 15 to 44	**75,716**	**6.7%**
Age at time of birth		
Under age 18	5,807	9.5
Aged 18 to 19	8,259	10.5
Aged 20 to 24	24,747	6.8
Aged 25 to 29	20,660	4.9
Aged 30 to 44	16,242	5.8
Wantedness status at conception		
Intended	47,078	5.7
Mistimed	17,778	8.6
Unwanted	10,860	8.0
Race and Hispanic origin		
Black, non-Hispanic	11,708	12.1
Hispanic	13,939	7.3
White, non-Hispanic	45,081	5.1
Education at interview		
Not a high school graduate	13,568	9.3
High school graduate or GED	25,706	6.3
Some college, no degree	20,736	6.2
Bachelor's degree or more	13,604	4.9
Timing of first prenatal visit		
Within first trimester	21,359	6.2
After first trimester or never	2,192	9.1
Any cigarette smoking during pregnancy		
No	20,541	6.1
Yes	2,980	8.8
Method of payment for delivery		
Any Medicaid or government assistance	8,280	9.7
All other	15,341	4.9

Note: Low birth weight is defined as 2,500 grams (5.5 pounds) or less. Education categories include only people aged 22 to 44. Source: National Center for Health Statistics, Fertility, Family Planning, and Reproductive Health of U.S. Women: Data from the 2002 National Survey of Family Growth, Vital and Health Statistics, Series 23, No. 25, 2005; Internet site http://www.cdc.gov/nchs/nsfg.htm

Amniocentesis Is Performed on Only 2 Percent of Births

Older women are much more likely to have amniocentesis.

Few births today could be called "natural." Most pregnant women participate in some kind of obstetric procedure either before or during childbirth. The most common procedure, electronic fetal monitoring, was performed during 85 percent of births in 2003. Sixty-seven percent of babies born in 2003 had ultrasound performed on them. Other procedures—such as induction and stimulation of labor—are performed on fewer than one-fourth of births. Amniocentesis is relatively rare, and occurs in fewer than 2 percent of births. But the rate of amniocentesis rises sharply with the age of the mother.

Some, but not all, congenital malformations are more common among older mothers. It is much more likely that an older mother will have a child with Down Syndrome, for example.

■ With the age of mothers rising, high-tech childbirth has become more common.

The incidence of some congenital anomalies rises sharply with age

(number of live births with Down Syndrome per 100,000 live births, by age, 2003)

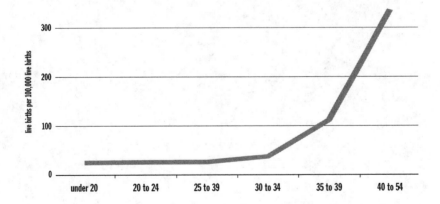

Table 10.18 Births by Obstetric Procedure and Age, 2003

(total number and percent distribution of live births in reporting states with selected obstetric procedures, and rate per 1,000 live births by age, 2003)

	number of births	percent with procedure
Total births in reporting states	**3,863,502**	**100.0%**
Electronic fetal monitoring	3,289,703	85.1
Ultrasound	2,592,258	67.1
Induction of labor	840,137	21.7
Stimulation of labor	645,075	16.7
Amniocentesis	66,901	1.7

	rate per 1,000 live births						
	total	under 20	20 to 24	25 to 29	30 to 34	35 to 39	40 to 54
Electronic fetal monitoring	854.2	866.6	862.5	856.6	848.3	837.8	825.6
Ultrasound	673.1	639.6	658.2	676.2	689.2	693.2	686.2
Induction of labor	206.0	203.2	210.2	213.9	203.7	190.7	184.4
Stimulation of labor	167.5	186.9	175.5	170.6	160.9	146.2	132.6
Amniocentesis	17.4	4.8	5.8	7.7	13.2	66.8	101.3

Note: Data exclude Pennsylvania and Washington.
Source: National Center for Health Statistics, Births: Final Data for 2003, National Vital Statistics Reports, Vol. 54, No. 2, 2005; Internet site http://www.cdc.gov/nchs/births.htm; calculations by New Strategist

Table 10.19 Births with Selected Congenital Anomalies by Age, 2003

(number of live births with selected congenital anomaly, and number per 100,000 live births, by age of mother, 2003)

	births with congenital anomaly	rate per 100,000 live births						
		total	under 20	20 to 24	25 to 29	30 to 34	35 to 39	40 to 54
Anencephalus	460	11.4	14.0	12.7	10.1	12.5	8.0	–
Spina bifida/meningocele	755	18.7	18.3	20.6	19.7	16.2	15.8	26.5
Hydrocephalus	847	22.2	28.4	23.5	20.5	20.9	20.1	24.2
Microcephalus	214	5.6	6.6	5.7	4.6	4.7	7.6	–
Other central nervous system anomalies	803	21.1	21.5	21.2	19.6	18.7	27.7	25.2
Heart malformations	4,916	128.9	107.6	118.9	123.1	131.9	150.9	247.4
Other circulatory/ respiratory anomalies	4,807	126.1	113.5	121.1	115.4	123.2	158.1	220.1
Rectal atresia/stenosis	298	7.8	6.1	8.6	6.7	7.6	9.5	–
Tracheo-esophageal fistula/ esophageal fistula	411	10.8	11.6	10.7	10.9	8.1	13.8	–
Omphalocele/gastroschisis	1,313	32.5	84.4	47.8	20.9	15.3	16.9	24.6
Other gastrointestinal anomalies	1,259	33.0	40.8	33.4	31.2	28.0	35.3	52.5
Malformed genitalia	3,038	79.7	72.9	76.5	84.4	78.8	82.4	84.8
Renal agenesis	533	14.0	14.2	13.8	13.3	15.7	12.5	–
Other urogenital anomalies	3,438	90.2	79.5	84.3	87.2	95.9	104.8	104.0
Cleft lip/palate	3,066	75.9	73.8	86.4	76.4	64.4	73.3	92.9
Polydactyly/syndactyly/adactyly	2,915	76.4	102.1	87.8	72.5	63.8	60.9	87.8
Clubfoot	2,198	57.6	64.6	65.3	58.4	49.0	51.2	55.5
Diaphragmatic hernia	436	11.4	9.1	10.8	12.0	11.0	14.1	–
Other musculoskeletal/ integumental anomalies	7,937	208.2	248.4	222.5	202.6	190.0	186.9	223.1
Down Syndrome	1,881	46.5	25.1	26.0	26.1	37.4	111.6	336.5
Other chromosomal anomalies	1,147	30.1	21.5	22.7	24.1	26.8	54.2	122.2

Note: "–" means no rate shown because fewer than 20 births.
Source: National Center for Health Statistics, Births: Final Data for 2003, National Vital Statistics Reports, Vol. 54, No. 2, 2005; Internet site http://www.cdc.gov/nchs/births.htm; calculations by New Strategist

Most Women Aged 15 to 44 Have Had at Least One Child

A smaller percentage of men have had children.

Among women aged 15 to 44, the 58 percent majority has had at least one child. Only 47 percent of their male counterparts have had children. The percentage of men and women who have had children rises with age to a peak of 78 and 85 percent, respectively, among those aged 40 to 44. Hispanics are most likely to have had children. Non-Hispanic whites are least likely to be parents.

Overall, 42 percent of women aged 15 to 44 have not yet had children, 18 percent have had one child, 22 percent have had two, and 18 percent have had three or more. Among women aged 40 to 44, only 15 percent have not had children, 18 percent have one, 32 percent have two, and 36 percent have three or more.

Education has a big influence on childbearing. Among women aged 15 to 44, only 54 percent of college graduates have had children compared with 91 percent of high school dropouts. Twenty-one percent of high school dropouts have had three or more children compared with only 3 percent of college graduates.

■ Among women, fundamentalist Protestants are most likely to have had children (63 percent), and those with no religion are least likely (47 percent).

Hispanics are more likely to have had children than blacks or non-Hispanic whites

(percent of women aged 15 to 44 who have had at least one child, by race and Hispanic origin, 2002)

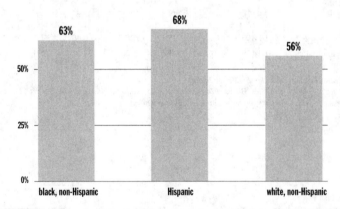

Table 10.20 Percentage of Men and Women Aged 15 to 44 Who Have Had Children, 2002

(total number of people aged 15 to 44 and percentage who have ever had a biological child, by selected characteristics and sex, 2002; numbers in thousands)

	men		women	
	total number	percent who have had a child	total number	percent who have had a child
Total aged 15 to 44	**61,147**	**46.7%**	**61,561**	**58.4%**
Aged 15 to 19	10,208	1.9	9,834	7.8
Aged 20 to 24	9,883	17.4	9,840	32.9
Aged 25 to 29	9,226	45.0	9,249	60.5
Aged 30 to 34	10,138	62.9	10,272	73.2
Aged 35 to 39	10,557	70.8	10,853	83.1
Aged 40 to 44	11,135	77.6	11,512	85.1
Marital or cohabiting status				
Currently married	25,808	78.7	28,327	81.9
Currently cohabiting	5,653	54.7	5,570	59.0
Never married, not cohabiting	25,412	7.2	21,568	20.2
Formerly married, not cohabiting	4,274	77.8	6,096	84.0
Race and Hispanic origin				
Black, non-Hispanic	6,940	49.6	8,250	63.3
Married	2,187	86.5	2,133	88.4
Unmarried	4,753	32.5	6,117	54.5
Hispanic	10,188	55.5	9,107	67.6
Married	4,349	85.6	4,138	88.6
Unmarried	5,839	33.0	4,969	50.1
White, non-Hispanic	38,738	43.9	39,498	55.8
Married	17,183	75.4	20,061	79.7
Unmarried	21,555	18.8	19,438	31.2
Education				
Not a high school graduate	6,355	73.3	5,627	91.1
High school graduate or GED	15,659	68.6	14,264	81.7
Some college, no degree	13,104	51.9	14,279	71.5
Bachelor's degree or more	11,901	47.8	13,551	53.5

Note: Education categories include only people aged 22 to 44.
Source: National Center for Health Statistics, Fertility, Contraception, and Fatherhood: Data on Men and Women from Cycle 6 of the 2002 National Survey of Family Growth, Vital and Health Statistics, Series 23, No. 26, 2006; Internet site http://www.cdc.gov/nchs/nsfg.htm

Table 10.21 Number of Children Ever Born to Women Aged 15 to 44 by Age, 2002

(total number of women aged 15 to 44, and percent distribution by number of children ever borne, by age, 2002; numbers in thousands)

| | total | | | number of children ever borne | | | | | |
| | | | | | one or more | | | | |
	number	percent	none	total	one	two	three	four or more
Total women aged 15 to 44	**61,561**	**100.0%**	**41.6%**	**58.4%**	**18.2%**	**21.8%**	**11.6%**	**6.8%**
Aged 15 to 19	9,834	100.0	92.2	7.8	7.0	0.8	–	0.0
Aged 20 to 24	9,840	100.0	67.1	33.0	19.3	10.0	2.8	0.9
Aged 25 to 29	9,249	100.0	39.5	60.6	23.7	20.9	10.3	5.7
Aged 30 to 34	10,272	100.0	26.8	73.2	22.2	29.0	14.7	7.3
Aged 35 to 39	10,853	100.0	16.9	83.1	19.2	34.9	18.5	10.5
Aged 40 to 44	11,512	100.0	15.0	85.1	18.0	31.6	20.7	14.8

Note: "–" means sample is too small to make a reliable estimate.
Source: National Center for Health Statistics, Fertility, Family Planning, and Reproductive Health of U.S. Women: Data from the 2002 National Survey of Family Growth, Vital and Health Statistics, Series 23, No. 25, 2005; Internet site http://www.cdc .gov/nchs/nsfg.htm

Table 10.22 Number of Children Fathered by Men Aged 15 to 44 by Age, 2002

(total number of men aged 15 to 44, and percent distribution by number of biological children fathered, by age, 2002; numbers in thousands)

| | total | | | number of biological children fathered | | | |
| | | | | | one or more | | |
	number	percent	none	total	one	two	three or more
Total men aged 15 to 44	**61,147**	**100.0%**	**53.3%**	**46.7%**	**17.1%**	**16.1%**	**13.5%**
Aged 15 to 19	10,208	100.0	98.1	1.9	1.6	–	–
Aged 20 to 24	9,883	100.0	82.6	17.4	11.3	4.5	1.6
Aged 25 to 29	9,226	100.0	55.0	45.0	20.2	15.2	9.6
Aged 30 to 34	10,138	100.0	37.1	62.9	26.9	22.8	13.1
Aged 35 to 39	10,557	100.0	29.2	70.8	22.4	27.0	21.4
Aged 40 to 44	11,135	100.0	22.4	77.6	19.9	25.0	32.7

Note: "–" means sample is too small to make a reliable estimate.
Source: National Center for Health Statistics, Fertility, Contraception, and Fatherhood: Data on Men and Women from Cycle 6 of the 2002 National Survey of Family Growth, Vital and Health Statistics, Series 23, No. 26, 2006; Internet site http://www.cdc .gov/nchs/nsfg.htm

Table 10.23 Number of Children Ever Borne by Mother's Marital Status, 2002

(total number of women aged 15 to 44, and percent distribution by number of children ever borne, by marital status, 2002; numbers in thousands)

| | total | | | number of children ever borne | | | | |
| | | | | | one or more | | | |
	number	percent	none	total	one	two	three	four or more
Total women aged 15 to 44	**61,561**	**100.0%**	**41.6%**	**58.4%**	**18.2%**	**21.8%**	**11.6%**	**6.8%**
Currently married	28,327	100.0	18.2	81.9	22.5	33.2	17.8	8.4
First marriage	23,082	100.0	20.1	79.9	23.2	33.3	15.8	7.6
Second or higher marriage	5,245	100.0	9.8	90.3	19.1	32.7	26.8	11.7
Currently cohabiting	5,570	100.0	41.1	59.0	21.5	14.7	11.5	11.3
Never married, not cohabiting	21,568	100.0	79.8	20.1	10.5	5.0	2.6	2.0
Formerly married, not cohabiting	6,096	100.0	16.0	83.9	22.5	34.4	14.3	12.7

Source: National Center for Health Statistics, Fertility, Family Planning, and Reproductive Health of U.S. Women: Data from the 2002 National Survey of Family Growth, Vital and Health Statistics, Series 23, No. 25, 2005; Internet site http://www.cdc .gov/nchs/nsfg.htm

Table 10.24 Number of Children Fathered by Father's Marital Status, 2002

(total number of men aged 15 to 44, and percent distribution by number of biological children fathered, by marital status, 2002; numbers in thousands)

| | total | | | number of biological children fathered | | | |
| | | | | | one or more | | |
	number	percent	none	total	one	two	three or more
Total men aged 15 to 44	**61,561**	**100.0%**	**53.3%**	**46.7%**	**17.1%**	**16.1%**	**13.5%**
Currently married	25,808	100.0	21.3	78.7	24.9	29.1	24.8
Currently cohabiting	5,653	100.0	45.3	54.7	25.3	13.7	15.7
Never married, not cohabiting	25,412	100.0	92.8	7.2	5.1	1.4	0.7
Formerly married, not cohabiting	4,274	100.0	22.2	77.8	30.5	28.1	19.2

Source: National Center for Health Statistics, Fertility, Contraception, and Fatherhood: Data on Men and Women from Cycle 6 of the 2002 National Survey of Family Growth, Vital and Health Statistics, Series 23, No. 26, 2006; Internet site http://www.cdc .gov/nchs/nsfg.htm

Table 10.25 Number of Children Ever Borne by Mother's Race and Hispanic Origin, 2002

(total number of women aged 15 to 44, and percent distribution by number of children ever borne, by race and Hispanic Origin, 2002; numbers in thousands)

| | total | | | number of children ever borne | | | | |
| | | | | | one or more | | | |
	number	percent	none	total	one	two	three	four or more
Total women aged 15 to 44	**61,561**	**100.0%**	**41.6%**	**58.4%**	**18.2%**	**21.8%**	**11.6%**	**6.8%**
Black, non-Hispanic	8,250	100.0	36.8	63.4	20.6	19.6	13.2	10.0
Hispanic	9,107	100.0	32.4	67.6	18.7	23.6	15.0	10.3
White, non-Hispanic	39,498	100.0	44.2	55.7	17.4	21.9	10.8	5.6

Source: National Center for Health Statistics, Fertility, Family Planning, and Reproductive Health of U.S. Women: Data from the 2002 National Survey of Family Growth, Vital and Health Statistics, Series 23, No. 25, 2005; Internet site http://www.cdc .gov/nchs/nsfg.htm

Table 10.26 Number of Children Fathered by Father's Race and Hispanic Origin, 2002

(total number of men aged 15 to 44, and percent distribution by number of biological children fathered, by race and Hispanic origin, 2002; numbers in thousands)

| | total | | | number of biological children fathered | | | |
| | | | | | one or more | | |
	number	percent	none	total	one	two	three or more
Total men aged 15 to 44	**61,147**	**100.0%**	**53.3%**	**46.7%**	**17.1%**	**16.1%**	**13.5%**
Black, non-Hispanic	6,940	100.0	50.5	49.6	17.9	15.6	16.1
Hispanic	10,188	100.0	44.5	55.5	17.3	17.4	20.8
White, non-Hispanic	38,738	100.0	56.1	43.9	17.1	16.1	10.7

Source: National Center for Health Statistics, Fertility, Contraception, and Fatherhood: Data on Men and Women from Cycle 6 of the 2002 National Survey of Family Growth, Vital and Health Statistics, Series 23, No. 26, 2006; Internet site http://www.cdc .gov/nchs/nsfg.htm

Table 10.27 Number of Children Ever Borne by Mother's Education, 2002

(total number of women aged 15 to 44, and percent distribution by number of children ever borne, by education, 2002; numbers in thousands)

| | total | | | number of children ever borne | | | | |
| | | | | | one or more | | | |
	number	percent	none	total	one	two	three	four or more
Total women aged 15 to 44	**61,561**	**100.0%**	**41.6%**	**58.4%**	**18.2%**	**21.8%**	**11.6%**	**6.8%**
Not a high school graduate	5,627	100.0	8.9	91.1	15.9	28.2	25.6	21.4
High school graduate or GED	14,264	100.0	18.4	81.6	22.1	30.6	18.1	10.8
Some college, no degree	14,279	100.0	28.6	71.5	22.0	29.7	12.2	7.6
Bachelor's degree or more	13,551	100.0	46.5	53.6	19.5	21.7	9.8	2.6

Note: Education categories include only people aged 22 to 44.
Source: National Center for Health Statistics, Fertility, Family Planning, and Reproductive Health of U.S. Women: Data from the 2002 National Survey of Family Growth, Vital and Health Statistics, Series 23, No. 25, 2005; Internet site http://www.cdc .gov/nchs/nsfg.htm

Table 10.28 Number of Children Fathered by Father's Education, 2002

(total number of men aged 15 to 44, and percent distribution by number of biological children, by education, 2002; numbers in thousands)

| | total | | | number of biological children fathered | | | |
| | | | | | one or more | | |
	number	percent	none	total	one	two	three or more
Total men aged 15 to 44	**61,147**	**100.0%**	**53.3%**	**46.7%**	**17.1%**	**16.1%**	**13.5%**
Not a high school graduate	6,355	100.0	26.7	73.3	21.3	20.3	31.8
High school graduate or GED	15,659	100.0	31.5	68.6	23.7	23.9	21.0
Some college, no degree	13,104	100.0	48.1	51.9	19.7	19.2	13.0
Bachelor's degree or more	11,901	100.0	52.2	47.8	19.3	18.3	10.2

Note: Education categories include only people aged 22 to 44.
Source: National Center for Health Statistics, Fertility, Contraception, and Fatherhood: Data on Men and Women from Cycle 6 of the 2002 National Survey of Family Growth, Vital and Health Statistics, Series 23, No. 26, 2006; Internet site http://www.cdc .gov/nchs/nsfg.htm

Table 10.29 Number of Children Ever Borne by Mother's Religion, 2002

(total number of women aged 15 to 44, and percent distribution by number of children ever borne, by religion raised, 2002; numbers in thousands)

| | total | | number of children ever borne | | | | | |
| | | | | one or more | | | | |
	number	percent	none	total	one	two	three	four or more
Total women aged 15 to 44	**61,561**	**100.0%**	**41.6%**	**58.4%**	**18.2%**	**21.8%**	**11.6%**	**6.8%**
No religion	4,773	100.0	53.3	46.7	21.3	15.1	7.4	2.9
Fundamentalist Protestant	3,620	100.0	37.4	62.6	16.8	19.6	17.3	8.9
Other Protestant	28,120	100.0	41.8	58.2	18.9	22.1	10.4	6.8
Catholic	21,517	100.0	38.7	61.3	17.0	23.2	13.4	7.7
Other religion	3,324	100.0	47.8	52.2	16.4	21.6	8.9	5.3

Source: National Center for Health Statistics, Fertility, Family Planning, and Reproductive Health of U.S. Women: Data from the 2002 National Survey of Family Growth, Vital and Health Statistics, Series 23, No. 25, 2005; Internet site http://www.cdc.gov/nchs/nsfg.htm

The Average Woman Expects to Have Two Children

Men and women agree on the number of children they want.

Women aged 15 to 44 have given birth to an average of 1.28 children. They expect to have an additional 0.99 children, for a total of 2.27. Plans can change as women age. Women aged 20 to 24 expect to have the greatest number of children, 2.44. But the figure declines with age as some women discover they cannot have as many children as they want.

The number of children women expect to have does not vary much by demographic characteristic. It is slightly higher for Hispanics (2.58) than blacks (2.34) or non-Hispanic whites (2.17). It is higher for the less educated (2.30) than for those with a college degree (2.08). Religion also makes a difference, with fundamentalist Protestants expecting 2.43 children and women without a religion expecting 1.88.

Men aged 15 to 44 expect to father 2.2 children, on average. As with women, Hispanic men expect to have the most (2.6) and non-Hispanic whites the least (2.0).

■ The two-child family is a well-established norm in the United States.

Women aged 15 to 44 expect to have one more child, on average

(average number of children borne and additional births expected among women aged 15 to 44, 2002)

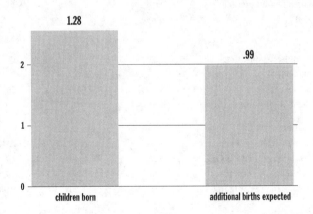

Table 10.30 Average Number of Children Ever Borne and Total Births Expected among Women, 2002

(average number of children ever borne by women aged 15 to 44, average number of additional births expected, and average number of total births expected, by selected characteristics, 2002)

	average number		
	children ever borne	additional births expected	total births expected
Total women aged 15 to 44	**1.28**	**0.99**	**2.27**
Aged 15 to 19	0.09	2.07	2.15
Aged 20 to 24	0.52	1.92	2.44
Aged 25 to 29	1.21	1.15	2.36
Aged 30 to 34	1.58	0.69	2.27
Aged 35 to 39	1.93	0.28	2.21
Aged 40 to 44	2.11	0.08	2.19
Marital status			
Currently married	1.80	0.60	2.40
First marriage	1.72	0.69	2.41
Second or higher marriage	2.15	0.22	2.37
Currently cohabiting	1.38	0.95	2.33
Never married, not cohabiting	0.39	1.70	2.09
Formerly married, not cohabiting	1.90	0.33	2.23
Fecundity status			
Surgically sterile			
Contraceptive	2.59	0.00	2.59
Noncontraceptive	1.65	0.00	1.65
Impaired fecundity	1.14	0.75	1.89
Fecund	0.85	1.39	2.24
Race and Hispanic origin			
Black, non-Hispanic	1.47	0.87	2.34
Hispanic	1.59	0.99	2.58
White, non-Hispanic	1.19	0.98	2.17
Education			
Not a high school graduate	2.50	0.44	2.94
High school graduate or GED	1.88	0.42	2.30
Some college, no degree	1.50	0.69	2.20
Bachelor's degree or more	1.04	1.04	2.08
Religion raised			
No religion	0.86	1.02	1.88
Fundamentalist Protestant	1.47	0.96	2.43
Other Protestant	1.25	0.99	2.23
Catholic	1.39	0.96	2.35
Other religion	1.14	1.24	2.38

Source: National Center for Health Statistics, Fertility, Family Planning, and Reproductive Health of U.S. Women: Data from the 2002 National Survey of Family Growth, Vital and Health Statistics, Series 23, No. 25, 2005; Internet site http://www.cdc.gov/nchs/nsfg.htm

Table 10.31 Average Number of Children Fathered and Total Children Expected among Men, 2002

(average number of biological children fathered by men aged 15 to 44, average number of additional children expected, and average number of total children expected, by selected characteristics, 2002)

	average number		
	biological children fathered	additional children expected	total children expected
Total men aged 15 to 44	**1.0**	**1.2**	**2.2**
Aged 15 to 19	0.0	2.0	2.0
Aged 20 to 24	0.3	2.0	2.3
Aged 25 to 29	0.8	1.5	2.4
Aged 30 to 34	1.2	0.9	2.1
Aged 35 to 39	1.5	0.5	2.1
Aged 40 to 44	1.9	0.3	2.2
Marital status			
Currently married	1.7	0.7	2.5
Currently cohabiting	1.1	0.9	2.0
Never married, not cohabiting	0.1	1.8	1.9
Formerly married, not cohabiting	1.6	0.6	2.2
Race and Hispanic origin			
Black, non-Hispanic	1.1	1.2	2.3
Hispanic	1.3	1.3	2.6
White, non-Hispanic	0.9	1.2	2.0
Education			
Not a high school graduate	1.8	0.8	2.6
High school graduate or GED	1.5	0.7	2.1
Some college, no degree	1.0	1.2	2.2
Bachelor's degree or more	0.9	1.1	2.0
Religion raised			
No religion	0.7	1.2	1.9
Fundamentalist Protestant	1.0	1.2	2.2
Other Protestant	1.0	1.1	2.1
Catholic	1.0	1.2	2.3
Other religion	0.9	1.3	2.1

Source: National Center for Health Statistics, Fertility, Contraception, and Fatherhood: Data on Men and Women from Cycle 6 of the 2002 National Survey of Family Growth, Vital and Health Statistics, Series 23, No. 26, 2006; Internet site http://www.cdc .gov/nchs/nsfg.htm

Births Outside of Marriage Are Common

Among women aged 15 to 44 with children, 42 percent have had a child out-of-wedlock.

Nonmarital childbearing has become commonplace among younger generations. The percentage of women who have had a child outside of wedlock is greatest among the youngest adults and falls with age.

Among women aged 15 to 44 who have had at least one child, the percentage who have had a child out-of-wedlock stands at 92 percent among 15-to-19-year-olds and falls with age to 29 percent among women aged 40 to 44. Eighty-one percent of black women have had a nonmarital birth compared with 51 percent of Hispanics and 30 percent of non-Hispanic whites.

Among all men aged 15 to 44, 19 percent have had at least one child outside of marriage. Among men who have had children, the figure is a larger 34 percent. Black men are more likely to have had a child out-of-wedlock (63 percent) than Hispanics (48 percent) or non-Hispanic whites (23 percent).

■ College graduates are much less likely to have had a child out-of-wedlock than those with less education.

Among men aged 15 to 44 with children, more than one-third have had a child out of wedlock

(percent distribution of men aged 15 to 44 who have had at least one child, by relationship with child's mother at first child's birth, 2002

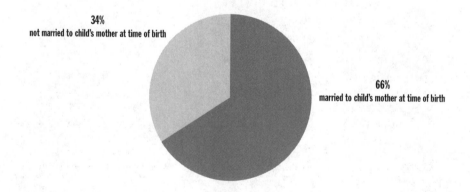

34%
not married to child's mother at time of birth

66%
married to child's mother at time of birth

Table 10.32 Women Who Have Ever Had a Nonmarital Birth, 2002

(number of women aged 15 to 44 who have had at least one live birth, and percent who have ever borne a child outside of wedlock, by selected characteristics, 2002; numbers in thousands)

	total	percent ever having nonmarital birth
Total women aged 15 to 44 who have had at least one birth	**35,938**	**42.2%**
Age at interview		
Aged 15 to 19	771	92.2
Aged 20 to 24	3,240	68.4
Aged 25 to 29	5,599	54.2
Aged 30 to 34	7,521	41.2
Aged 35 to 39	9,016	35.8
Aged 40 to 44	9,791	29.2
Race and Hispanic origin		
Black, non-Hispanic	5,218	80.9
Hispanic	6,159	50.6
White, non-Hispanic	22,047	30.1
Education		
Not a high school graduate	11,056	51.2
High school graduate or GED	13,770	39.6
Some college, no degree	6,532	40.8
Bachelor's degree or more	4,308	27.8
Religion raised		
No religion	2,229	49.3
Fundamentalist Protestant	2,266	47.0
Other Protestant	16,359	43.4
Catholic	13,189	39.6
Other religion	1,736	32.4
Family structure at age 14		
Living with both parents	25,468	35.1
Other	10,471	59.4

Note: Education categories include only people aged 22 to 44.
Source: National Center for Health Statistics, Fertility, Family Planning, and Reproductive Health of U.S. Women: Data from the 2002 National Survey of Family Growth, Vital and Health Statistics, Series 23, No. 25, 2005; Internet site http://www.cdc.gov/nchs/nsfg.htm

Table 10.33 Men Who Have Ever Had a Biological Child Outside of Marriage, 2002

(total number of men aged 15 to 44, percent who have had at least one biological child outside of marriage, and percent with paternity established for at least one child, by selected characteristics, 2002; numbers in thousands)

	total	percent with at least one biological child outside of marriage	percent with paternity established for at least one child
Total men aged 15 to 44	**61,147**	**18.5%**	**14.0%**
Age			
Aged 15 to 19	10,208	1.7	1.5
Aged 20 to 24	9,883	12.8	10.9
Aged 25 to 29	9,226	24.8	21.7
Aged 30 to 44	31,830	23.9	16.7
Marital or cohabiting status			
Currently married	25,808	21.2	15.3
First marriage	21,409	19.1	14.1
Second or higher marriage	4,399	31.8	20.9
Currently cohabiting	5,653	49.9	42.6
Never married, not cohabiting	25,412	7.2	5.7
Formerly married, not cohabiting	4,274	27.9	18.0
Race and Hispanic origin			
Black, non-Hispanic	6,940	36.1	29.1
Hispanic	10,188	29.2	23.1
White, non-Hispanic	38,738	12.4	8.9
Education			
Not a high school graduate	6,355	46.9	33.5
High school graduate or GED	15,659	30.6	23.4
Some college, no degree	13,104	17.0	13.3
Bachelor's degree or more	11,901	5.9	3.9

Note: Education categories include only people aged 22 to 44.
Source: National Center for Health Statistics, Fertility, Contraception, and Fatherhood: Data on Men and Women from Cycle 6 of the 2002 National Survey of Family Growth, Vital and Health Statistics, Series 23, No. 26, 2006; Internet site http://www.cdc.gov/nchs/nsfg.htm

Table 10.34 Women's Marital Status at First Child's Birth, 2002

(number of women aged 15 to 44 who have had at least one live birth, and percent distribution by marital or cohabiting status with child's father at time of delivery of first birth, by selected characteristics, 2002; numbers in thousands)

	total		married to child's father at delivery	premarital first birth		
					living with child's father at delivery	not married or living with child's father at delivery
	number	percent		total		
Total women aged 15 to 44 with at least one birth	**35,938**	**100.0%**	**60.4%**	**39.6%**	**12.4%**	**27.2%**
Age of mother at first birth						
Under age 18	5,069	100.0	21.4	78.7	18.5	60.2
Aged 18 to 19	5,984	100.0	36.6	63.5	20.7	42.8
Aged 20 to 24	12,289	100.0	63.2	36.8	13.4	23.4
Aged 25 to 29	8,039	100.0	81.9	18.1	5.3	12.8
Aged 30 to 44	4,558	100.0	89.2	10.8	4.6	6.2
Race and Hispanic origin of mother						
Black, non-Hispanic	5,218	100.0	21.3	78.7	15.0	63.7
Hispanic	6,159	100.0	50.9	49.1	22.4	26.7
White, non-Hispanic	22,047	100.0	72.7	27.3	9.1	18.2
Education of mother						
Not a high school graduate	11,056	100.0	52.1	47.9	15.2	32.7
High school grad. or GED	13,770	100.0	63.0	37.0	10.6	26.4
Some college, no degree	6,532	100.0	61.4	38.6	12.3	26.3
Bachelor's degree or more	4,308	100.0	73.5	26.5	9.4	17.1

Note: Education categories include only people aged 22 to 44.
Source: National Center for Health Statistics, Fertility, Family Planning, and Reproductive Health of U.S. Women: Data from the 2002 National Survey of Family Growth, Vital and Health Statistics, Series 23, No. 25, 2005; Internet site http://www.cdc .gov/nchs/nsfg.htm

Table 10.35 Men's Marital Status at First Child's Birth, 2002

(number of men aged 15 to 44 who have fathered at least one biological child and percent distribution by marital or cohabiting status with child's mother at first child's birth, by selected characteristics, 2002; numbers in thousands)

| | total | | currently or formerly married to child's mother | premarital first birth | | |
| | | | | total | cohabiting with child's mother | living alone or apart from child's mother |
	number	percent				
Total men aged 15 to 44 with at least one biological child	**28,554**	**100.0%**	**66.2%**	**33.8%**	**18.2%**	**15.6%**
Age of father at first birth						
Under age 18	1,227	100.0	36.0	64.0	23.2	40.8
Aged 18 to 19	3,147	100.0	38.4	61.6	27.6	34.1
Aged 20 to 24	10,113	100.0	52.2	47.8	27.1	20.7
Aged 25 to 29	8,162	100.0	81.9	18.1	11.4	6.8
Aged 30 to 44	5,905	100.0	89.6	10.5	6.2	4.2
Race and Hispanic origin of father						
Black, non-Hispanic	3,439	100.0	36.7	63.3	24.2	39.1
Hispanic	5,652	100.0	51.7	48.4	32.1	16.2
White, non-Hispanic	16,998	100.0	77.2	22.8	12.4	10.4
Religion raised						
None	1,841	100.0	72.3	27.7	10.8	16.9
Fundamentalist Protestant	1,334	100.0	54.0	46.0	18.2	27.9
Other Protestant	13,150	100.0	70.9	29.1	14.7	14.4
Catholic	10,512	100.0	59.8	40.2	25.2	15.0
Other religion	1,624	100.0	74.7	25.3	9.1	16.2

Source: National Center for Health Statistics, Fertility, Contraception, and Fatherhood: Data on Men and Women from Cycle 6 of the 2002 National Survey of Family Growth, Vital and Health Statistics, Series 23, No. 26, 2006; Internet site http://www.cdc.gov/nchs/nsfg.htm

Nearly One-Third of Women Have Had an Unwanted or Mistimed Birth

Less educated women are much more likely to have had an unwanted or mistimed birth.

Most births are wanted, but a substantial 31 percent of women aged 15 to 44 have had an unwanted or mistimed birth. The younger a woman was when she first had sexual intercourse, the more likely she has had an unwanted or mistimed birth. Forty-five percent of black women compared with only 26 percent of non-Hispanic whites have had an unwanted or mistimed birth. Fully 61 percent of high school dropouts say they have had an unwanted or mistimed birth compared with only 18 percent of college graduates.

Among all births in the past five years to women aged 15 to 44, 65 percent were intended at conception, 21 percent were mistimed, and 14 percent were unwanted. Among births to women under age 18, only 12 percent were intended. Among births to women aged 30 to 44, fully 78 percent were intended.

■ Among women who had an unintended pregnancy in the past few years and were not using contraception, 46 percent thought they could not get pregnant and 31 percent did not expect to have sex.

Most births are wanted by both mother and father

(percent distribution of births to women aged 15 to 44 in the past five years, by couple agreement on intendedness of birth, 2002)

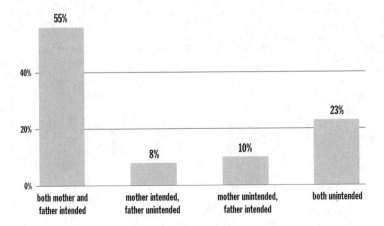

Table 10.36 Women Who Have Ever Had an Unwanted or Mistimed Birth, 2002

(number of women aged 15 to 44, and percentage who have ever had an unwanted or mistimed birth, by selected characteristics, 2002; numbers in thousands)

	total		unwanted or mistimed		
	number	percent	total	unwanted	mistimed
Total women aged 15 to 44	**61,561**	**100.0%**	**30.8%**	**12.4%**	**23.2%**
Under age 20	9,834	100.0	6.9	1.8	5.2
Aged 20 to 24	9,840	100.0	22.3	6.9	17.7
Aged 25 to 44	41,887	100.0	38.3	16.2	28.8
Age at first sexual intercourse					
Under age 16	10,475	100.0	54.7	26.2	39.8
Aged 16	6,678	100.0	47.4	17.8	37.5
Aged 17	6,262	100.0	38.4	13.4	29.9
Aged 18	5,539	100.0	30.6	14.4	22.4
Aged 19	3,291	100.0	33.9	17.6	21.7
Aged 20 or older	8,817	100.0	22.2	7.4	17.5
Race and Hispanic origin					
Black, non-Hispanic	8,250	100.0	44.9	24.7	30.2
Hispanic	9,107	100.0	40.1	18.1	28.8
White, non-Hispanic	39,498	100.0	26.0	8.7	20.8
Education					
Not a high school graduate	4,850	100.0	61.2	30.7	44.4
High school graduate or GED	12,725	100.0	49.5	21.0	38.0
Some college, no degree	12,276	100.0	37.5	16.2	27.2
Bachelor's degree or more	12,037	100.0	18.2	5.4	14.2

Note: Education categories include only people aged 22 to 44.
Source: National Center for Health Statistics, Fertility, Family Planning, and Reproductive Health of U.S. Women: Data from the 2002 National Survey of Family Growth, Vital and Health Statistics, Series 23, No. 25, 2005; Internet site http://www.cdc .gov/nchs/nsfg.htm

Table 10.37   Unintended Pregnancies Resulting in Live Births by Why Contraception Was Not Used, 2002

(number of women aged 15 to 44 who had an unintended pregnancy leading to a live birth in January 1999 or later and who were not using a method of contraception at the time of pregnancy, and percent distribution by reason for not using contraception, by selected characteristics, 2002; numbers in thousands)

	total		did not think you could get pregnant	did not expect to have sex	did not really mind it if you got pregnant	male partner didn't want to use birth control	male partner didn't want you to use birth control	worried about side effects of birth control
	number	percent						
Women having unintended pregnancy leading to live birth	**2,200**	**100.0%**	**45.6%**	**30.9%**	**17.3%**	**7.7%**	**5.6%**	**5.4%**
Age at birth								
Under age 25	1,242	100.0	49.1	32.9	15.6	6.3	7.6	3.6
Aged 25 or older	957	100.0	41.0	28.2	19.6	9.5	3.0	7.8
Marital status at birth								
Married	1,035	100.0	48.2	22.0	23.9	7.6	4.7	4.1
Cohabiting	402	100.0	57.4	15.1	16.5	11.4	9.2	10.2
Neither married, not cohabiting	763	100.0	35.8	51.2	8.8	5.9	4.7	4.7
Race and Hispanic origin								
Black, non-Hispanic	451	100.0	34.6	45.6	10.8	7.4	–	6.5
Hispanic	633	100.0	50.0	26.8	13.2	8.8	6.8	6.1
White, non-Hispanic	997	100.0	45.6	28.2	23.3	7.5	–	5.1
Education								
High school graduate or less	1,104	100.0	42.3	32.4	17.7	6.2	5.3	5.2
Some college or more	683	100.0	49.5	23.7	23.3	8.7	–	5.7

Note: Education categories include only people aged 22 to 44. "–" means sample is too small to make a reliable estimate. Figures will not sum to 100 because more than one reason may have been given.
Source: National Center for Health Statistics, Fertility, Family Planning, and Reproductive Health of U.S. Women: Data from the 2002 National Survey of Family Growth, Vital and Health Statistics, Series 23, No. 25, 2005; Internet site http://www.cdc .gov/nchs/nsfg.htm

Table 10.38 Births by Wantedness Status and Mother's Age, 2002

(number of births in past five years to women aged 15 to 44, and percent distribution by wantedness status at conception, by age at birth, 2002; numbers in thousands)

| | total | | | | mistimed | | |
	number	percent	intended	unwanted	total	less than two years too soon	two or more years too soon
Total births	**21,018**	**100.0%**	**64.9%**	**14.1%**	**20.8%**	**8.0%**	**12.1%**
Under age 18	921	100.0	11.9	25.4	62.7	7.0	53.3
Aged 18 to 19	1,294	100.0	28.6	18.6	52.9	10.4	41.4
Aged 20 to 24	5,553	100.0	55.8	17.2	26.9	9.4	16.3
Aged 25 to 29	5,726	100.0	73.0	10.4	16.3	8.8	7.6
Aged 30 to 44	7,524	100.0	78.2	12.6	9.0	6.1	2.4

Source: National Center for Health Statistics, Fertility, Family Planning, and Reproductive Health of U.S. Women: Data from the 2002 National Survey of Family Growth, Vital and Health Statistics, Series 23, No. 25, 2005; Internet site http://www.cdc.gov/nchs/nsfg.htm

Table 10.39 Children by Wantedness Status and Father's Age, 2002

(number of children fathered in past five years by men aged 15 to 44, and percent distribution by wantedness status at conception, by father's age at child's birth, 2002; numbers in thousands)

| | total | | wanted | unwanted | mistimed | did not know about child until after birth |
	number	percent				
Total children	**19,962**	**100.0%**	**65.2%**	**8.6%**	**24.8%**	**1.2%**
Under age 18	209	100.0	31.2	–	52.8	–
Aged 18 to 19	630	100.0	39.5	11.2	38.4	11.0
Aged 20 to 24	3,790	100.0	48.2	7.1	41.4	3.3
Aged 25 to 29	5,648	100.0	65.0	6.1	28.7	–
Aged 30 to 44	9,685	100.0	74.4	10.5	14.5	–

Note: "–" means sample is too small to make a reliable estimate.
Source: National Center for Health Statistics, Fertility, Contraception, and Fatherhood: Data on Men and Women from Cycle 6 of the 2002 National Survey of Family Growth, Vital and Health Statistics, Series 23, No. 26, 2006; Internet site http://www.cdc.gov/nchs/nsfg.htm

Table 10.40 **Births by Wantedness Status and Mother's Marital Status at Birth, 2002**

(number of births in past five years to women aged 15 to 44, and percent distribution by wantedness status at conception, by marital status at birth, 2002; numbers in thousands)

	total				mistimed		
	number	percent	intended	unwanted	total	less than two years too soon	two or more years too soon
Total births	**21,018**	**100.0%**	**64.9%**	**14.1%**	**20.8%**	**8.0%**	**12.1%**
Married	13,534	100.0	76.6	9.0	14.1	8.4	5.3
Cohabiting	2,998	100.0	48.8	18.1	33.2	8.2	24.2
Never married, not cohabiting	3,510	100.0	35.3	28.5	36.1	5.4	28.9
Formerly married, not cohabiting	976	100.0	58.2	21.2	20.1	10.7	9.0

Source: National Center for Health Statistics, Fertility, Family Planning, and Reproductive Health of U.S. Women: Data from the 2002 National Survey of Family Growth, Vital and Health Statistics, Series 23, No. 25, 2005; Internet site http://www.cdc .gov/nchs/nsfg.htm

Table 10.41 **Children by Wantedness Status and Father's Marital Status at Birth, 2002**

(number of children fathered in past five years by men aged 15 to 44, and percent distribution by wantedness status at conception, by father's marital status at child's birth, 2002; numbers in thousands)

	total		wanted	unwanted	mistimed	did not know about child until after birth
	number	percent				
Total children	**19,962**	**100.0%**	**65.2%**	**8.6%**	**24.8%**	**1.2%**
Married to child's mother	14,267	100.0	69.9	7.4	22.4	–
Cohabiting with child's mother	3,955	100.0	61.1	10.5	28.4	–
Living alone or apart from child's mother	1,740	100.0	36.3	14.0	36.2	13.5

Note: "–" means sample is too small to make a reliable estimate.
Source: National Center for Health Statistics, Fertility, Contraception, and Fatherhood: Data on Men and Women from Cycle 6 of the 2002 National Survey of Family Growth, Vital and Health Statistics, Series 23, No. 26, 2006; Internet site http://www.cdc .gov/nchs/nsfg.htm

Table 10.42 Births by Wantedness Status and Birth Order, 2002

(number of births in past five years to women aged 15 to 44, and percent distribution by wantedness status at conception, by birth order, 2002; numbers in thousands)

	total				mistimed		
	number	percent	intended	unwanted	total	less than two years too soon	two or more years too soon
Total births	**21,018**	**100.0%**	**64.9%**	**14.1%**	**20.8%**	**8.0%**	**12.1%**
First birth	8,481	100.0	63.9	8.5	27.6	8.3	18.3
Second birth	7,116	100.0	71.4	11.3	17.2	8.2	8.6
Third or higher birth	5,421	100.0	57.9	26.6	14.8	7.2	7.0

Source: National Center for Health Statistics, Fertility, Family Planning, and Reproductive Health of U.S. Women: Data from the 2002 National Survey of Family Growth, Vital and Health Statistics, Series 23, No. 25, 2005; Internet site http://www.cdc .gov/nchs/nsfg.htm

Table 10.43 Births by Wantedness Status and Mother's Race and Hispanic Origin, 2002

(number of births in past five years to women aged 15 to 44, and percent distribution by wantedness status at conception, by race and Hispanic origin, 2002; numbers in thousands)

| | total | | intended | unwanted | mistimed | | |
	number	percent			total	less than two years too soon	two or more years too soon
Total births	**21,018**	**100.0%**	**64.9%**	**14.1%**	**20.8%**	**8.0%**	**12.1%**
Black, non-Hispanic	2,818	100.0	49.1	26.2	24.6	4.9	19.1
Hispanic	4,242	100.0	56.4	16.8	26.5	10.7	14.2
White, non-Hispanic	12,309	100.0	70.9	10.7	18.1	7.9	9.9

Source: National Center for Health Statistics, Fertility, Family Planning, and Reproductive Health of U.S. Women: Data from the 2002 National Survey of Family Growth, Vital and Health Statistics, Series 23, No. 25, 2005; Internet site http://www.cdc.gov/nchs/nsfg.htm

Table 10.44 Children Fathered by Wantedness Status and Father's Race and Hispanic Origin, 2002

(number of children fathered in past five years by men aged 15 to 44, and percent distribution by wantedness status at conception, by father's race and Hispanic origin, 2002; numbers in thousands)

| | total | | wanted | unwanted | mistimed | did not know about child until after birth |
	number	percent				
Total children	**19,962**	**100.0%**	**65.2%**	**8.6%**	**24.8%**	**1.2%**
Black, non-Hispanic	2,151	100.0	55.8	9.0	32.7	2.5
Hispanic	4,460	100.0	57.5	12.3	27.6	2.6
White, non-Hispanic	11,390	100.0	67.3	7.6	24.8	–

Note: "–" means sample is too small to make a reliable estimate.
Source: National Center for Health Statistics, Fertility, Contraception, and Fatherhood: Data on Men and Women from Cycle 6 of the 2002 National Survey of Family Growth, Vital and Health Statistics, Series 23, No. 26, 2006; Internet site http://www.cdc.gov/nchs/nsfg.htm

Table 10.45 Births by Wantedness Status and Mother's Education, 2002

(number of births in past five years to women aged 22 to 44, and percent distribution by wantedness status at conception, by education, 2002; numbers in thousands)

	total				mistimed		
	number	percent	intended	unwanted	total	less than two years too soon	two or more years too soon
Total births	**18,998**	**100.0%**	**69.3%**	**13.4%**	**17.1%**	**8.0%**	**8.7%**
Not a high school graduate	3,023	100.0	57.7	19.1	22.7	7.2	15.1
High school grad. or GED	5,823	100.0	64.1	16.1	19.7	7.5	11.6
Some college, no degree	5,194	100.0	66.5	13.9	19.3	10.8	8.1
Bachelor's degree or more	4,957	100.0	85.3	6.0	8.5	6.3	1.8

Source: National Center for Health Statistics, Fertility, Family Planning, and Reproductive Health of U.S. Women: Data from the 2002 National Survey of Family Growth, Vital and Health Statistics, Series 23, No. 25, 2005; Internet site http://www.cdc .gov/nchs/nsfg.htm

Table 10.46 Children Fathered by Wantedness Status and Father's Education, 2002

(number of children fathered in past five years by men aged 15 to 44, and percent distribution by wantedness status at conception, by father's education, 2002; numbers in thousands)

	total		wanted	unwanted	mistimed	did not know about child until after birth
	number	percent				
Total children	**19,962**	**100.0%**	**65.2%**	**8.6%**	**24.8%**	**1.2%**
Not a high school graduate	3,051	100.0	57.3	15.5	26.1	–
High school grad. or GED	6,641	100.0	56.4	9.1	32.6	1.2
Some college, no degree	4,947	100.0	65.7	5.9	27.2	–
Bachelor's degree or more	4,478	100.0	86.9	6.5	6.6	–

Note: Education categories include only people aged 22 to 44. "–" means sample is too small to make a reliable estimate.
Source: National Center for Health Statistics, Fertility, Contraception, and Fatherhood: Data on Men and Women from Cycle 6 of the 2002 National Survey of Family Growth, Vital and Health Statistics, Series 23, No. 26, 2006; Internet site http://www.cdc .gov/nchs/nsfg.htm

Table 10.47 Births by Wantedness Status and Mother's Religion, 2002

(number of births in past five years to women aged 15 to 44, and percent distribution by wantedness status at conception, by mother's religion, 2002; numbers in thousands)

	total				mistimed		
	number	percent	intended	unwanted	total	less than two years too soon	two or more years too soon
Total births	**21,018**	**100.0%**	**64.9%**	**14.1%**	**20.8%**	**8.0%**	**12.1%**
No religion	1,423	100.0	61.4	16.4	22.2	6.0	16.2
Fundamentalist Protestant	1,391	100.0	55.0	20.1	24.9	8.2	14.9
Other Protestant	9,101	100.0	64.7	13.3	21.8	8.8	12.4
Catholic	7,777	100.0	66.4	13.9	19.3	7.7	10.8
Other religion	1,239	100.0	72.3	12.4	15.3	6.0	9.3

Source: National Center for Health Statistics, Fertility, Family Planning, and Reproductive Health of U.S. Women: Data from the 2002 National Survey of Family Growth, Vital and Health Statistics, Series 23, No. 25, 2005; Internet site http://www.cdc .gov/nchs/nsfg.htm

Table 10.48 Births by Couple Agreement on Intendedness of Birth, 2002

(number of births in the past five years to women aged 15 to 44, and percent distribution by couple agreement on intendedness of birth, by selected characteristics, 2002; numbers in thousands)

	total		both intended	mother intended, father unintended	mother unintended, father intended	both unintended
	number	percent				
Total births	21,018	100.0%	55.2%	8.1%	10.1%	22.6%
Age of mother at birth						
Under age 18	921	100.0	9.2	1.9	16.1	64.6
Aged 18 to 19	1,294	100.0	20.7	7.7	13.6	54.4
Aged 20 to 24	5,553	100.0	44.6	9.2	12.2	29.4
Aged 25 to 29	5,726	100.0	61.5	9.7	9.7	15.3
Aged 30 to 44	7,524	100.0	69.8	6.8	7.4	12.6
Marital status at birth						
Married	13,534	100.0	68.8	6.5	8.0	13.6
Cohabiting	2,998	100.0	37.1	10.2	14.3	34.3
Never married, not cohabiting	3,510	100.0	21.6	11.4	12.0	48.1
Formerly married, not cohabiting	976	100.0	43.1	10.8	19.0	21.0
Birth order						
First birth	8,481	100.0	53.9	8.0	9.7	24.3
Second birth	7,116	100.0	64.3	6.5	8.7	18.3
Third or higher birth	5,421	100.0	45.3	10.3	12.5	25.8
Race and Hispanic origin of mother						
Black, non-Hispanic	2,818	100.0	39.4	7.9	15.5	31.5
Hispanic	4,242	100.0	48.7	7.2	15.4	26.2
White, non-Hispanic	12,309	100.0	60.9	8.0	7.7	19.0
Education at interview						
Not a high school graduate	3,023	100.0	46.4	10.0	15.1	24.1
High school graduate or GED	5,823	100.0	51.2	11.2	10.8	22.0
Some college, no degree	5,194	100.0	57.1	6.8	9.1	22.7
Bachelor's degree or more	4,957	100.0	78.7	5.6	5.0	8.4

Note: Education categories include only people aged 22 to 44. Figures will not sum to 100 because "unknown" intent is not shown.
Source: National Center for Health Statistics, Fertility, Family Planning, and Reproductive Health of U.S. Women: Data from the 2002 National Survey of Family Growth, Vital and Health Statistics, Series 23, No. 25, 2005; Internet site http://www.cdc .gov/nchs/nsfg.htm

Most Women Wait Two or More Years between First and Second Births

Only 4 percent have the second birth within a year of the first.

American women plan their families by spacing their childbearing. Among women aged 15 to 44 who have had at least two children, fully 70 percent waited at least two years before having their second child. A substantial 30 percent waited four years or more before having number two.

Some women, of course, do not have any choice about having child number two or three right away. The rate of twin, triplet, and higher-order births has climbed over the past few years. The twin birth rate rose 39 percent between 1990 and 2003. The triplet and higher-order birth rate more than doubled during those years.

■ Fertility treatments have boosted the rate of twin and higher-order births, especially among older women.

Multiple births are more common among older women

(number of triplet or higher-order births per 100,000 live births, by age, 2003)

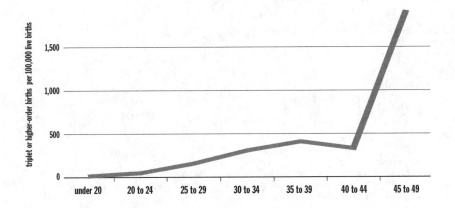

Table 10.49 Timing of Second Delivery Relative to First, 2002

(percent distribution of women aged 15 to 44 who have had at least two live births by number of months from first birth to second birth, by selected characteristics, 2002)

	total	interval between first and second deliveries				
		less than 12 months	13 to 24 months	25 to 36 months	37 to 48 months	49 or more months
Total women aged 15 to 44 who have had at least two deliveries	100.0%	4.1%	26.1%	24.0%	15.8%	30.2%
Age at first birth						
Under age 18	100.0	6.4	26.4	21.0	15.3	31.0
Aged 18 to 19	100.0	4.0	20.4	23.5	14.4	37.7
Aged 20 to 24	100.0	4.5	26.1	22.9	15.5	31.1
Aged 25 to 29	100.0	1.7	27.8	28.0	15.6	27.0
Aged 30 to 44	100.0	3.5	33.7	24.9	21.6	16.3
Race and Hispanic origin						
Black, non-Hispanic	100.0	5.9	23.8	23.0	14.1	33.1
Hispanic	100.0	5.5	24.7	19.3	17.3	33.0
White, non-Hispanic	100.0	2.8	27.5	25.3	16.2	28.3
Education						
Not a high school graduate	100.0	7.3	31.4	20.3	13.0	28.0
High school graduate or GED	100.0	4.4	22.7	22.5	15.5	34.9
Some college, no degree	100.0	3.3	26.4	24.6	15.9	29.7
Bachelor's degree or more	100.0	1.1	26.1	28.0	18.5	26.3
Religion raised						
No religion	100.0	3.7	33.3	18.6	16.6	27.7
Fundamentalist Protestant	100.0	3.8	29.6	24.3	16.9	31.7
Other Protestant	100.0	3.6	26.6	26.6	14.1	29.1
Catholic	100.0	5.0	24.2	21.3	14.2	28.8
Other religion	100.0	1.8	23.9	24.8	19.3	30.2

Note: A delivery may consist of multiple births.
Source: National Center for Health Statistics, Fertility, Family Planning, and Reproductive Health of U.S. Women: Data from the 2002 National Survey of Family Growth, Vital and Health Statistics, Series 23, No. 25, 2005; Internet site http://www.cdc .gov/nchs/nsfg.htm; calculations by New Strategist

Table 10.50 Twin and Higher-Order Multiple Births, 1990 and 2003

(number of twin births per 1,000 live births, and number of triplet and higher-order multiple births per 100,000 live births, by age, race, and Hispanic origin, 1990 and 2003; percent change, 1990–2003)

	twin births (number per 1,000 live births)			triplet and higher-order births (number per 100,000 live births)		
	2003	1990	percent change 1990–2003	2003	1990	percent change 1990–2003
Total	**31.5**	**22.6**	**39.4%**	**187.4**	**72.8**	**157.4%**
Under age 20	15.3	14.3	7.0	12.8	15.9	–19.5
Aged 20 to 24	22.4	19.2	16.7	48.4	32.4	49.4
Aged 25 to 29	29.6	23.5	26.0	158.9	73.9	115.0
Aged 30 to 34	39.2	27.6	42.0	309.1	126.3	144.7
Aged 35 to 39	47.8	30.2	58.3	409.5	156.8	161.2
Aged 40 to 44	51.3	24.7	107.7	330.7	–	–
Aged 45 to 49	189.2	23.8	695.0	1,919.6	–	–
Aged 50 to 54	374.6	344.8	8.6	–	–	–
Race and Hispanic origin						
Asian	25.7	16.4	56.7	111.7	43.1	159.2
Black	34.4	26.5	29.8	108.4	46.9	131.1
Hispanic	21.3	18.0	18.3	85.9	39.5	117.5
White, non-Hispanic	35.2	22.9	53.7	255.0	89.8	184.0

Note: "–" means data are not available or sample is too small to make a reliable estimate.
Source: National Center for Health Statistics, Health United States 2005; Internet site http://www.cdc.gov/nchs/hus.htm; calculations by New Strategist

Breastfeeding Is Increasing

Two-thirds of newborns are breastfed.

More babies are being breastfed as doctors and nutritionists encourage the practice. The percentage of newborns who are breastfed increased from 53 to 67 percent between 1989–91 and 1999–2001.

The likelihood of breastfeeding varies by the mother's demographic characteristics. Older mothers are much more likely to breastfeed than younger ones, for example. Only 54 percent of babies born between 1997 and 2002 to women under age 20 were breastfed compared with 78 percent of those born to women aged 30 to 44. Black babies are least likely to be breastfed (47 percent), Hispanic babies most (75 percent). Education plays perhaps the biggest role in determining breastfeeding, with 84 percent of babies born to college graduates being breastfed versus only 50 percent of babies born to women who did not graduate from high school.

■ Only 17 percent of babies are breastfed for one year or more.

Breastfeeding is more likely for babies born to college graduates

(percent of singleton babies born to women aged 15 to 44 between 1997 and 2002 who were breastfed, by education of mother, 2002)

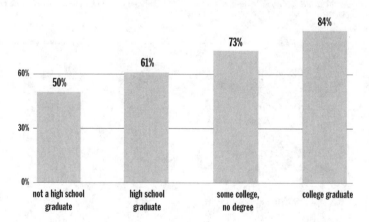

Table 10.51　Breastfeeding Trends, 1989–91 and 1999–2001

(percent of babies born to women aged 15 to 44 during specified years who were breastfed, by selected charac-teristics, 1989–91 and 1999–01; percentage point change, 1989–91 to 1999–01)

| | percent breastfed | | |
	1999–2001	1989–91	percentage point change
Total babies	**66.5%**	**53.3%**	**13.2**
Age at time of birth			
Under age 20	47.3	34.7	12.6
Aged 20 to 24	59.3	44.3	15.0
Aged 25 to 29	63.5	56.4	7.1
Aged 30 to 44	80.0	66.0	14.0
Race and Hispanic origin			
Black, non-Hispanic	45.3	22.4	22.9
Hispanic	76.0	57.0	19.0
White, non-Hispanic	68.7	58.4	10.3
Education at interview			
Not a high school graduate	46.6	36.5	10.1
High school graduate or GED	61.6	45.5	16.1
Some college, no degree	75.6	61.4	14.2
Bachelor's degree or more	81.3	80.6	0.7
Region			
Northeast	66.9	53.5	13.4
Midwest	61.9	49.6	12.3
South	60.9	43.6	17.3
West	78.9	69.5	9.4

Source: National Center for Health Statistics, Health United States 2005; Internet site http://www.cdc.gov/nchs/hus.htm; calculations by New Strategist

Table 10.52 Breastfeeding by Selected Characteristics, 2002

(number of singleton babies born to women aged 15 to 44 between 1997 and 2000, and percent distribution by duration of breastfeeding, by selected characteristics, 2002; numbers in thousands)

	total number	total percent	not breastfed at all	total breastfed	duration of breastfeeding 2 months or less	3 to 5 months	6 to 11 months	12 months or more
Total babies	16,475	100.0%	33.3%	66.8%	18.7%	13.1%	17.6%	17.3%
Age at time of birth								
Under age 18	743	100.0	46.1	54.0	23.0	9.0	10.5	11.5
Aged 18 to 19	1,108	100.0	46.5	53.5	20.6	13.6	8.6	10.8
Aged 20 to 24	4,297	100.0	43.5	56.5	17.2	12.6	15.9	10.9
Aged 25 to 29	4,501	100.0	32.2	67.8	22.5	13.4	18.2	13.7
Aged 30 to 44	5,826	100.0	22.5	77.5	16.0	13.8	21.1	26.8
Marital or cohabiting status at time of birth								
Married	10,560	100.0	26.0	74.0	18.7	14.2	19.8	21.3
Cohabiting	3,683	100.0	42.8	57.3	21.5	13.8	12.6	9.4
Neither	2,232	100.0	48.5	51.5	17.0	9.8	14.5	10.3
Wantedness status at conception								
Intended	10,812	100.0	30.1	69.9	18.5	13.8	18.7	18.8
Mistimed	3,328	100.0	36.1	63.9	20.3	14.4	15.1	14.1
Unwanted	2,335	100.0	43.9	56.2	17.2	8.1	16.1	14.8
Maternity leave for this birth								
Not employed during pregnancy	6,925	100.0	32.9	67.1	15.8	11.5	16.1	23.7
Employed during pregnancy	9,527	100.0	33.5	66.5	20.8	14.3	18.8	12.7
Took six weeks leave or less	2,536	100.0	42.3	57.7	26.2	8.7	14.0	8.8
Took longer than six weeks leave	4,116	100.0	29.6	70.4	19.6	17.9	21.0	11.9
No leave taken	2,849	100.0	31.0	69.0	17.9	14.1	19.8	17.2
Race and Hispanic origin								
Black, non-Hispanic	2,322	100.0	53.4	46.7	15.3	11.3	13.5	6.5
Hispanic	3,283	100.0	25.3	74.7	23.5	13.3	20.0	17.9
White, non-Hispanic	9,735	100.0	31.3	68.7	18.6	13.1	18.0	19.0
Education at interview								
Not a high school graduate	2,416	100.0	50.5	49.5	15.3	8.5	15.1	10.7
High school graduate or GED	5,148	100.0	39.1	60.9	17.0	13.0	13.6	17.4
Some college, no degree	4,235	100.0	27.1	72.9	22.1	12.5	19.4	18.9
Bachelor's degree or more	3,660	100.0	16.5	83.5	19.7	16.9	25.0	21.9
Region of residence at interview								
Northeast	2,060	100.0	33.2	66.8	13.8	11.1	22.8	19.1
Midwest	3,921	100.0	33.7	66.3	19.8	12.4	15.9	18.3
South	6,455	100.0	40.3	59.7	18.7	13.2	14.5	13.2
West	4,039	100.0	21.5	78.5	20.1	14.8	21.7	21.9

Note: Education categories include only people aged 22 to 44.
Source: National Center for Health Statistics, Fertility, Family Planning, and Reproductive Health of U.S. Women: Data from the 2002 National Survey of Family Growth, Vital and Health Statistics, Series 23, No. 25, 2005; Internet site http://www.cdc.gov/nchs/nsfg.htm

Most Working Women Take Maternity Leave

Some are not offered leave, however.

Among employed women aged 15 to 44 who gave birth between 1997 and 2002, a substantial 70 percent took maternity leave. That leaves 30 percent who did not take maternity leave for one reason or another. For 8 percent, maternity leave was not necessary because, for example, they were schoolteachers and had their baby during summer break. Four percent did not take leave because they would have been fired or were part-time workers without leave benefits. Seventeen percent did not take leave for other reasons. This group includes women who quit their job after childbirth, could not afford to take leave, or worked right after delivery.

Most women aged 15 to 44 who gave birth between 1997 and 2002 paid for their most recent delivery with private insurance. A substantial 33 percent paid for their most recent delivery with Medicaid or government assistance, including the majority of blacks and Hispanics.

■ The women least likely to take maternity leave are younger, Hispanic, and lacking a high school diploma.

Medicaid or government assistance pays for one-third of deliveries

(percent distribution of live births to women aged 15 to 44 between 1997 and 2002, by method of payment for most recent delivery, 2002)

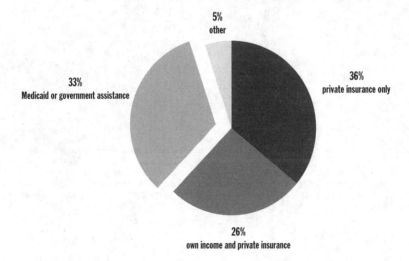

5%
other

36%
private insurance only

33%
Medicaid or government assistance

26%
own income and private insurance

Table 10.53 Use of Maternity Leave, 2002

(percent distribution of employed women aged 15 to 44 who had a live birth in January 1997 or later by use of maternity leave for most recent birth, by selected characteristics, 2002; numbers in thousands)

	total employed	took maternity leave	did not take leave total	not needed	not offered	other reasons
Employed women aged 15 to 44 who had a live birth	**100.0%**	**70.0%**	**29.8%**	**8.0%**	**4.4%**	**17.4%**
Age at time of birth						
Under age 20	100.0	51.3	48.7	12.6	13.9	22.2
Aged 20 to 24	100.0	60.7	39.1	8.0	6.6	24.5
Aged 25 to 29	100.0	74.8	25.2	5.3	3.0	16.9
Aged 30 to 44	100.0	74.4	25.6	9.4	2.7	13.6
Marital or cohabiting status at time of birth						
Married	100.0	72.4	27.6	8.8	2.8	16.1
Cohabiting	100.0	62.1	37.9	8.2	8.0	21.7
Never married, not cohabiting	100.0	62.9	37.1	5.8	8.1	23.3
Formerly married, not cohabiting	100.0	78.3	21.9	5.9	5.3	10.7
Birth order						
First birth	100.0	67.6	32.5	8.0	2.9	21.6
Second birth	100.0	73.6	26.4	7.2	5.8	13.4
Third or higher birth	100.0	69.4	30.6	9.8	4.7	16.2
Race and Hispanic origin						
Black, non-Hispanic	100.0	76.4	23.8	4.6	6.1	13.1
Hispanic	100.0	60.0	39.7	9.9	8.7	21.0
White, non-Hispanic	100.0	70.8	29.0	8.1	3.0	17.9
Education at interview						
Not a high school graduate	100.0	48.9	51.4	7.6	13.0	30.8
High school graduate or GED	100.0	72.2	27.8	7.7	3.9	16.1
Some college, no degree	100.0	71.8	28.4	5.6	4.3	18.4
Bachelor's degree or more	100.0	75.8	24.2	10.6	1.1	12.5

Note: Women who did not need maternity leave are those whose job schedules allowed them to deliver during a break, such as teachers during the summer; women who worked at home; and women who decided to quit their job after delivery. Women who were not offered maternity leave are those who would have been fired if they had taken leave and those whose job benefits did not include leave, such as part-time workers. Women reporting "other reasons" are those who quit their job before delivery, who could not afford to take leave, or who worked right after delivery. Education categories incude only people aged 22 to 44.
Source: National Center for Health Statistics, Fertility, Family Planning, and Reproductive Health of U.S. Women: Data from the 2002 National Survey of Family Growth, Vital and Health Statistics, Series 23, No. 25, 2005; Internet site http://www.cdc .gov/nchs/nsfg.htm

Table 10.54 Method of Payment for Most Recent Delivery, 2002

(number of women aged 15 to 44 who had a live birth in January 1997 or later, and percent distribution by method of payment for most recent delivery, by selected characteristics, 2002; numbers in thousands)

	total number	total percent	private insurance only	own income and private insurance	Medicaid or government assistance	all other
Total women aged 15 to 44 with a live birth	18,167	100.0%	36.0%	25.6%	33.4%	5.1%
Age at time of birth						
Under age 18	696	100.0	21.1	–	65.3	11.7
Aged 18 to 19	891	100.0	19.3	6.4	66.1	8.2
Aged 20 to 24	4,322	100.0	23.1	16.2	53.7	7.0
Aged 25 to 29	4,847	100.0	36.9	24.7	34.8	3.6
Aged 30 to 44	7,411	100.0	46.2	36.1	13.8	3.9
Marital status at time of birth						
Married	12,027	100.0	42.7	34.6	18.2	4.6
Cohabiting	2,412	100.0	20.2	8.9	66.3	4.5
Never married, not cohabiting	2,871	100.0	20.5	5.7	65.7	8.1
Formerly married, not cohabiting	858	100.0	37.4	12.7	46.7	3.1
Wantedness status at conception						
Intended	12,034	100.0	39.8	29.5	26.0	4.7
Mistimed	3,487	100.0	23.6	19.0	50.3	7.2
Unwanted	2,646	100.0	34.7	16.4	44.9	3.9
Race and Hispanic origin						
Black, non-Hispanic	2,352	100.0	31.5	10.3	54.8	3.5
Hispanic	3,656	100.0	28.8	9.5	54.1	7.6
White, non-Hispanic	10,748	100.0	38.8	35.1	21.9	4.3
Education at interview						
Not a high school graduate	2,298	100.0	22.2	3.2	67.1	7.5
High school graduate or GED	5,238	100.0	35.6	21.5	39.4	3.5
Some college, no degree	4,626	100.0	38.4	32.6	24.6	4.3
Bachelor's degree or more	4,299	100.0	47.5	43.1	5.0	4.4
Metropolitan residence						
Metropolitan, central city	9,704	100.0	40.8	29.6	25.6	4.0
Metropolitan, suburban	5,695	100.0	34.5	16.8	43.6	5.0
Nonmetropolitan	2,769	100.0	21.8	29.5	39.9	8.9

Note: "All other" are those paying with own funds only. Education categories include only people aged 22 to 44.
Source: National Center for Health Statistics, Fertility, Family Planning, and Reproductive Health of U.S. Women: Data from the 2002 National Survey of Family Growth, Vital and Health Statistics, Series 23, No. 25, 2005; Internet site http://www.cdc.gov/nchs/nsfg.htm

Most Men and Women Think Out-of-Wedlock Childbearing Is OK

Fundamentalist Protestant men are most disapproving.

American attitudes toward out-of-wedlock childbearing have changed over the years. Overall, 59 percent of men and 70 percent of women aged 15 to 44 think it is OK for an unmarried woman to have a child. Regardless of demographic characteristic, the majority of men and women think out-of-wedlock childbearing is acceptable, with a few exceptions. Among men, only 37 percent of fundamentalist Protestants think it is OK to have a child out-of-wedlock. A larger 49 percent of their female counterparts agree. Nonmarital childbearing is acceptable to only 45 percent of men (but 57 percent of women) for whom religion is very important.

Parenting is regarded almost universally as a rewarding experience. Ninety-four percent of men and women aged 15 to 44 agree that "the rewards of being a parent are worth it, despite the cost and the work it takes." There are few differences in this attitude by demographic characteristic.

■ Men and women who have not yet had children are slightly less likely than parents to agree that the rewards of parenting are worth the sacrifice.

The rewards of parenting are worth the sacrifice

(percent of people aged 15 to 44 who agree with the statement, "The rewards of being a parent are worth it, despite the cost and the work it takes," by sex and parenthood status, 2002)

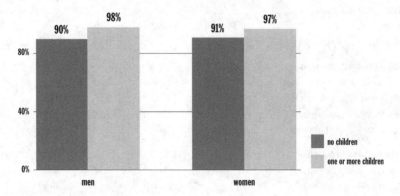

Table 10.55 Attitude toward Out-of-Wedlock Childbearing, 2002

"It is okay for an unmarried female to have a child."

(percent of people aged 15 to 44 who agree with statement, by selected characteristics and sex, 2002)

	percent agreeing	
	men	women
Total aged 15 to 44	**58.9%**	**69.6%**
Aged 15 to 19	49.9	64.8
Aged 20 to 24	63.9	74.7
Aged 25 to 29	64.0	76.0
Aged 30 to 44	58.7	67.5
Marital status		
Currently married	52.7	64.8
Currently cohabiting	75.7	82.2
Never married, not cohabiting	60.0	71.0
Formerly married, not cohabiting	66.8	74.7
Ever fathered/delivered a nonmarital birth		
Yes	60.6	77.0
No	58.5	67.1
Race and Hispanic origin		
Black, non-Hispanic	56.7	62.8
Hispanic	49.5	64.8
White, non-Hispanic	62.1	72.6
Education		
Not a high school graduate	50.7	65.6
High school graduate or GED	60.2	69.6
Some college, no degree	62.7	71.7
Bachelor's degree or more	62.6	71.5
Current religion		
No religion	73.2	85.5
Fundamentalist Protestant	36.9	48.5
Other Protestant	55.1	65.8
Catholic	58.6	71.5
Other religion	57.9	71.5
Importance of religion		
Very important	45.0	57.2
Somewhat important	62.4	79.2
Not important	73.5	86.1
Family structure at age 14		
Living with both parents	56.8	67.7
Other	64.8	74.0

Source: National Center for Health Statistics, Fertility, Contraception, and Fatherhood: Data on Men and Women from Cycle 6 of the 2002 National Survey of Family Growth, Vital and Health Statistics, Series 23, No. 26, 2006; Internet site http://www.cdc .gov/nchs/nsfg.htm

Table 10.56 Attitude toward the Rewards of Parenthood, 2002

"The rewards of being a parent are worth it,
despite the cost and the work it takes."

(percent of people aged 15 to 44 who agree with statement, by selected characteristics and sex, 2002)

	percent agreeing	
	men	women
Total aged 15 to 44	**93.8%**	**94.2%**
Aged 15 to 24	91.4	93.4
Aged 25 to 29	95.2	93.9
Aged 30 to 44	94.9	94.9
Marital status		
Currently married	97.6	96.0
First marriage	97.6	96.8
Second or later marriage	97.9	92.4
Currently cohabiting	91.0	92.6
Never married, not cohabiting	90.4	92.3
Formerly married, not cohabiting	94.4	94.7
Number of children		
No children	90.1	91.1
One or more children	97.9	96.5
Race and Hispanic origin		
Black, non-Hispanic	92.4	93.8
Hispanic	93.8	93.7
White, non-Hispanic	94.0	94.7
Education		
Not a high school graduate	94.4	93.5
High school graduate or GED	94.7	94.0
Some college, no degree	95.3	95.4
Bachelor's degree or more	94.1	95.1
Current religion		
No religion	88.4	90.4
Fundamentalist Protestant	96.2	98.2
Other Protestant	95.1	95.1
Catholic	94.8	94.4
Other religion	94.7	92.8
Importance of religion		
Very important	95.1	95.3
Somewhat important	95.6	95.1
Not important	89.9	90.3

Source: National Center for Health Statistics, Fertility, Contraception, and Fatherhood: Data on Men and Women from Cycle 6 of the 2002 National Survey of Family Growth, Vital and Health Statistics, Series 23, No. 26, 2006; Internet site http://www.cdc .gov/nchs/nsfg.htm

11

Caring for Children

■ The lives of the nation's children are becoming more diverse now that divorce, working parents, and day care are common.

■ Fewer children live with both parents. The percentage of American children who live with both parents fell from 85 to 67 percent between 1970 and 2005.

■ Adoption is rare. Although 33 percent of women aged 18 to 44 have considered adopting a child, only 1 percent have actually done so.

■ Caring for other people's children is common. Thirteen percent of women aged 18 to 44 have lived with and cared for a child to whom they did not give birth.

■ Many fathers live apart from their children. Among men aged 15 to 44 who have children under age 19, fully 27 percent live separately from some or all of their children.

■ Fathers have doubts about their parenting skills. Among men living with their children, only 46 percent say they are doing a "very good" job as a father.

■ Most parents work. Among married couples with children under age 18, the 61 percent majority are dual-income couples.

■ Relatives provide much childcare. Among working women with children under age 13, the most popular childcare provider is one of the child's grandparents or another relative, used by 35 percent in the past four weeks.

■ Traditional sex roles are out. Only about one-third of men and women aged 15 to 44 agree that traditional sex roles—where the man earns the living and the woman takes care of the home and family—are best.

Only 67 Percent of Children Live with Both Parents

Among blacks, the figure is just 36 percent.

The percentage of American children who live with both parents fell from 85 to 67 percent during the past 25 years. At the same time, the percentage of children who live with only their mother only climbed from 11 to 23 percent.

Asian children are most likely to live with both parents, and 82 percent do so. Among non-Hispanic whites, 76 percent live with both parents. For Hispanics, the proportion is a slightly smaller 65 percent. A minority of black children lives with both parents, while nearly half (49 percent) live with only their mother.

Slightly fewer than 6 percent of children live with their grandparents. Among those who live with a grandparent, the 56 percent majority also lives with their mother or with both parents. Just 39 percent of those living with a grandparent do not also have a parent in the home.

■ The living arrangements of children have become more diverse, and black children have the most diverse living arrangements of all.

Asian children are most likely to live with both parents

(percent of children under age 18 living with both parents, by race and Hispanic origin, 2005)

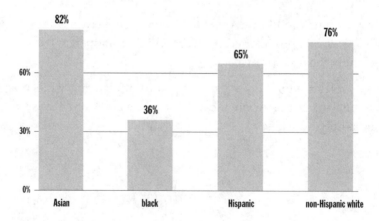

Table 11.1 Living Arrangements of Children, 1970 to 2005

(number and percent distribution of children under age 18 by living arrangement, 1970 to 2005; numbers in thousands)

	total		children living with			
	number	percent	both parents	mother only	father only	neither parent
Total children						
2005	73,523	100.0%	67.4%	23.4%	4.7%	4.5%
2000	72,012	100.0	69.1	22.4	4.2	4.2
1995	70,254	100.0	68.7	23.5	3.5	4.3
1990	64,137	100.0	72.5	21.6	3.1	2.8
1985	62,475	100.0	73.9	20.9	2.5	2.7
1980	63,427	100.0	76.7	18.0	1.7	3.7
1975	66,087	100.0	80.3	15.5	1.5	2.7
1970	69,162	100.0	85.2	10.8	1.1	2.9

Source: Bureau of the Census, Families and Living Arrangements, Historical Time Series, Internet site http://www.census.gov/population/www/socdemo/hh-fam.html; calculations by New Strategist

Table 11.2 Children Living with Grandparents, 1970 to 2005

(number and percent distribution of children living in the home of a grandparent by presence of parent, 1970 to 2005; numbers in thousands)

		grandchildren living in grandparents' home				
			with parent(s) present			
	total children	total	both parents	mother only	father only	without parents present
2005	73,523	4,136	486	1,817	239	1,591
2000	72,012	3,842	531	1,732	220	1,359
1990	64,137	3,155	467	1,563	191	935
1980	63,369	2,306	310	922	86	988
1970	69,276	2,214	363	817	78	957
Percent distribution by living arrangement						
2005	100.0%	5.6%	0.7%	2.5%	0.3%	2.2%
2000	100.0	5.3	0.7	2.4	0.3	1.9
1990	100.0	4.9	0.7	2.4	0.3	1.5
1980	100.0	3.6	0.5	1.5	0.1	1.6
1970	100.0	3.2	0.5	1.2	0.1	1.4
Percent distribution of children living with a grandparent by presence of parent in the home						
2005	–	100.0%	11.8%	43.9%	5.8%	38.5%
2000	–	100.0	13.8	45.1	5.7	35.4
1990	–	100.0	14.8	49.5	6.1	29.6
1980	–	100.0	13.4	40.0	3.7	42.8
1970	–	100.0	16.4	36.9	3.5	43.2

Note: "–" means not applicable.
Source: Bureau of the Census, Families and Living Arrangements, Historical Time Series, Internet site http://www.census.gov/population/www/socdemo/hh-fam.html; calculations by New Strategist

Table 11.3 Living Arrangements of Children by Race and Hispanic Origin, 2005

(number and percent distribution of children under age 18 by living arrangement, race, and Hispanic origin of child, 2005; numbers in thousands)

	total	Asian	black	Hispanic	non-Hispanic white
Total children	**73,523**	**3,413**	**12,251**	**14,248**	**43,122**
Living with both parents	49,573	2,797	4,394	9,225	32,754
Living with mother only	17,172	385	6,052	3,612	7,065
Living with father only	3,486	131	603	678	2,048
Living with neither parent	3,293	100	1,202	733	1,256
PERCENT DISTRIBUTION BY LIVING ARRANGEMENT					
Total children	**100.0%**	**100.0%**	**100.0%**	**100.0%**	**100.0%**
Living with both parents	67.4	82.0	35.9	64.7	76.0
Living with mother only	23.4	11.3	49.4	25.4	16.4
Living with father only	4.7	3.8	4.9	4.8	4.7
Living with neither parent	4.5	2.9	9.8	5.1	2.9
PERCENT DISTRIBUTION BY RACE AND HISPANIC ORIGIN					
Total children	**100.0%**	**4.6%**	**16.7%**	**19.4%**	**58.7%**
Living with both parents	100.0	5.6	8.9	18.6	66.1
Living with mother only	100.0	2.2	35.2	21.0	41.1
Living with father only	100.0	3.8	17.3	19.4	58.7
Living with neither parent	100.0	3.0	36.5	22.3	38.1

Note: Numbers will not add to total because each racial group includes those identifying themselves as being of the race alone and those identifying themselves as being of the race in combination with other races. Hispanics may be of any race. Non-Hispanic whites include only those identifying themselves as being white alone and not Hispanic.
Source: Bureau of the Census, Current Population Survey Annual Social and Economic Supplement, America's Families and Living Arrangements: 2005, detailed tables, Internet site http://www.census.gov/population/www/socdemo/hh-fam/cps2005.html; calculations by New Strategist

Many Households Have Stepchildren or Adopted Children

Householders with adopted children are better educated.

Among the nation's 45 million households with children of the householder present, 89 percent include only biological children. A substantial 11 percent include adopted or stepchildren—7 percent include stepchildren and 4 percent include adopted children.

Adopted children are less likely to be white than biological or stepchildren. While 71 percent of biological children are white, the figure is just 64 percent among adopted children. Seventeen percent of adopted children are of a different race than the householder.

Parents of adopted children are much better educated than the parents of stepchildren. Thirty-three percent of the householders of adopted children have a college degree. This compares with only 16 percent of the householders of stepchildren.

Thirteen percent of adopted children are foreign born, versus 4 percent of biological and stepchildren. Among foreign-born adopted children, the most common country of birth is Korea, which accounts for 24 percent of the total. Russia accounts for another 10 percent.

■ Divorce and the fertility problems caused by delayed childbearing are creating more diverse families.

More than one in ten households include adopted or stepchildren

(percent distribution of households with children under age 18, by relationship of child to householder, 2000)

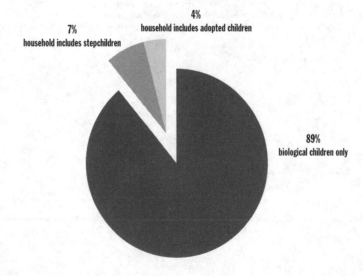

7%
household includes stepchildren

4%
household includes adopted children

89%
biological children only

Table 11.4 Households by Relationship of Children in Household to Householder, 2000

(number and percent distribution of households by presence of biological, step, and adopted children of any age, 2000; numbers in thousands)

	number	percent distribution
Total households with children of householder present	**45,490**	**100.0%**
HOUSEHOLDS BY TYPE OF CHILDREN PRESENT		
Total households with children of householder	**45,490**	**100.0%**
Biological children only	40,658	89.4
Other relationships	4,832	10.6
Biological children and stepchildren	1,660	3.6
Stepchildren only	1,485	3.3
Adopted children only	817	1.8
Adopted and biological children	808	1.8
Biological children, adopted children, and stepchildren	32	0.1
Adopted and stepchildren	30	0.1
HOUSEHOLDS BY NUMBER OF ADOPTED CHILDREN PRESENT		
Total households with adopted children	**1,687**	**100.0%**
One adopted child	1,383	82.0
Two adopted children	248	14.7
Three or more adopted children	56	3.3

Source: Adopted Children and Stepchildren: 2000, Census 2000 Special Reports, CENSR-GRV, 2003 Internet site http://www .census.gov/population/www/cen2000/phc-t21.html

Table 11.5 Biological, Step, and Adopted Children by Race and Hispanic Origin of Householder, 2000

(number and percent distribution of biological, step, and adopted children of the householder by race and Hispanic origin, 2000; numbers in thousands)

	total	biological	step	adopted
RACE OF CHILD				
Total children under age 18	**64,652**	**59,774**	**3,292**	**1,586**
American Indian alone	663	598	40	26
Asian alone	2,225	2,069	39	117
Black alone	8,568	7,911	403	254
White alone	45,859	42,359	2,482	1,018
Other race	7,337	6,837	329	172
HISPANIC ORIGIN OF CHILD				
Total children under age 18	**64,652**	**59,774**	**3,292**	**1,586**
Hispanic	9,814	9,720	479	216
Non-Hispanic white	42,413	37,958	2,262	918
CHILD AND HOUSEHOLDER RACE/HISPANIC DIFFERENCE				
Total children under age 18	**64,652**	**59,774**	**3,292**	**1,586**
Child is of different race than householder	4,638	4,011	356	271
Child is of different Hispanic origin than householder	1,708	1,385	218	105
PERCENT DISTRIBUTION				
RACE OF CHILD				
Total children under age 18	**100.0%**	**100.0%**	**100.0%**	**100.0%**
American Indian alone	1.0	1.0	1.2	1.6
Asian alone	3.4	3.5	1.2	7.4
Black alone	13.3	13.2	12.2	16.0
White alone	70.9	70.9	75.4	64.2
Other race	11.3	11.4	10.0	10.8
HISPANIC ORIGIN OF CHILD				
Total children under age 18	**100.0**	**100.0**	**100.0**	**100.0**
Hispanic	15.2	16.3	14.6	13.6
Non-Hispanic white	65.6	63.5	68.7	57.9
CHILD AND HOUSEHOLDER RACE/HISPANIC DIFFERENCE				
Total children under age 18	**100.0%**	**100.0%**	**100.0%**	**100.0%**
Child is of different race than householder	7.2	6.7	10.8	17.1
Child is of different Hispanic origin than householder	2.6	2.3	6.6	6.6

Source: Adopted Children and Stepchildren: 2000, Census 2000 Special Reports, CENSR-GRV, 2003, Internet site http://www .census.gov/population/www/cen2000/phc-t21.html; calculations by New Strategist

Table 11.6 Biological, Step, and Adopted Children by Education of Householder, 2000

(number and percent distribution of biological, step, and adopted children of the householder by educational attainment of householder, 2000; numbers in thousands)

	total	biological	step	adopted
Total children under age 18	**64,652**	**59,774**	**3,292**	**1,586**
Not a high school graduate	11,536	10,742	568	227
High school graduate	17,300	15,808	1,133	359
Some college	19,315	17,769	1,075	471
Bachelor's degree or more	16,501	15,455	517	530
Bachelor's degree	10,274	9,631	354	288
Graduate or professional school degree	6,227	5,824	162	241

PERCENT DISTRIBUTION BY EDUCATIONAL ATTAINMENT OF HOUSEHOLDER

Total children under age 18	**100.0%**	**100.0%**	**100.0%**	**100.0%**
Not a high school graduate	17.8	18.0	17.3	14.3
High school graduate	26.8	26.4	34.4	22.6
Some college	29.9	29.7	32.6	29.7
Bachelor's degree or more	25.5	25.9	15.7	33.4
Bachelor's degree	15.9	16.1	10.8	18.2
Graduate or professional school degree	9.6	9.7	4.9	15.2

Source: Adopted Children and Stepchildren: 2000, Census 2000 Special Reports, CENSR-GRV, 2003, Internet site http://www.census.gov/population/www/cen2000/phc-t21.html; calculations by New Strategist

Table 11.7 Biological, Step, and Adopted Children by Nativity, 2000

(number and percent distribution of biological, step, and adopted children of the householder by nativity, 2000; numbers in thousands)

	total	biological	step	adopted
Total children under age 18	**64,652**	**59,774**	**3,292**	**1,586**
Native	62,007	57,461	3,160	1,387
Foreign-born	2,645	2,313	133	199
Total children under age 18	**100.0%**	**100.0%**	**100.0%**	**100.0%**
Native	95.9	96.1	96.0	87.4
Foreign-born	4.1	3.9	4.0	12.6

Source: Adopted Children and Stepchildren: 2000, Census 2000 Special Reports, CENSR-GRV, 2003, Internet site http://www.census.gov/population/www/cen2000/phc-t21.html; calculations by New Strategist

Table 11.8 Adopted Children by Place of Birth, 2000

(number and percent distribution of adopted children under age 18 by place of birth, 2000; numbers in thousands)

	number	percent
Total adopted children of householder	**1,586**	**100.0%**
Native-born	1,387	87.4
Foreign-born	199	12.6
Foreign-born	**199**	**100.0**
Europe	37	18.5
Russia	20	9.9
Romania	6	3.1
Ukraine	2	1.2
Asia	98	49.4
China	21	10.6
India	8	3.9
Korea	48	23.9
Phillippines	6	3.2
Vietnam	4	2.2
Africa	3	1.6
Latin America	58	29.2
Central America	32	16.3
Guatemala	7	3.7
Mexico	18	9.1
El Salvador	2	1.1
South America	20	10.2
Colombia	7	3.5
North America	2	0.8

Source: Adopted Children and Stepchildren: 2000, Census 2000 Special Reports, CENSR-GRV, 2003, Internet site http://www.census.gov/population/www/cen2000/phc-t21.html; calculations by New Strategist

Many Women Consider Adoption, Few Adopt

One-third of women aged 18 to 44 have considered adoption.

Although 33 percent of women aged 18 to 44 have considered adopting a child, only 3 percent have actually taken steps to adopt and just 1 percent have adopted. The percentage of Americans who actually adopted a child rises with age, to 3 percent among women aged 40 to 44.

Not surprisingly, the percentage of women who have adopted a child is highest among those with fertility problems. Among women with impaired fecundity, more than half have considered adoption and 3.5 percent have adopted. Among women who have used infertility services, 57 percent have considered adoption and 5 percent have adopted.

Nearly half the women actively seeking to adopt would prefer a child under age 2, but most would accept a child under age 12. Seventy percent would accept two or more siblings. Most say race does not matter, nor does the sex of the child. Only 30 percent would accept a child with a severe disability, however.

■ With so many women considering adoption, but so few actually adopting, the barriers to adoption appear large.

Only 1 percent of women have adopted a child

(percent of women aged 18 to 44 who have considered adopting or have adopted a child, 2002)

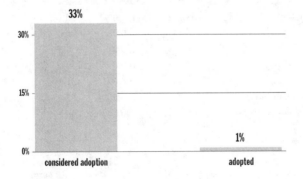

Table 11.9 Women Who Have Ever Considered Adoption or Adopted by Age, 2002

(total number of women aged 18 to 44 and percent who have ever considered adoption, taken steps to adopt, or adopted a child, by age, 2002; numbers in thousands)

	total		considered adoption	taken steps to adopt	adopted
	number	percent			
Total women aged 18 to 44	**55,742**	**100.0%**	**33.1%**	**3.4%**	**1.1%**
Aged 18 to 24	13,855	100.0	27.3	0.9	–
Aged 25 to 29	9,249	100.0	32.6	1.7	–
Aged 30 to 34	10,272	100.0	34.1	4.6	0.7
Aged 35 to 39	10,853	100.0	38.5	5.3	1.6
Aged 40 to 44	11,512	100.0	34.6	4.9	2.9

Note: The category "considered adoption" includes those who have adopted children, those who have ever considered adoption, and those who are currently seeking to adopt. "–" means sample is too small to make a reliable estimate.
Source: National Center for Health Statistics, Fertility, Family Planning, and Reproductive Health of U.S. Women: Data from the 2002 National Survey of Family Growth, Vital and Health Statistics, Series 23, No. 25, 2005; Internet site http://www.cdc .gov/nchs/nsfg.htm

Table 11.10 Women Who Have Ever Considered Adoption or Adopted by Marital Status, 2002

(total number of women aged 18 to 44 and percent who have ever considered adoption, taken steps to adopt, or adopted a child, by marital status, 2002; numbers in thousands)

	total		considered adoption	taken steps to adopt	adopted
	number	percent			
Total aged 18 to 44	**55,742**	**100.0%**	**33.1%**	**3.4%**	**1.1%**
Married	28,323	100.0	35.2	4.4	1.6
First marriage	23,078	100.0	34.3	3.9	1.3
Second or later marriage	5,245	100.0	39.0	6.8	3.2
Cohabiting	5,452	100.0	32.1	2.4	–
Never married, not cohabiting	15,871	100.0	27.6	1.8	0.7
Formerly married, not cohabiting	6,096	100.0	38.8	3.6	0.8

Note: The category "considered adoption" includes those who have adopted children, those who have ever considered adoption, and those who are currently seeking to adopt. "–" means sample is too small to make a reliable estimate.
Source: National Center for Health Statistics, Fertility, Family Planning, and Reproductive Health of U.S. Women: Data from the 2002 National Survey of Family Growth, Vital and Health Statistics, Series 23, No. 25, 2005; Internet site http://www.cdc .gov/nchs/nsfg.htm

Table 11.11 Women Who Have Ever Considered Adoption or Adopted by Number of Children Ever Borne, 2002

(total number of women aged 18 to 44, and percent who have ever considered adoption, taken steps to adopt, or adopted a child, by number of children ever born, 2002; numbers in thousands)

	total		considered adoption	taken steps to adopt	adopted
	number	percent			
Total aged 18 to 44	**55,742**	**100.0%**	**33.1%**	**3.4%**	**1.1%**
No births	19,993	100.0	35.4	2.6	1.4
One birth	11,015	100.0	32.3	4.3	0.6
Two births	13,390	100.0	31.2	3.1	1.2
Three or more births	11,343	100.0	32.3	4.4	1.0

Note: The category "considered adoption" includes those who have adopted children, those who have ever considered adoption, and those who are currently seeking to adopt.
Source: National Center for Health Statistics, Fertility, Family Planning, and Reproductive Health of U.S. Women: Data from the 2002 National Survey of Family Growth, Vital and Health Statistics, Series 23, No. 25, 2005; Internet site http://www.cdc .gov/nchs/nsfg.htm

Table 11.12 Women Who Have Ever Considered Adoption or Adopted by Fecundity Status, 2002

(total number of women aged 18 to 44 and percent who have ever considered adoption, taken steps to adopt, or adopted a child, by fecundity status and use of infertility services, 2002; numbers in thousands)

	total		considered adoption	taken steps to adopt	adopted
	number	percent			
Total aged 18 to 44	**55,742**	**100.0%**	**33.1%**	**3.4%**	**1.1%**
Fecundity status					
Surgically sterile	14,439	100.0	32.7	5.3	1.7
Impaired fecundity	7,063	100.0	51.8	9.1	3.5
Fecund	32,240	100.0	29.5	1.4	0.4
Use of infertility services					
Yes	7,306	100.0	57.1	11.5	5.1
No	48,436	100.0	29.5	2.2	0.5

Note: The category "considered adoption" includes those who have adopted children, those who have ever considered adoption, and those who are currently seeking to adopt.
Source: National Center for Health Statistics, Fertility, Family Planning, and Reproductive Health of U.S. Women: Data from the 2002 National Survey of Family Growth, Vital and Health Statistics, Series 23, No. 25, 2005; Internet site http://www.cdc .gov/nchs/nsfg.htm

Table 11.13 Women Who Have Ever Considered Adoption or Adopted by Race and Hispanic Origin, 2002

(total number of women aged 18 to 44 and percent who have ever considered adoption, taken steps to adopt, or adopted a child, by race and Hispanic origin, 2002; numbers in thousands)

	total		considered adoption	taken steps to adopt	adopted
	number	percent			
Total aged 18 to 44	**55,742**	**100.0%**	**33.1%**	**3.4%**	**1.1%**
Black, non-Hispanic	7,399	100.0	35.2	4.5	1.4
Hispanic	8,194	100.0	30.8	3.0	0.3
White, non-Hispanic	35,936	100.0	33.6	3.3	1.3

Note: The category "considered adoption" includes those who have adopted children, those who have ever considered adoption, and those who are currently seeking to adopt.
Source: National Center for Health Statistics, Fertility, Family Planning, and Reproductive Health of U.S. Women: Data from the 2002 National Survey of Family Growth, Vital and Health Statistics, Series 23, No. 25, 2005; Internet site http://www.cdc .gov/nchs/nsfg.htm

Table 11.14 Women Who Have Ever Considered Adoption or Adopted by Education, 2002

(total number of women aged 18 to 44 and percent who have ever considered adoption, taken steps to adopt, or adopted a child, by education, 2002; numbers in thousands)

	total		considered adoption	taken steps to adopt	adopted
	number	percent			
Total aged 18 to 44	**55,742**	**100.0%**	**33.1%**	**3.4%**	**1.1%**
Not a high school graduate	5,627	100.0	23.8	2.3	0.7
High school graduate or GED	14,264	100.0	32.6	4.1	1.8
Some college, no degree	14,279	100.0	36.8	3.8	0.9
Bachelor's degree or more	13,551	100.0	37.1	4.2	1.5

Note: The category "considered adoption" includes those who have adopted children, those who have ever considered adoption, and those who are currently seeking to adopt. Education categories include only people aged 22 to 44.
Source: National Center for Health Statistics, Fertility, Family Planning, and Reproductive Health of U.S. Women: Data from the 2002 National Survey of Family Growth, Vital and Health Statistics, Series 23, No. 25, 2005; Internet site http://www.cdc .gov/nchs/nsfg.htm

Table 11.15 Preferences of Women Seeking to Adopt, 2002

(percent of women aged 18 to 44 who are currently seeking to adopt a child not already known to them who would prefer or accept selected attributes, 2002)

	prefer	would accept
Total aged 18 to 44 seeking to adopt	100.0%	100.0%
Sex of child		
Boy	28.9	95.0
Girl	34.6	97.2
Indifferent	36.5	–
Race of child		
Black	10.0	86.9
White	20.1	91.4
Other race	16.9	94.9
Indifferent	52.2	–
Age of child		
Under age 2	49.2	94.1
Aged 2 to 5	22.3	78.7
Aged 6 to 12	16.1	58.6
Aged 13 or older	–	30.9
Indifferent	7.6	–
Disability status		
No disability	55.1	100.0
With a mild disability	21.6	89.0
With a severe disabilitiy	–	30.3
Indifferent	22.8	–
Number of children		
Single child	56.3	100.0
Two or more siblings	27.3	74.6
Indifferent	16.5	–

Note: "–" means sample is too small to make a reliable estimate or not applicable.
Source: National Center for Health Statistics, Fertility, Family Planning, and Reproductive Health of U.S. Women: Data from the 2002 National Survey of Family Growth, Vital and Health Statistics, Series 23, No. 25, 2005; Internet site http://www.cdc .gov/nchs/nsfg.htm

Table 11.16 Men Who Have Ever Adopted a Child, 2002

(percentage of men aged 18 to 44 who have ever adopted a child, by selected characteristics, 2002)

	percent who have ever adopted a child
Total men aged 18 to 44	**2.1%**
Age	
Aged 18 to 24	–
Aged 25 to 29	1.0
Aged 30 to 34	3.2
Aged 35 to 39	3.8
Aged 40 to 44	3.5
Marital status	
Currently married	4.0
Currently cohabiting	1.6
Never married, not cohabiting	–
Formerly married, not cohabiting	2.9
Race and Hispanic origin	
Black, non-Hispanic	2.4
Hispanic	1.9
White, non-Hispanic	2.0
Education	
Not a high school graduate	2.5
High school graduate or GED	4.0
Some college, no degree	1.8
Bachelor's degree or more	2.0

Note: "–" means sample is too small to make a reliable estimate.
Source: National Center for Health Statistics, Fertility, Contraception, and Fatherhood: Data on Men and Women from Cycle 6 of the 2002 National Survey of Family Growth, Vital and Health Statistics, Series 23, No. 26, 2006; Internet site http://www.cdc.gov/nchs/nsfg.htm

Many Women Care for Children to Whom They Did Not Give Birth

The percentage rises sharply with age.

Thirteen percent of women aged 18 to 44 have lived with and cared for a child to whom they did not give birth. By age, the proportion peaks at 19 percent among women aged 40 to 44.

Women in second or later marriages are most likely to have cared (or be caring) for someone else's child, with 29 percent having done so. Ten percent of women married two or more times have cared for a stepchild.

There are large differences by education in caring for the children of others. Fully 21 percent of women without a high school diploma have cared for someone else's child, and 10 percent have cared for the child of a blood relative. Among women with a college degree, only 8 percent have cared for someone else's child.

■ Fewer than 2 percent of women have cared for a child unrelated to them.

The experience of caring for the children of others falls with education

(percent of women aged 18 to 44 who have ever lived with and cared for a child to whom they did not give birth, by education, 2002)

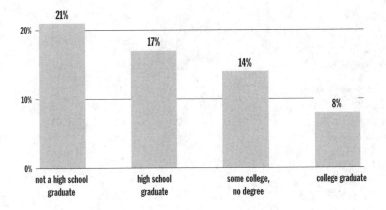

Table 11.17 Women Caring for Children to Whom They Did Not Give Birth, 2002

(percent of women aged 18 to 44 who have ever lived with and cared for a child to whom they did not give birth, by child's relationship with woman when child first began living with woman, by selected characteristics, 2002; numbers in thousands)

	lived with and cared for a child to whom they did not give birth				
	any child	stepchild	child of relative by blood	child related in some other way	unrelated child
Total women aged 18 to 44	**12.6%**	**2.8%**	**4.5%**	**4.7%**	**1.6%**
Age					
Aged 18 to 19	3.9	0.0	2.1	1.8	–
Aged 20 to 24	5.8	0.5	2.3	2.6	0.6
Aged 25 to 29	9.1	1.8	4.1	2.8	0.7
Aged 30 to 34	14.1	4.1	4.5	5.6	1.2
Aged 35 to 39	17.4	4.0	5.5	6.9	2.1
Aged 40 to 44	18.6	4.1	6.7	6.2	3.8
Marital status					
Married	14.3	4.4	4.5	4.7	1.9
First marriage	11.0	3.1	4.0	3.3	1.6
Second or later marriage	28.6	10.2	6.6	11.2	3.1
Cohabiting	15.2	–	4.8	9.5	1.1
Never married, not cohabiting	7.6	–	3.9	2.8	1.3
Formerly married, not cohabiting	15.8	4.3	6.3	5.4	1.9
Parity					
No births	8.3	0.9	2.4	3.3	2.1
One birth	14.3	4.6	4.3	4.8	1.3
Two births	14.7	4.5	5.9	5.1	1.3
Three or more births	16.2	2.2	6.9	6.6	1.7
Race and Hispanic origin					
Black, non-Hispanic	18.9	3.0	9.7	6.2	1.5
Hispanic	11.9	2.2	5.8	3.4	1.2
White, non-Hispanic	11.5	3.0	3.0	4.6	1.8
Education					
Not a high school graduate	21.1	2.2	10.0	8.5	1.8
High school graduate or GED	16.8	3.7	5.8	6.4	2.2
Some college, no degree	13.8	3.7	5.2	5.1	1.5
Bachelor's degree or more	8.4	2.6	2.1	2.2	2.0

Note: Numbers may not sum to "any child" total because woman may have lived with and cared for more than one child. "–" means sample is too small to make a reliable estimate.
Source: National Center for Health Statistics, Fertility, Family Planning, and Reproductive Health of U.S. Women: Data from the 2002 National Survey of Family Growth, Vital and Health Statistics, Series 23, No. 25, 2005; Internet site http://www.cdc .gov/nchs/nsfg.htm

Twenty-Seven Percent of Fathers Live Apart from Their Children

The majority of black men live apart from some of their children.

Among men aged 15 to 44 who have children under age 19, fully 27 percent live separately from some or all of their children. Fourteen percent do not live with any of their children, and 12 percent live with some but not others.

By race and Hispanic origin, the percentage of men living apart from their children ranges from 19 percent among non-Hispanic whites to 53 percent among blacks. The least-educated men are most likely to live separately from their children. Among men without a high school diploma, 35 percent live apart from some or all of their children. Among college graduates the proportion is just 14 percent.

Child support is paid regularly by 76 percent of the men who live apart from their children. Only 15 percent say they do not contribute child support. The median amount of child support paid in the past 12 months stood at $4,250 in 2002.

■ Most men who do not live with some or all of their children live apart from only one child.

Most fathers living apart from their children pay child support regularly

(percent distribution of men aged 15 to 44 who live apart from one or more children under age 19, by frequency of child support payments in past 12 months, 2002)

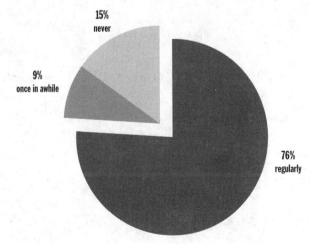

15% never

9% once in awhile

76% regularly

Table 11.18 Father's Living Arrangements with Children, 2002

(number of men aged 15 to 44 who have biological or adopted children under age 19, and percent distribution by living arrangement with children, by selected characteristics, 2002; numbers in thousands)

	total		living with children	not living with children	living with some but not others
	number	percent			
Total men aged 15 to 44 with children	**27,821**	**100.0%**	**73.4%**	**14.3%**	**12.4%**
Aged 15 to 24	1,832	100.0	65.8	23.2	11.1
Aged 25 to 29	4,107	100.0	77.4	13.9	8.7
Aged 30 to 44	21,882	100.0	73.3	13.6	13.2
Marital status					
Currently married	20,133	100.0	83.7	6.0	10.3
First marriage	16,400	100.0	90.2	4.8	5.0
Second or later marriage	3,733	100.0	55.2	11.5	33.3
Currently cohabiting	3,046	100.0	60.0	13.5	26.5
Never married, not cohabiting	1,592	100.0	34.8	54.1	11.2
Formerly married, not cohabiting	3,049	100.0	38.9	48.5	12.6
Race and Hispanic origin					
Black, non-Hispanic	3,292	100.0	47.0	25.5	27.5
Hispanic	5,542	100.0	65.8	18.4	15.8
White, non-Hispanic	16,596	100.0	80.8	11.0	8.2
Education					
Not a high school graduate	4,480	100.0	64.8	16.9	18.3
High school graduate or GED	10,456	100.0	71.4	14.8	13.9
Some college, no degree	6,650	100.0	73.8	13.6	12.7
Bachelor's degree or more	5,600	100.0	85.7	10.4	4.0
Labor force status					
Full-time	22,506	100.0	75.9	12.2	11.9
Part-time	2,291	100.0	67.4	19.0	13.5
Other	3,014	100.0	59.0	25.9	15.2
Childhood living arrangement under age 19					
Intact	19,552	100.0	76.0	12.9	11.2
Not intact	8,269	100.0	67.3	17.6	15.2

Note: Education categories include only people aged 22 to 44.
Source: National Center for Health Statistics, Fertility, Contraception, and Fatherhood: Data on Men and Women from Cycle 6 of the 2002 National Survey of Family Growth, Vital and Health Statistics, Series 23, No. 26, 2006; Internet site http://www.cdc .gov/nchs/nsfg.htm

Table 11.19 Fathers by Number of Children with Whom They Live, 2002

(number of men aged 15 to 44 who live with one or more of their biological or adopted children under age 19, and percent distribution by number of children with whom they live, by selected characteristics, 2002; numbers in thousands)

	total		father lives with		
	number	percent	one child	two children	three or more children
Total men aged 15 to 44 living with one or more children	**23,856**	**100.0%**	**34.7%**	**39.3%**	**26.0%**
Aged 15 to 24	1,408	100.0	49.8	37.0	13.2
Aged 25 to 29	3,537	100.0	37.7	35.4	27.0
Aged 30 to 44	18,912	100.0	33.0	40.2	26.8
Marital status					
Currently married	18,918	100.0	30.4	42.7	27.0
First marriage	15,614	100.0	31.3	44.1	24.7
Second or later marriage	3,304	100.0	26.3	36.0	37.7
Currently cohabiting	2,636	100.0	41.9	28.8	29.2
Never married, not cohabiting	731	100.0	59.4	24.8	15.8
Formerly married, not cohabiting	1,571	100.0	62.8	23.5	13.8
Race and Hispanic origin					
Black, non-Hispanic	2,452	100.0	36.5	33.0	30.5
Hispanic	4,520	100.0	29.3	37.2	33.4
White, non-Hispanic	14,774	100.0	36.0	42.7	21.4
Education					
Not a high school graduate	3,722	100.0	30.0	36.4	33.5
High school graduate or GED	8,912	100.0	34.2	39.4	26.5
Some college, no degree	5,748	100.0	34.3	39.3	26.5
Bachelor's degree or more	5,020	100.0	38.0	41.8	20.3
Labor force status					
Full-time	19,757	100.0	35.3	39.8	24.9
Part-time	1,855	100.0	27.9	47.0	25.2
Other	2,234	100.0	34.4	28.6	37.0

Note: Education categories include only people aged 22 to 44.
Source: National Center for Health Statistics, Fertility, Contraception, and Fatherhood: Data on Men and Women from Cycle 6 of the 2002 National Survey of Family Growth, Vital and Health Statistics, Series 23, No. 26, 2006; Internet site http://www.cdc.gov/nchs/nsfg.htm

Table 11.20 Fathers by Number of Children with Whom They Do Not Live, 2002

(number of men aged 15 to 44 who do not live with one or more of their biological or adopted children under age 19, and percent distribution by number of children with whom they do not live, by selected characteristics, 2002; numbers in thousands)

	total		father does not live with		
	number	percent	one child	two children	three or more children
Total men aged 15 to 44 not living with one or more children	**7,405**	**100.0%**	**60.3%**	**26.8%**	**12.9%**
Aged 15 to 29	1,555	100.0	62.5	25.2	12.3
Aged 30 to 44	5,850	100.0	59.7	27.3	13.0
Marital status					
Currently married	3,285	100.0	63.3	23.4	13.3
First marriage	1,612	100.0	55.9	26.8	17.3
Second or later marriage	1,673	100.0	70.5	20.2	9.3
Currently cohabiting	1,219	100.0	52.4	35.7	12.0
Never married, not cohabiting	1,038	100.0	72.5	19.3	8.3
Formerly married, not cohabiting	1,863	100.0	53.5	31.3	15.3
Race and Hispanic origin					
Black, non-Hispanic	1,745	100.0	55.5	28.2	16.3
Hispanic	1,897	100.0	48.4	33.6	18.1
White, non-Hispanic	3,190	100.0	69.9	20.3	9.8
Education					
Not a high school graduate	1,577	100.0	55.8	25.0	19.2
High school graduate or GED	2,992	100.0	59.4	29.5	11.0
Some college or more	2,545	100.0	62.5	26.8	10.8
Labor force status					
Full-time	5,186	100.0	60.9	26.7	12.5
Other	1,823	100.0	58.5	27.2	14.3

Note: Education categories include only people aged 22 to 44.
Source: National Center for Health Statistics, Fertility, Contraception, and Fatherhood: Data on Men and Women from Cycle 6 of the 2002 National Survey of Family Growth, Vital and Health Statistics, Series 23, No. 26, 2006; Internet site http://www.cdc .gov/nchs/nsfg.htm

Table 11.21 Frequency of Child Support Payments by Fathers, 2002

(number of men aged 15 to 44 with children under age 19 with whom they do not live, and percent distribution by frequency of child support payments in past 12 months, by selected characteristics, 2002; numbers in thousands)

	total		frequency of child support payments		
	number	percent	regularly	once in a while	never
Total men aged 15 to 44 with children under age 19 living elsewhere	**7,405**	**100.0%**	**75.8%**	**8.9%**	**15.3%**
Aged 15 to 29	1,555	100.0	73.8	7.6	18.6
Aged 30 to 44	5,850	100.0	76.3	9.3	14.5
Marital status					
Currently married	3,285	100.0	79.0	7.2	13.8
First marriage	1,612	100.0	73.4	7.7	18.9
Second or later marriage	1,673	100.0	84.4	6.8	8.8
Currently cohabiting	1,219	100.0	63.0	16.9	20.1
Never married, not cohabiting	1,038	100.0	66.9	10.0	23.1
Formerly married, not cohabiting	1,863	100.0	83.3	6.1	10.6
Number of own children not living with respondent					
One child	4,466	100.0	75.1	9.6	15.3
Two or more children	2,939	100.0	76.7	7.9	15.4
Race and Hispanic origin					
Black, non-Hispanic	1,745	100.0	80.4	8.3	11.3
Hispanic	1,897	100.0	77.9	10.2	11.9
White, non-Hispanic	3,190	100.0	77.1	6.3	16.6
Education					
Not a high school graduate	1,577	100.0	67.5	12.3	20.2
High school graduate or GED	2,992	100.0	75.5	6.8	17.7
Some college or more	2,545	100.0	81.3	8.3	10.4
Labor force status					
Full-time	5,186	100.0	78.9	6.2	14.9
Other	2,219	100.0	68.4	15.3	16.3

Note: Education categories include only people aged 22 to 44.
Source: National Center for Health Statistics, Fertility, Contraception, and Fatherhood: Data on Men and Women from Cycle 6 of the 2002 National Survey of Family Growth, Vital and Health Statistics, Series 23, No. 26, 2006; Internet site http://www.cdc.gov/nchs/nsfg.htm

Table 11.22 Amount of Child Support Payments Made by Fathers, 2002

(number of men aged 15 to 44 who have children under age 19 with whom they do not live, median amount of child support paid in past 12 months, and percent distribution by amount paid, by selected characteristics, 2002; numbers in thousands)

	median amount of child support paid in past 12 months	percent distribution by amount paid				
		total	less than $3,000	$3,001 to $5,000	$5,001 to $9,000	more than $9,000
Total men aged 15 to 44 with children under age 19 living elsewhere	$4,250	100.0%	36.0%	22.9%	23.5%	17.6%
Aged 15 to 29	4,000	100.0	39.6	23.0	22.0	15.5
Aged 30 to 44	4,500	100.0	35.1	22.8	24.0	18.1
Marital status						
Currently married	4,500	100.0	36.7	21.4	26.1	15.9
First marriage	4,000	100.0	45.2	17.4	23.3	14.1
Second or later marriage	5,000	100.0	30.5	24.3	28.1	17.1
Currently cohabiting	3,000	100.0	53.1	22.0	12.1	12.9
Never married, not cohabiting	4,160	100.0	38.6	21.4	19.3	20.7
Formerly married, not cohabiting	5,040	100.0	23.3	26.6	28.5	21.7
Number of own children not living with respondent						
One child	3,600	100.0	42.1	29.0	17.9	11.0
Two or more children	6,000	100.0	26.0	12.7	32.9	28.4
Race and Hispanic origin						
Black, non-Hispanic	4,250	100.0	36.2	23.7	22.0	18.1
Hispanic	4,000	100.0	38.6	22.2	25.8	13.4
White, non-Hispanic	5,000	100.0	29.1	24.4	25.9	20.6
Education						
Not a high school graduate	3,000	100.0	50.5	17.5	24.3	7.7
High school graduate or GED	4,500	100.0	36.2	25.4	23.2	15.2
Some college or more	5,000	100.0	27.6	22.7	23.9	25.7
Labor force status						
Full-time	4,500	100.0	34.5	23.3	24.5	17.7
Other	3,600	100.0	40.5	21.7	20.7	17.1

Source: National Center for Health Statistics, Fertility, Contraception, and Fatherhood: Data on Men and Women from Cycle 6 of the 2002 National Survey of Family Growth, Vital and Health Statistics, Series 23, No. 26, 2006; Internet site http://www.cdc.gov/nchs/nsfg.htm

Fathers Who Live Apart from Their Children Are Not Satisfied with Visits

Nonresident fathers are much less likely to take part in activities with children.

Fathers who do not live with their children do not get much satisfaction from their visits with the kids. Among men living apart from their children, the level of satisfaction they get from visits on a scale of 1 (very dissatisfied) to 10 (very satisfied) was just 4.6.

Nonresident fathers miss out on a lot of family activities. Among men not living with their children under age 5, nearly half say they have not played with their children at all in the past four weeks. Only 10 percent play with them every day. Among men living with their children under age 5, fully 81 percent say they play with them every day.

The lack of contact with their children makes nonresident fathers doubt their parenting skills. Only 27 percent of fathers who do not live with one or more of their children say they are doing a "very good" job as a father. Twenty percent say they are "not very good" or "bad" as fathers. Among fathers living with their children, a larger 46 percent (but still a minority) say they are doing a "very good" job. Fewer than 1 percent say they are doing a bad job.

■ Sixty-four percent of fathers living with their children aged 5 to 18 say they talk to them about things every day versus only 8 percent of fathers who do not live with their children.

Many men do not think they are doing a good job as a father

(percent of men aged 15 to 44 with children who think they are doing a "very good" job as a father, by living arrangement with children, 2002)

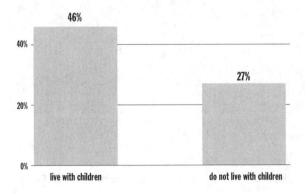

Table 11.23 Father's Satisfaction with Child Visitation, 2002

(number of men aged 15 to 44 with children under age 19 with whom they do not live, percent having contact with own children living elsewhere, percent distribution of those in contact with children by satisfaction with visits on a scale of 1 (very dissatisfied) to 10 (very satisfied), and average level of satisfaction, by selected characteristics, 2002; numbers in thousands)

	number	percent having contact with their children	percent distribution by level of satisfaction with visits						average satisfaction level
			total	1 to 2	3 to 4	5 to 6	7 to 8	9 to 10	
Total men aged 15 to 44 with children not living with them	**7,405**	**73.6%**	**100.0%**	**41.1%**	**9.7%**	**16.5%**	**10.6%**	**22.2%**	**4.6**
Aged 15 to 29	1,555	80.3	100.0	38.5	4.6	16.7	11.6	28.5	5.2
Aged 30 to 44	5,850	71.8	100.0	41.8	11.0	16.4	10.3	20.5	4.4
Marital status									
Currently married	3,285	71.5	100.0	41.6	9.9	19.3	6.8	22.4	4.5
First marriage	1,612	72.1	100.0	29.0	7.2	19.3	10.5	33.9	5.7
Second or later marriage	1,673	70.9	100.0	53.6	12.4	19.3	3.3	11.4	3.3
Currently cohabiting	1,219	60.0	100.0	48.2	9.2	17.2	5.3	20.1	4.1
Never married, not cohabiting	1,038	84.4	100.0	39.3	6.5	14.1	16.0	24.1	5.0
Formerly married, not cohabiting	1,863	80.0	100.0	36.8	11.4	12.2	17.7	22.0	4.9
Race and Hispanic origin									
Black, non-Hispanic	1,745	89.5	100.0	39.1	10.6	13.8	10.6	25.9	4.9
Hispanic	1,897	61.7	100.0	41.8	5.2	13.5	7.3	32.3	5.1
White, non-Hispanic	3,190	73.9	100.0	43.4	13.1	15.9	11.4	16.2	4.2
Education									
Not a high school graduate	1,577	59.0	100.0	40.0	4.2	10.2	9.5	36.1	5.3
High school graduate or GED	2,992	75.5	100.0	42.7	10.8	18.7	9.5	18.3	4.3
Some college or more	2,545	78.9	100.0	41.9	11.9	18.4	12.1	15.8	4.3

Note: Education categories include only people aged 22 to 44.
Source: National Center for Health Statistics, Fertility, Contraception, and Fatherhood: Data on Men and Women from Cycle 6 of the 2002 National Survey of Family Growth, Vital and Health Statistics, Series 23, No. 26, 2006; Internet site http://www.cdc.gov/nchs/nsfg.htm

Table 11.24 Fathers Eating Meals with Children under Age 5, 2002

(number of men aged 15 to 44 with children under age 5, and percent distribution by frequency of feeding and eating meals with their children in past four weeks, by living arrangement with children and selected characteristics, 2002; numbers in thousands)

	total		frequency of feeding and eating meals			
	number	percent	not at all	about once a week or less	several times a week	everyday
LIVING WITH CHILDREN						
Total men aged 15 to 44 with children under age 5	**13,995**	**100.0%**	**1.9%**	**2.8%**	**21.5%**	**73.8%**
Aged 15 to 29	5,015	100.0	3.6	4.6	19.9	71.9
Aged 30 to 44	8,979	100.0	0.9	1.8	22.4	74.9
Race and Hispanic origin						
Black, non-Hispanic	1,446	100.0	–	3.3	32.1	62.7
Hispanic	2,931	100.0	3.5	8.6	23.9	64.1
White, non-Hispanic	8,472	100.0	1.3	0.8	19.8	78.1
Education						
High school graduate or less	7,158	100.0	2.8	4.4	22.5	70.3
Some college or more	6,565	100.0	0.4	0.6	20.4	78.6
NOT LIVING WITH CHILDREN						
Total men aged 15 to 44 with children under age 5	**1,938**	**100.0**	**52.8**	**20.0**	**18.5**	**8.7**
Aged 15 to 29	1,108	100.0	47.3	19.0	25.1	8.7
Aged 30 to 44	830	100.0	59.5	21.4	10.5	8.7
Race and Hispanic origin						
Black, non-Hispanic	451	100.0	44.5	32.4	14.1	9.0
Hispanic	859	100.0	60.5	18.6	13.8	7.1
White, non-Hispanic	504	100.0	–	–	–	–
Education						
High school graduate or less	1,263	100.0	61.1	17.1	13.7	8.2
Some college or more	574	100.0	39.3	24.4	27.3	9.0

Note: Men who live with their children may also have children living elsewhere; those men are represented under both categories. Education categories include only people aged 22 to 44. "–" means sample is too small to make a reliable estimate.
Source: National Center for Health Statistics, Fertility, Contraception, and Fatherhood: Data on Men and Women from Cycle 6 of the 2002 National Survey of Family Growth, Vital and Health Statistics, Series 23, No. 26, 2006; Internet site http://www.cdc.gov/nchs/nsfg.htm

Table 11.25 Fathers Eating Meals with Children Aged 5 to 18, 2002

(number of men aged 15 to 44 with children aged 5 to 18, and percent distribution by frequency of eating meals with their children in past four weeks, by living arrangement with children and selected characteristics, 2002; numbers in thousands)

	total		frequency of feeding and eating meals			
	number	percent	not at all	about once a week or less	several times a week	everyday
LIVING WITH CHILDREN						
Total men aged 15 to 44 with children aged 5 to 18	**18,251**	**100.0%**	**1.9%**	**3.8%**	**22.8%**	**71.6%**
Aged 15 to 29	2,401	100.0	3.9	7.5	19.1	69.4
Aged 30 to 44	15,850	100.0	1.6	3.2	23.3	71.9
Race and Hispanic origin						
Black, non-Hispanic	1,993	100.0	8.7	9.9	27.3	54.0
Hispanic	3,460	100.0	2.2	6.0	21.0	70.8
White, non-Hispanic	11,140	100.0	0.8	2.2	24.7	72.2
Education						
Not a high school graduate	3,097	100.0	3.3	6.5	19.5	70.7
High school graduate or GED	7,218	100.0	1.1	2.7	25.4	70.8
Some college or more	7,677	100.0	1.7	3.2	21.9	73.2
NOT LIVING WITH CHILDREN						
Total men aged 15 to 44 with children aged 5 to 18	**6,273**	**100.0**	**56.8**	**24.7**	**15.1**	**3.4**
Aged 15 to 29	789	100.0	54.3	20.6	17.7	7.3
Aged 30 to 44	5,485	100.0	57.2	25.3	14.7	2.8
Race and Hispanic origin						
Black, non-Hispanic	1,480	100.0	52.2	36.2	6.6	5.0
Hispanic	1,403	100.0	66.6	18.7	10.2	4.5
White, non-Hispanic	2,898	100.0	53.7	23.7	20.4	2.1
Education						
Not a high school graduate	1,387	100.0	73.5	13.4	9.7	3.5
High school graduate or GED	2,662	100.0	54.1	28.7	12.8	4.5
Some college or more	2,205	100.0	50.1	27.3	21.3	1.3

Note: Men who live with their children may also have children living elsewhere; those men are represented under both categories. Education categories include only people aged 22 to 44.
Source: National Center for Health Statistics, Fertility, Contraception, and Fatherhood: Data on Men and Women from Cycle 6 of the 2002 National Survey of Family Growth, Vital and Health Statistics, Series 23, No. 26, 2006; Internet site http://www.cdc.gov/nchs/nsfg.htm

Table 11.26 Fathers Bathing, Diapering, and Dressing Children under Age 5, 2002

(number of men aged 15 to 44 with children under age 5, and percent distribution by frequency of bathing, diapering, and dressing their children in past four weeks, by living arrangement with children and selected characteristics, 2002; numbers in thousands)

| | total | | frequency of bathing, diapering, dressing | | | |
	number	percent	not at all	about once a week or less	several times a week	everyday
LIVING WITH CHILDREN						
Total men aged 15 to 44 with children under age 5	**13,995**	**100.0%**	**8.4%**	**9.3%**	**29.9%**	**52.5%**
Aged 15 to 29	5,015	100.0	10.0	13.9	28.2	47.9
Aged 30 to 44	8,979	100.0	7.4	6.7	30.8	55.0
Race and Hispanic origin						
Black, non-Hispanic	1,446	100.0	8.9	3.1	34.1	53.9
Hispanic	2,931	100.0	16.3	18.2	33.7	31.8
White, non-Hispanic	8,472	100.0	5.1	7.4	26.4	61.1
Education						
High school graduate or less	7,158	100.0	12.3	12.5	33.7	41.6
Some college or more	6,565	100.0	3.2	5.7	25.7	65.4
NOT LIVING WITH CHILDREN						
Total men aged 15 to 44 with children under age 5	**1,938**	**100.0**	**55.9**	**18.1**	**18.3**	**7.7**
Aged 15 to 29	1,108	100.0	49.0	16.6	24.6	9.8
Aged 30 to 44	830	100.0	64.4	19.9	10.5	5.2
Race and Hispanic origin						
Black, non-Hispanic	451	100.0	51.3	28.1	10.4	10.2
Hispanic	859	100.0	63.0	14.4	15.8	6.8
White, non-Hispanic	504	100.0	–	–	–	–
Education						
High school graduate or less	1,263	100.0	63.3	14.5	15.2	7.0
Some college or more	574	100.0	44.8	23.1	25.2	6.9

Note: Men who live with their children may also have children living elsewhere; those men are represented under both categories. Education categories include only people aged 22 to 44. "–" means sample is too small to make a reliable estimate.
Source: National Center for Health Statistics, Fertility, Contraception, and Fatherhood: Data on Men and Women from Cycle 6 of the 2002 National Survey of Family Growth, Vital and Health Statistics, Series 23, No. 26, 2006; Internet site http://www.cdc .gov/nchs/nsfg.htm

Table 11.27 Fathers Playing with Children under Age 5, 2002

(number of men aged 15 to 44 with children under age 5, and percent distribution by frequency of playing with their children in past four weeks, by living arrangement with children and selected characteristics, 2002; numbers in thousands)

	total		frequency of playing			
	number	percent	not at all	about once a week or less	several times a week	everyday
LIVING WITH CHILDREN						
Total men aged 15 to 44 with children under age 5	**13,995**	**100.0%**	**0.9%**	**1.4%**	**16.6%**	**81.1%**
Aged 15 to 29	5,015	100.0	–	2.5	16.7	79.8
Aged 30 to 44	8,979	100.0	–	0.8	16.6	81.8
Race and Hispanic origin						
Black, non-Hispanic	1,446	100.0	–	–	19.3	77.8
Hispanic	2,931	100.0	–	4.0	21.9	71.9
White, non-Hispanic	8,472	100.0	–	–	13.2	86.1
Education						
High school graduate or less	7,158	100.0	–	2.3	20.7	75.8
Some college or more	6,565	100.0	–	–	12.1	87.1
NOT LIVING WITH CHILDREN						
Total men aged 15 to 44 with children under age 5	**1,938**	**100.0**	**48.6**	**17.4**	**24.0**	**10.0**
Aged 15 to 29	1,108	100.0	45.2	12.5	30.4	11.9
Aged 30 to 44	830	100.0	52.9	23.4	16.1	7.7
Race and Hispanic origin						
Black, non-Hispanic	451	100.0	32.5	24.1	30.0	13.4
Hispanic	859	100.0	59.5	16.5	15.8	8.2
White, non-Hispanic	504	100.0	–	–	–	–
Education						
High school graduate or less	1,263	100.0	57.2	12.7	21.1	9.1
Some college or more	574	100.0	35.8	25.1	30.8	8.4

Note: Men who live with their children may also have children living elsewhere; those men are represented under both categories. Education categories include only people aged 22 to 44. "–" means sample is too small to make a reliable estimate.
Source: National Center for Health Statistics, Fertility, Contraception, and Fatherhood: Data on Men and Women from Cycle 6 of the 2002 National Survey of Family Growth, Vital and Health Statistics, Series 23, No. 26, 2006; Internet site http://www.cdc .gov/nchs/nsfg.htm

Table 11.28 Fathers Reading to Children under Age 5, 2002

(number of men aged 15 to 44 with children under age 5, and percent distribution by frequency of reading to their children in past four weeks, by living arrangement with children and selected characteristics, 2002; numbers in thousands)

| | total | | frequency of reading | | | |
	number	percent	not at all	about once a week or less	several times a week	everyday
LIVING WITH CHILDREN						
Total men aged 15 to 44 with children under age 5	**13,995**	**100.0%**	**17.2%**	**26.5%**	**31.0%**	**25.3%**
Aged 15 to 29	5,015	100.0	20.8	31.5	26.4	21.3
Aged 30 to 44	8,979	100.0	15.2	23.8	33.5	27.6
Race and Hispanic origin						
Black, non-Hispanic	1,446	100.0	10.8	37.5	25.7	25.9
Hispanic	2,931	100.0	36.0	26.3	22.8	14.8
White, non-Hispanic	8,472	100.0	11.7	23.0	35.1	30.2
Education						
High school graduate or less	7,158	100.0	24.6	30.6	25.3	19.5
Some college or more	6,565	100.0	8.3	22.3	37.4	32.0
NOT LIVING WITH CHILDREN						
Total men aged 15 to 44 with children under age 5	**1,938**	**100.0**	**61.0**	**22.0**	**12.2**	**4.9**
Aged 15 to 29	1,108	100.0	58.8	21.1	13.0	7.1
Aged 30 to 44	830	100.0	63.6	23.0	11.2	2.2
Race and Hispanic origin						
Black, non-Hispanic	451	100.0	55.3	20.3	14.6	9.9
Hispanic	859	100.0	68.0	20.8	8.1	3.2
White, non-Hispanic	504	100.0	–	–	–	–
Education						
High school graduate or less	1,263	100.0	69.5	15.4	9.6	5.6
Some college or more	574	100.0	43.8	36.7	15.4	4.2

Note: Men who live with their children may also have children living elsewhere; those men are represented under both categories. Education categories include only people aged 22 to 44. "–" means sample is too small to make a reliable estimate.
Source: National Center for Health Statistics, Fertility, Contraception, and Fatherhood: Data on Men and Women from Cycle 6 of the 2002 National Survey of Family Growth, Vital and Health Statistics, Series 23, No. 26, 2006; Internet site http://www.cdc .gov/nchs/nsfg.htm

Table 11.29 Fathers Taking Children Aged 5 to 18 to and from Activities, 2002

(number of men aged 15 to 44 with children aged 5 to 18, and percent distribution by frequency of taking their children to or from their activities in past four weeks, by living arrangement with children and selected characteristics, 2002; numbers in thousands)

	total		frequency of taking to or from activities			
	number	percent	not at all	about once a week or less	several times a week	everyday
LIVING WITH CHILDREN						
Total men aged 15 to 44 with children aged 5 to 18	**18,251**	**100.0%**	**19.4%**	**26.9%**	**34.9%**	**18.8%**
Aged 15 to 29	2,401	100.0	25.5	25.7	37.1	11.7
Aged 30 to 44	15,850	100.0	18.5	27.1	34.6	19.8
Race and Hispanic origin						
Black, non-Hispanic	1,993	100.0	22.0	30.2	28.1	19.7
Hispanic	3,460	100.0	23.8	23.4	27.5	25.4
White, non-Hispanic	11,140	100.0	17.7	28.6	36.6	17.0
Education						
Not a high school graduate	3,097	100.0	28.3	27.8	22.0	21.9
High school graduate or GED	7,218	100.0	22.9	27.1	32.1	17.9
Some college or more	7,677	100.0	11.3	26.8	43.3	18.7
NOT LIVING WITH CHILDREN						
Total men aged 15 to 44 with children aged 5 to 18	**6,273**	**100.0**	**73.2**	**19.9**	**5.0**	**1.9**
Aged 15 to 29	789	100.0	76.1	12.8	6.6	–
Aged 30 to 44	5,485	100.0	72.8	20.9	4.7	1.6
Race and Hispanic origin						
Black, non-Hispanic	1,480	100.0	66.3	21.1	9.2	3.4
Hispanic	1,403	100.0	79.2	15.6	2.9	–
White, non-Hispanic	2,898	100.0	71.9	23.0	4.0	–
Education						
Not a high school graduate	1,387	100.0	84.1	11.0	3.8	–
High school graduate or GED	2,662	100.0	69.1	24.0	4.3	2.6
Some college or more	2,205	100.0	71.9	20.8	6.5	–

Note: Men who live with their children may also have children living elsewhere; those men are represented under both categories. Education categories include only people aged 22 to 44. "–" means sample is too small to make a reliable estimate.
Source: National Center for Health Statistics, Fertility, Contraception, and Fatherhood: Data on Men and Women from Cycle 6 of the 2002 National Survey of Family Growth, Vital and Health Statistics, Series 23, No. 26, 2006; Internet site http://www.cdc.gov/nchs/nsfg.htm

Table 11.30 Fathers Talking with Children Aged 5 to 18, 2002

(number of men aged 15 to 44 with children aged 5 to 18, and percent distribution by frequency of talking with their children about things that happened during the day in past four weeks, by living arrangement with children and selected characteristics, 2002; numbers in thousands)

	total		frequency of talking with children			
	number	percent	not at all	about once a week or less	several times a week	everyday
LIVING WITH CHILDREN						
Total men aged 15 to 44 with children aged 5 to 18	**18,251**	**100.0%**	**2.5%**	**10.4%**	**23.6%**	**63.6%**
Aged 15 to 29	2,401	100.0	6.6	11.9	23.6	57.9
Aged 30 to 44	15,850	100.0	1.9	10.2	23.6	64.4
Race and Hispanic origin						
Black, non-Hispanic	1,993	100.0	5.2	12.7	22.5	59.6
Hispanic	3,460	100.0	4.6	19.7	23.5	52.2
White, non-Hispanic	11,140	100.0	1.8	6.6	24.3	67.4
Education						
Not a high school graduate	3,097	100.0	7.0	14.2	17.3	61.5
High school graduate or GED	7,218	100.0	0.7	14.6	25.8	59.0
Some college or more	7,677	100.0	1.8	4.6	24.0	69.7
NOT LIVING WITH CHILDREN						
Total men aged 15 to 44 with children aged 5 to 18	**6,273**	**100.0**	**42.2**	**31.4**	**18.3**	**8.1**
Aged 15 to 29	789	100.0	44.7	26.0	14.9	14.4
Aged 30 to 44	5,485	100.0	41.8	32.2	18.8	7.2
Race and Hispanic origin						
Black, non-Hispanic	1,480	100.0	31.9	37.1	22.2	8.9
Hispanic	1,403	100.0	59.2	20.3	12.1	8.5
White, non-Hispanic	2,898	100.0	37.5	36.6	18.0	8.0
Education						
Not a high school graduate	1,387	100.0	61.5	20.5	14.4	3.7
High school graduate or GED	2,662	100.0	36.9	34.6	19.4	9.1
Some college or more	2,205	100.0	36.7	34.8	19.5	9.0

Note: Men who live with their children may also have children living elsewhere; those men are represented under both categories. Education categories include only people aged 22 to 44.
Source: National Center for Health Statistics, Fertility, Contraception, and Fatherhood: Data on Men and Women from Cycle 6 of the 2002 National Survey of Family Growth, Vital and Health Statistics, Series 23, No. 26, 2006; Internet site http://www.cdc.gov/nchs/nsfg.htm

Table 11.31 Fathers Helping Children Aged 5 to 18 with Homework, 2002

(number of men aged 15 to 44 with children aged 5 to 18, and percent distribution by frequency of helping their children with homework or checking that they did homework in past four weeks, by living arrangement with children and selected characteristics, 2002; numbers in thousands)

	total		frequency of helping with or checking homework			
	number	percent	not at all	about once a week or less	several times a week	everyday
LIVING WITH CHILDREN						
Total men aged 15 to 44 with children aged 5 to 18	**18,251**	**100.0%**	**18.2%**	**24.3%**	**28.8%**	**28.7%**
Aged 15 to 29	2,401	100.0	18.9	23.2	28.9	29.0
Aged 30 to 44	15,850	100.0	18.1	24.5	28.7	28.7
Race and Hispanic origin						
Black, non-Hispanic	1,993	100.0	17.4	31.8	18.6	32.2
Hispanic	3,460	100.0	17.9	22.0	24.9	35.2
White, non-Hispanic	11,140	100.0	19.1	22.5	31.9	26.5
Education						
Not a high school graduate	3,097	100.0	26.5	16.2	22.4	34.9
High school graduate or GED	7,218	100.0	19.8	24.5	27.7	28.0
Some college or more	7,677	100.0	13.1	27.2	32.9	26.9
NOT LIVING WITH CHILDREN						
Total men aged 15 to 44 with children aged 5 to 18	**6,273**	**100.0**	**73.6**	**18.2**	**4.8**	**3.4**
Aged 15 to 29	789	100.0	70.9	17.2	4.4	7.5
Aged 30 to 44	5,485	100.0	74.0	18.4	4.8	2.8
Race and Hispanic origin						
Black, non-Hispanic	1,480	100.0	71.5	15.2	9.0	4.3
Hispanic	1,403	100.0	76.0	18.5	1.2	4.3
White, non-Hispanic	2,898	100.0	72.4	20.6	5.1	1.9
Education						
Not a high school graduate	1,387	100.0	86.1	10.5	2.3	–
High school graduate or GED	2,662	100.0	70.3	20.9	3.9	5.0
Some college or more	2,205	100.0	69.5	20.0	7.4	3.0

Note: Men who live with their children may also have children living elsewhere; those men are represented under both categories. Education categories include only people aged 22 to 44. "–" means sample is too small to make a reliable estimate.
Source: National Center for Health Statistics, Fertility, Contraception, and Fatherhood: Data on Men and Women from Cycle 6 of the 2002 National Survey of Family Growth, Vital and Health Statistics, Series 23, No. 26, 2006; Internet site http://www.cdc .gov/nchs/nsfg.htm

Table 11.32 Father's Attendance at Religious Services with Children Aged 5 to 18, 2002

(number of men aged 15 to 44 with children aged 5 to 18, and percent distribution by frequency of attendance at religious services with their children in past 12 months, by living arrangement with children and selected characteristics, 2002; numbers in thousands)

	total		frequency of attendance		
	number	percent	not at all	less than once a month	once a month or more
LIVING WITH CHILDREN					
Total men aged 15 to 44 with children aged 5 to 18	**18,251**	**100.0%**	**32.9%**	**25.0%**	**42.2%**
Aged 15 to 29	2,401	100.0	43.5	20.6	35.8
Aged 30 to 44	15,850	100.0	31.3	25.6	43.1
Race and Hispanic origin					
Black, non-Hispanic	1,993	100.0	25.4	23.6	51.0
Hispanic	3,460	100.0	27.5	29.3	43.2
White, non-Hispanic	11,140	100.0	36.0	24.3	39.6
Education					
Not a high school graduate	3,097	100.0	43.9	20.3	35.9
High school graduate or GED	7,218	100.0	36.9	24.7	38.4
Some college or more	7,677	100.0	23.9	27.5	48.6
Importance of religion					
Very important	8,309	100.0	13.4	19.4	67.2
Somewhat important	5,853	100.0	34.8	34.8	30.4
Not important	4,090	100.0	69.9	22.1	8.1
NOT LIVING WITH CHILDREN					
Total men aged 15 to 44 with children aged 5 to 18	**6,273**	**100.0**	**64.2**	**24.1**	**11.7**
Aged 15 to 29	789	100.0	70.7	15.1	14.2
Aged 30 to 44	5,485	100.0	63.2	25.4	11.4
Race and Hispanic origin					
Black, non-Hispanic	1,480	100.0	54.3	36.3	9.5
Hispanic	1,403	100.0	73.0	12.0	15.0
White, non-Hispanic	2,898	100.0	63.8	25.9	10.4
Education					
Not a high school graduate	1,387	100.0	71.5	16.0	12.5
High school graduate or GED	2,662	100.0	65.7	23.3	11.0
Some college or more	2,205	100.0	58.1	30.5	11.3
Importance of religion					
Very important	3,263	100.0	55.3	26.1	18.5
Somewhat important	1,514	100.0	62.5	31.1	6.4
Not important	1,487	100.0	84.4	13.0	–

Note: Men who live with their children may also have children living elsewhere; those men are represented under both categories. Education categories include only people aged 22 to 44. "–" means sample is too small to make a reliable estimate.
Source: National Center for Health Statistics, Fertility, Contraception, and Fatherhood: Data on Men and Women from Cycle 6 of the 2002 National Survey of Family Growth, Vital and Health Statistics, Series 23, No. 26, 2006; Internet site http://www.cdc.gov/nchs/nsfg.htm

Table 11.33 Fathers' Rating of Job of Fatherhood, 2002

(number of men aged 15 to 44 with children under age 19, and percent distribution by how good a job they think they do as a father, by living arrangement with children and selected characteristics, 2002; numbers in thousands)

	total		how good a job you do as a father			
	number	percent	very good	good	okay	not very good or bad
LIVING WITH CHILDREN						
Total men aged 15 to 44 with children under age 19	**23,856**	**100.0%**	**46.4%**	**43.5%**	**9.7%**	**0.4%**
Aged 15 to 24	1,408	100.0	60.6	33.4	6.0	–
Aged 25 to 29	3,537	100.0	52.8	37.1	10.1	–
Aged 30 to 44	18,912	100.0	44.1	45.5	9.9	0.5
Race and Hispanic origin						
Black, non-Hispanic	2,452	100.0	50.8	33.1	15.8	–
Hispanic	4,520	100.0	42.8	42.2	14.3	–
White, non-Hispanic	14,774	100.0	47.4	45.0	7.5	–
Education						
Not a high school graduate	3,722	100.0	44.0	42.2	12.7	–
High school grad. or GED	8,912	100.0	42.3	46.8	10.7	–
Some college or more	10,768	100.0	50.2	41.6	8.0	–
NOT LIVING WITH CHILDREN						
Total men aged 15 to 44 with children under age 19	**7,405**	**100.0**	**26.7**	**29.1**	**24.0**	**20.2**
Aged 15 to 24	627	100.0	21.2	38.2	23.1	17.5
Aged 25 to 29	928	100.0	32.7	20.0	22.2	25.1
Aged 30 to 44	5,850	100.0	26.3	29.5	24.4	19.8
Race and Hispanic origin						
Black, non-Hispanic	1,745	100.0	29.2	28.3	27.1	15.4
Hispanic	1,897	100.0	25.5	31.0	25.2	18.3
White, non-Hispanic	3,190	100.0	29.3	27.9	21.0	21.8
Education						
Not a high school graduate	1,577	100.0	18.8	34.5	23.1	23.6
High school grad. or GED	2,992	100.0	30.3	23.7	25.1	20.9
Some college or more	2,545	100.0	28.0	31.4	22.5	18.2

Note: Men who live with their children may also have children living elsewhere; those men are represented under both categories. Education categories include only people aged 22 to 44. "–" means sample is too small to make a reliable estimate.
Source: National Center for Health Statistics, Fertility, Contraception, and Fatherhood: Data on Men and Women from Cycle 6 of the 2002 National Survey of Family Growth, Vital and Health Statistics, Series 23, No. 26, 2006; Internet site http://www.cdc .gov/nchs/nsfg.htm

Most Mothers Work

Even among women with children under age 1, the majority is in the labor force.

Among married couples with children under age 18, the 61 percent majority are dual-income couples. Seventy-one percent of women heading single-parent families have jobs, as do 83 percent of men who head single-parent families.

Among women with children under age 18, fully 71 percent were in the labor force in 2005. Fifty percent are employed full-time.

Fifty-five percent of women who have given birth in the past year are in the labor force, and 35 percent are full-time workers. The new mothers most likely to work are those aged 30 to 44 (59 percent), those with only one child (60 percent), non-Hispanic whites (60 percent), and those with graduate degrees (70 percent).

■ With most parents working, day care has become the norm in childhood.

Women with school-aged children are most likely to work

(percent of women in the labor force by presence and age of children at home, 2005)

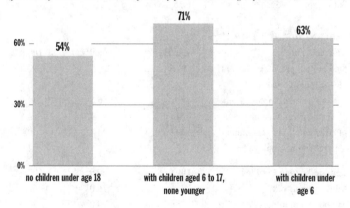

Table 11.34 Labor Force Status of Parents with Children under Age 18, 2005

(number and percent distribution of people aged 16 or older with own children under age 18 by family type, labor force status, and age of children, 2005; numbers in thousands)

		with children under age 18	
	total	aged 6 to 17, none younger	under age 6
NUMBER			
Married couples	**24,942**	**13,781**	**11,161**
One or both parents employed	24,218	13,350	10,868
Mother employed	16,501	9,990	6,511
Both parents employed	15,298	9,210	6,089
Mother employed, not father	1,203	780	422
Father employed, not mother	7,716	3,360	4,357
Neither parent employed	724	431	293
Female-headed families	**8,347**	**5,147**	**3,200**
Mother employed	5,943	3,913	2,030
Mother not employed	2,404	1,233	1,170
Male-headed families	**2,113**	**1,274**	**839**
Father employed	1,756	1,056	700
Father not employed	357	218	139
PERCENT DISTRIBUTION			
Married couples	**100.0%**	**100.0%**	**100.0%**
One or both parents employed	97.1	96.9	97.4
Mother employed	66.2	72.5	58.3
Both parents employed	61.3	66.8	54.6
Mother employed, not father	4.8	5.7	3.8
Father employed, not mother	30.9	24.4	39.0
Neither parent employed	2.9	3.1	2.6
Female-headed families	**100.0**	**100.0**	**100.0**
Mother employed	71.2	76.0	63.4
Mother not employed	28.8	24.0	36.6
Male-headed families	**100.0**	**100.0**	**100.0**
Father employed	83.1	82.9	83.4
Father not employed	16.9	17.1	16.6

Source: Bureau of Labor Statistics, Employment Characteristics of Families, Internet site http://www.bls.gov/news.release/ famee.t04.htm

Table 11.35 Labor Force Status of Women by Presence of Children, 2005

(number and percent distribution of women by labor force status and presence and age of own children under age 18 at home, 2005; numbers in thousands)

	civilian population	civilian labor force				not in labor force
		total	employed			
			total	full-time	part-time	
Total women	**116,931**	**69,118**	**65,756**	**49,158**	**16,599**	**47,813**
No children under age 18	80,514	43,461	41,462	31,019	10,444	37,053
With children under age 18	36,417	25,657	24,294	18,139	6,155	10,760
Children aged 6 to 17, none younger	20,348	15,572	14,887	11,468	3,419	4,776
Children under age 6	16,070	10,085	9,407	6,671	2,736	5,985
Children under age 3	9,365	5,470	5,077	3,501	1,576	3,895
Children under age 1	3,233	1,740	1,600	1,092	508	1,493
Total women	**100.0%**	**59.1%**	**56.2%**	**42.0%**	**14.2%**	**40.9%**
No children under age 18	100.0	54.0	51.5	38.5	13.0	46.0
With children under age 18	100.0	70.5	66.7	49.8	16.9	29.5
Children aged 6 to 17, none younger	100.0	76.5	73.2	56.4	16.8	23.5
Children under age 6	100.0	62.8	58.5	41.5	17.0	37.2
Children under age 3	100.0	58.4	54.2	37.4	16.8	41.6
Children under age 1	100.0	53.8	49.5	33.8	15.7	46.2

Source: Bureau of Labor Statistics, Employment Characteristics of Families, Internet site http://www.bls.gov/news.release/ famee.t05.htm and http://www.bls.gov/news.release/famee.t06.htm; calculations by New Strategist

Table 11.36 Labor Force Status of Women Aged 15 to 44 Who Gave Birth in Past Year, 2004

(percent distribution of women aged 15 to 44 who gave birth in past year by selected characateristics and labor force status, 2004)

	total	in labor force total	full-time	part-time	unemployed	not in labor force
Women aged 15 to 44 who gave birth in past year	**100.0%**	**54.6%**	**34.8%**	**13.9%**	**5.9%**	**45.4%**
Aged 15 to 19	100.0	40.1	13.1	16.3	10.7	59.9
Aged 20 to 24	100.0	52.7	31.5	12.6	8.7	47.3
Aged 25 to 29	100.0	55.1	37.4	13.3	4.4	44.9
Aged 30 to 44	100.0	59.1	40.5	14.4	4.1	40.9
Marital status						
Married, husband present	100.0	55.3	38.9	13.3	3.0	44.7
Divorced or widowed	100.0	54.8	33.0	14.3	7.5	45.2
Never married	100.0	53.8	26.9	15.2	11.7	46.2
Children ever borne and age						
One child	100.0	59.8	41.4	12.7	5.7	40.2
Aged 15 to 19	100.0	44.4	17.7	17.4	9.4	55.6
Aged 20 to 24	100.0	55.6	35.6	11.4	8.6	44.4
Aged 25 to 29	100.0	65.0	48.3	13.9	2.8	35.0
Aged 30 to 44	100.0	67.0	53.0	10.6	3.4	33.0
Two or more children	100.0	51.3	30.5	14.7	6.1	48.7
Aged 15 to 19	100.0	34.3	6.9	14.8	12.5	65.7
Aged 20 to 24	100.0	50.0	27.5	13.7	8.8	50.0
Aged 25 to 29	100.0	48.2	29.8	12.9	5.5	51.8
Aged 30 to 44	100.0	55.9	35.6	16.0	4.4	44.1
Race and Hispanic origin						
Asian	100.0	34.9	26.2	8.1	0.6	65.1
Black	100.0	55.2	35.3	6.2	13.8	44.8
Hispanic	100.0	48.3	32.4	10.0	6.0	51.7
White, non-Hispanic	100.0	59.5	36.7	18.1	4.7	40.5
Education						
Not a high school graduate	100.0	35.6	16.5	10.4	8.7	64.4
High school graduate or GED	100.0	52.3	32.6	12.9	6.8	47.7
College, one year or more	100.0	63.4	43.2	15.8	4.4	36.6
No degree	100.0	58.6	36.2	17.5	4.9	41.4
Associate's degree	100.0	75.6	49.9	16.9	8.7	24.4
Bachelor's degree	100.0	60.1	43.1	14.3	2.7	39.9
Graduate or prof. degree	100.0	70.0	53.4	14.3	2.3	30.0

Source: Bureau of the Census, Fertility of American Women: June 2004, Current Population Reports, P20–555, 2005; Internet site http://www.census.gov/population/www/socdemo/fertility.html

Working Women Depend on a Variety of Childcare Arrangements

Most popular is care by grandparents or other relatives.

Among working women with children under age 13, the most popular childcare provider is one of the child's grandparents or another relative, used by 35 percent in the past four weeks. Ranking second is a day care center, used by 23 percent. Seventeen percent of working mothers have nonrelatives caring for their children.

Unmarried mothers are most likely to depend on relatives for childcare, and 46 percent do so. Also, the younger the child, the more likely the mother depends on relatives for care. Among women with children aged 1 to 5, 44 percent have used relatives for care in the past four weeks versus only 24 percent of women with children aged 6 to 12. Depending on relatives for childcare does not vary by education, but the use of day care centers increases greatly with the educational level of the mother. Thirty-one percent of working women with a bachelor's degree used a day care center in the past four weeks versus only 10 percent of those who did not graduate from high school.

■ Grandparents and other relatives provide an enormous amount of childcare for the nation's working parents.

Women with a college degree are most likely to use day care centers

(percent of working women aged 15 to 44 with children under age 13 using a day care center as their childcare arrangement during past four weeks, by education, 2002)

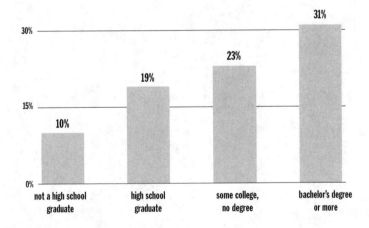

Table 11.37 **Childcare Arrangements during Past Month by Mother's Work Status, 2002**

(percent of working women aged 15 to 44 who live with at least one child under age 13 and have used selected childcare arrangements during past four weeks, by full- or part-time work status, 2002; numbers in thousands)

	total working mothers	work full-time	work part-time
All childcare arrangements	**100.0%**	**100.0%**	**100.0%**
Grandparent or other relative	35.1	36.4	31.8
Day care center or preschool	22.6	24.0	19.0
Nonrelative	16.7	16.3	17.7
Before- or after-school care	10.0	11.8	5.2
Other parent or stepparent	7.3	7.5	7.0
Kindergarten or school	6.9	6.8	7.3
Child's brother or sister	5.6	6.3	3.6
Family day care	3.8	4.2	2.7
Other arrangement	4.0	4.8	1.8

Note: Figures will not sum to 100 because more than one childcare arrangement may have been used. "Other arrangement" includes federally funded Head Start program, child cares for self, and "other" arrangements.
Source: National Center for Health Statistics, Fertility, Family Planning, and Reproductive Health of U.S. Women: Data from the 2002 National Survey of Family Growth, Vital and Health Statistics, Series 23, No. 25, 2005; Internet site http://www.cdc .gov/nchs/nsfg.htm

Table 11.38 Childcare Arrangements during Past Month by Age of Child, 2002

(percent of working women aged 15 to 44 who live with at least one child under age 13 and have used selected childcare arrangements during the past four weeks, by age of youngest child at home, 2002; numbers in thousands)

	total working mothers	age of youngest child		
		under 1	1 to 5	6 to 12
All childcare arrangements	**100.0%**	**100.0%**	**100.0%**	**100.0%**
Grandparent or other relative	35.1	37.2	43.8	24.3
Day care center or preschool	22.6	20.4	36.4	6.5
Nonrelative	16.7	22.0	21.2	10.2
Before- or after-school care	10.0	3.2	8.6	13.0
Other parent or stepparent	7.3	4.6	8.8	6.2
Kindergarten or school	6.9	3.4	10.1	3.8
Child's brother or sister	5.6	0.7	4.3	8.1
Family day care	3.8	5.0	5.5	1.4
Other arrangement	4.0	2.1	3.7	4.7

Note: Figures will not sum to 100 because more than one childcare arrangement may have been used. "Other arrangement" includes federally funded Head Start program, child cares for self, and "other" arrangements.
Source: National Center for Health Statistics, Fertility, Family Planning, and Reproductive Health of U.S. Women: Data from the 2002 National Survey of Family Growth, Vital and Health Statistics, Series 23, No. 25, 2005; Internet site http://www.cdc .gov/nchs/nsfg.htm

Table 11.39 Childcare Arrangements during Past Month by Mother's Marital Status, 2002

(percent of working women aged 15 to 44 who live with at least one child under age 13 and have used selected childcare arrangements during the past four weeks, by marital status, 2002; numbers in thousands)

	total working mothers	currently married	currently cohabiting	never married, not cohabiting	formerly married, not cohabiting
All childcare arrangements	**100.0%**	**100.0%**	**100.0%**	**100.0%**	**100.0%**
Grandparent or other relative	35.1	31.5	38.3	46.4	39.4
Day care center or preschool	22.6	22.7	17.2	25.3	22.9
Nonrelative	16.7	15.4	19.2	21.3	17.0
Before- or after-school care	10.0	8.2	11.6	11.1	15.9
Other parent or stepparent	7.3	4.8	13.7	6.3	15.9
Kindergarten or school	6.9	6.7	9.1	5.0	8.2
Child's brother or sister	5.6	3.7	2.9	5.0	15.8
Family day care	3.8	3.3	5.3	6.7	2.4
Other arrangement	4.0	3.5	1.9	4.8	6.5

Note: Figures will not sum to 100 because more than one childcare arrangement may have been used. "Other arrangement" includes federally funded Head Start program, child cares for self, and "other" arrangements.
Source: National Center for Health Statistics, Fertility, Family Planning, and Reproductive Health of U.S. Women: Data from the 2002 National Survey of Family Growth, Vital and Health Statistics, Series 23, No. 25, 2005; Internet site http://www.cdc .gov/nchs/nsfg.htm

Table 11.40 Childcare Arrangements during Past Month by Mother's Race and Hispanic Origin, 2002

(percent of working women aged 15 to 44 who live with at least one child under age 13 and have used selected childcare arrangements during the past four weeks, by race and Hispanic origin, 2002; numbers in thousands)

	total working mothers	non-Hispanic black	Hispanic	non-Hispanic white
All childcare arrangements	**100.0%**	**100.0%**	**100.0%**	**100.0%**
Grandparent or other relative	35.1	33.4	34.8	35.7
Day care center or preschool	22.6	27.1	15.3	24.1
Nonrelative	16.7	9.6	16.5	17.9
Before- or after-school care	10.0	15.3	6.9	9.2
Other parent or stepparent	7.3	8.4	5.5	7.3
Kindergarten or school	6.9	6.4	4.4	7.4
Child's brother or sister	5.6	4.5	4.6	6.2
Family day care	3.8	4.8	2.8	3.6
Other arrangement	4.0	6.2	2.5	3.8

Note: Figures will not sum to 100 because more than one childcare arrangement may have been used. "Other arrangement" includes federally funded Head Start program, child cares for self, and "other" arrangements.
Source: National Center for Health Statistics, Fertility, Family Planning, and Reproductive Health of U.S. Women: Data from the 2002 National Survey of Family Growth, Vital and Health Statistics, Series 23, No. 25, 2005; Internet site http://www.cdc .gov/nchs/nsfg.htm

Table 11.41 Childcare Arrangements during Past Month by Mother's Education, 2002

(percent of working women aged 15 to 44 who live with at least one child under age 13 and have used selected childcare arrangements during the past four weeks, by education, 2002; numbers in thousands)

	total working mothers	not a high school graduate	high school graduate	some college, no degree	bachelor's degree or more
All childcare arrangements	**100.0%**	**100.0%**	**100.0%**	**100.0%**	**100.0%**
Grandparent or other relative	35.1	33.5	35.9	33.8	34.1
Day care center or preschool	22.6	9.7	18.8	23.4	30.8
Nonrelative	16.7	17.3	16.5	14.7	20.1
Before- or after-school care	10.0	4.6	8.7	10.8	14.3
Other parent or stepparent	7.3	2.8	6.2	9.6	7.2
Kindergarten or school	6.9	1.4	5.7	6.8	11.6
Child's brother or sister	5.6	4.7	5.3	6.5	5.0
Family day care	3.8	3.8	2.6	4.2	4.3
Other arrangement	4.0	3.1	3.6	4.3	4.7

Note: Figures will not sum to 100 because more than one childcare arrangement may have been used. "Other arrangement" includes federally funded Head Start program, child cares for self, and "other" arrangements.
Source: National Center for Health Statistics, Fertility, Family Planning, and Reproductive Health of U.S. Women: Data from the 2002 National Survey of Family Growth, Vital and Health Statistics, Series 23, No. 25, 2005; Internet site http://www.cdc .gov/nchs/nsfg.htm

Table 11.42 Childcare Arrangements during Past Month by Metropolitan Residence, 2002

(percent of working women aged 15 to 44 who live with at least one child under age 13 and have used sing selected childcare arrangements during the past four weeks, by metropolitan residence, 2002; numbers in thousands)

	total working mothers	metropolitan		nonmetropolitan
		central city	suburbs	
All childcare arrangements	**100.0%**	**100.0%**	**100.0%**	**100.0%**
Grandparent or other relative	35.1	35.8	33.2	36.4
Day care center or preschool	22.6	23.0	25.3	16.9
Nonrelative	16.7	16.6	18.6	13.6
Before- or after-school care	10.0	10.6	10.9	6.3
Other parent or stepparent	7.3	7.3	8.1	5.9
Kindergarten or school	6.9	7.6	6.1	6.2
Child's brother or sister	5.6	5.8	4.0	7.7
Family day care	3.8	3.6	3.4	4.9
Other arrangement	4.0	4.2	4.0	3.1

Note: Figures will not sum to 100 because more than one childcare arrangement may have been used. "Other arrangement" includes federally funded Head Start program, child cares for self, and "other" arrangements.
Source: National Center for Health Statistics, Fertility, Family Planning, and Reproductive Health of U.S. Women: Data from the 2002 National Survey of Family Growth, Vital and Health Statistics, Series 23, No. 25, 2005; Internet site http://www.cdc .gov/nchs/nsfg.htm

Few Young and Middle-Aged Adults Believe in Traditional Sex Roles

Most think working women can have just as good a relationship with their children as women who do not work.

Only about one-third of men and women aged 15 to 44 agree that traditional sex roles—where the man earns the living and the woman takes care of the home and family—are best. Those most likely to subscribe to traditional roles are fundamentalist Protestants.

Seventy-three percent of men and 83 percent of women think working women can establish just as warm a relationship with their children as mothers who do not work. Regardless of demographic characteristic, the majority of 15-to-44-year-olds agree. And most also think it is more important for a man to spend a lot of time with his family than to be successful in his career.

■ Young and middle-aged men and women want to have it all—a successful family life and a career.

Fundamentalist Protestant men are the most traditional

(percent of men aged 15 to 44 agreeing with the statement, "It is much better for everyone if the man earns the main living and the women takes care of the home and family," by current religion, 2002)

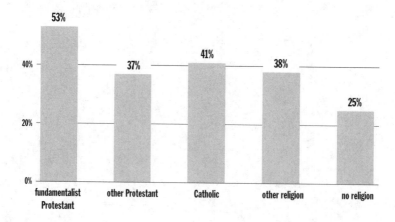

Table 11.43 Attitude toward Traditional Sex Roles by Sex, 2002

"It is much better for everyone if the man earns the main living
and the woman takes care of the home and family."

(percent of people aged 15 to 44 agreeing with statement, by selected characteristics and sex, 2002)

	percent agreeing	
	men	women
Total aged 15 to 44	**36.6%**	**33.5%**
Aged 15 to 24	37.6	27.4
Aged 25 to 29	36.1	34.4
Aged 30 to 44	36.3	36.9
Marital status		
Currently married	39.7	39.7
Currently cohabiting	42.6	32.0
Never married, not cohabiting	33.2	25.8
Formerly married, not cohabiting	30.7	33.5
Number of children ever borne or fathered		
None	32.9	23.9
One or more	40.9	40.3
Race and Hispanic origin		
Black, non-Hispanic	35.5	31.2
Hispanic	57.9	49.2
White, non-Hispanic	31.1	30.1
Education		
Not a high school graduate	59.0	55.9
High school graduate or GED	34.9	37.5
Some college, no degree	33.8	34.9
Bachelor's degree or more	27.7	25.9
Current religion		
No religion	25.2	24.6
Fundamentalist Protestant	52.7	44.2
Other Protestant	37.1	34.8
Catholic	40.5	34.4
Other religion	37.7	29.1
Importance of religion		
Very important	48.6	41.5
Somewhat important	33.8	26.6
Not important	23.9	23.9

Source: National Center for Health Statistics, Fertility, Contraception, and Fatherhood: Data on Men and Women from Cycle 6 of the 2002 National Survey of Family Growth, Vital and Health Statistics, Series 23, No. 26, 2006; Internet site http://www.cdc.gov/nchs/nsfg.htm

Table 11.44 Attitude toward Working Women by Sex, 2002

"A working woman can establish just as warm and secure a relationship with her children as a mother who does not work."

(percent of people aged 15 to 44 agreeing with statement, by selected characteristics and sex, 2002)

	percent agreeing	
	men	women
Total aged 15 to 44	**72.6%**	**83.2%**
Aged 15 to 24	75.0	84.1
Aged 25 to 29	71.5	84.8
Aged 30 to 44	71.4	82.2
Marital status		
Currently married	71.1	81.2
Currently cohabiting	67.9	86.2
Never married, not cohabiting	75.2	85.2
Formerly married, not cohabiting	72.4	82.5
Number of children ever borne or fathered		
None	74.8	84.2
One or more	70.2	62.4
Race and Hispanic origin		
Black, non-Hispanic	80.3	88.0
Hispanic	67.9	76.2
White, non-Hispanic	73.2	84.1
Education		
Not a high school graduate	66.5	74.7
High school graduate or GED	71.2	84.2
Some college, no degree	72.0	82.1
Bachelor's degree or more	75.5	84.5
Current religion		
No religion	74.1	84.4
Fundamentalist Protestant	69.0	84.9
Other Protestant	74.0	82.9
Catholic	71.1	83.0
Other religion	70.4	81.6
Importance of religion		
Very important	69.4	80.5
Somewhat important	75.5	86.8
Not important	73.6	84.2

Source: National Center for Health Statistics, Fertility, Contraception, and Fatherhood: Data on Men and Women from Cycle 6 of the 2002 National Survey of Family Growth, Vital and Health Statistics, Series 23, No. 26, 2006; Internet site http://www.cdc .gov/nchs/nsfg.htm

Table 11.45 Attitude toward Working Men by Sex, 2002

"It is more important for a man to spend a lot of time with his family than to be successful at his career."

(percent of people aged 15 to 44 agreeing with statement, by selected characteristics and sex, 2002)

	percent agreeing	
	men	women
Total aged 15 to 44	**76.3%**	**72.1%**
Aged 15 to 24	71.4	68.5
Aged 25 to 29	73.1	73.4
Aged 30 to 44	80.4	74.0
Marital status		
Currently married	82.2	76.4
Currently cohabiting	71.6	64.8
Never married, not cohabiting	71.1	68.7
Formerly married, not cohabiting	78.6	71.4
Number of children ever borne or fathered		
None	72.9	71.5
One or more	80.4	72.5
Race and Hispanic origin		
Black, non-Hispanic	69.4	62.6
Hispanic	68.2	67.2
White, non-Hispanic	80.1	75.1
Education		
Not a high school graduate	72.0	63.4
High school graduate or GED	75.3	69.2
Some college, no degree	78.8	74.1
Bachelor's degree or more	83.3	81.3
Current religion		
No religion	73.6	72.0
Fundamentalist Protestant	81.0	69.9
Other Protestant	80.4	74.1
Catholic	72.2	70.2
Other religion	75.1	69.6
Importance of religion		
Very important	80.9	74.7
Somewhat important	74.3	69.1
Not important	72.6	70.7

Source: National Center for Health Statistics, Fertility, Contraception, and Fatherhood: Data on Men and Women from Cycle 6 of the 2002 National Survey of Family Growth, Vital and Health Statistics, Series 23, No. 26, 2006; Internet site http://www.cdc .gov/nchs/nsfg.htm

Appendix

National Survey of Family Growth

The National Survey of Family Growth (NSFG) is a survey of Americans' sexual and reproductive behavior taken every few years by the National Center for Health Statistics. It is based on interviews administered in person by trained interviewers in the respondent's home. The Cycle 6 (2002) data are based on a nationally representative sample of the household population. Interviews were carried out between March 2002 and March 2003.

The NSFG data are collected through computer-assisted interviewing, with questionnaires programmed into laptop computers. Interviewers administered most of the questions, but some of the more sensitive questions were asked using audio computer assisted self-interviewing. This mode of interviewing is a more private method of data collection because it allows the respondent to hear the questions and response choices over headphones or read them on the computer screen and enter a response into the computer without the interviewer knowing what the response is.

The 2002 NSFG survey updates previous such surveys taken in 1973, 1976, 1982, 1988, and 1995. In 1973 and 1976, the NSFG interviewed only ever-married women aged 15 to 44. In 1982 the survey expanded to include all women aged 15 to 44. Men aged 15 to 44 were included for the first time in the 2002 survey.

• **Cycle 6 (2002)** The National Center for Health Statistics conducted cycle 6 of the NSFG with the participation and funding support of nine other programs of the U.S. Department of Health and Human Services. Cycle 6 was based on an area probability sample. The sample represents the household population of the United States, 15 to 44 years of age. The survey sample is designed to produce national data, not estimates for individual states. The contractor for the survey, the Survey Research Center of the University of Michigan, hired and trained over 200 female interviewers for the NSFG. In-person interviews were completed with 12,571 respondents 15 to 44 years of age—7,643 females and 4,928 males. The interviews were voluntary and confidential. Signed parental consent and signed respondent assent was obtained for unmarried respondents aged 15 to 17. The response rate was 79 percent overall—80 percent for females and 78 percent for males. The interview for males averaged about 60 minutes in length, while that for females averaged about 80 minutes. The male and female questionnaires were similar but not identical. Consequently, some 2002 data are available for females but not for males and vice versa.

• **Cycles 1–5** The National Center for Health Statistics conducted cycles 1 through 5 of the NSFG in 1973, 1976, 1982, 1988, and 1995. These surveys were based on personal interviews conducted in the homes of a national sample of women 15 to 44 years of age in the civilian, noninstitutionalized population of the United States. The main purpose of the

1973 to 1995 surveys was to provide reliable national data on marriage, divorce, contraception, infertility, and the health of women and infants in the United States.

More than 360 studies in academic journals and National Center for Health Statistics reports have been published using NSFG data. NSFG statistics have also been cited in thousands of newspaper, magazine, and newsletter articles over the years.

Contact information:
National Survey of Family Growth Staff
Division of Vital Statistics
National Center for Health Statistics
Centers for Disease Control and Prevention
3311 Toledo Road, Floor 7
Hyattsville, Maryland 20782
telephone: (301) 458-4222
e-mail: NSFG@cdc.gov
web site: www.cdc.gov/nchs/nsfg.htm

Bibliography

Bureau of Labor Statistics

Internet site http://www.bls.gov

— Employment Characteristics of Families; Internet site http://www.bls.gov/news.release/famee.toc.htm

Bureau of the Census

Internet site http://www.census.gov/

— *Adopted Children and Stepchildren: 2000*, Census 2000 Special Reports, CENSR-GRV, 2003; Internet site http://www.census.gov/population/www/cen2000/phc-t21.html

— America's Families and Living Arrangements: 2005, detailed tables; Internet site http://www.census.gov/population/www/socdemo/hh-fam/cps2005.html

— Families and Living Arrangements, Historical Time Series; Internet site http://www.census.gov/population/www/socdemo/hh-fam.html

— Fertility of American Women, Historical Time Series Tables; Internet site http://www.census.gov/population/www/socdemo/fertility.html#hist

—*Fertility of American Women: June 2004*, detailed tables, Current Population Reports, P20-555; Internet site http://www.census.gov/population/www/socdemo/fertility.html

— *Number, Timing, and Duration of Marriages and Divorces: 2001*, Current Population Reports, P70–97, 2005; Internet site http://www.census.gov/population/www/socdemo/marr-div.html

— *Statistical Abstract of the United States: 2006;* Internet site http://www.census.gov/prod/www/statistical-abstract.html

Centers for Disease Control and Prevention

Internet site http://www.cdc.gov

— "Abortion Surveillance—United States, 2002," *Mortality and Morbidity Weekly Report*, Vol. 54/SS07, November 25, 2005; Internet site http://www.cdc.gov/mmwr/preview/mmwrhtml/ss5407a1.htm

— *HIV/AIDS Surveillance Report, 2004*, Vol. 16, 2005; Internet site http://www.cdc.gov/hiv/topics/surveillance/resources/reports/2004report/default.htm

— Sexually Transmitted Disease Surveillance, 2004; Internet site http://www.cdc.gov/std/stats/toc2004.htm

National Center for Health Statistics

Internet site http://www.cdc.gov/nchs

— *Births: Final Data for 2003*, National Vital Statistics Report, Vol. 54, No. 2, 2005; Internet site http://www.cdc.gov/nchs/births.htm

— Births: Final Data for 2004, Health E-Stats, 2006; Internet site http://www.cdc.gov/nchs/products/pubs/pubd/hestats/finalbirths04/finalbirths04.htm

—*Births: Preliminary Data for 2004*, National Vital Statistics Reports, Vol. 54, No. 8, 2005; Internet site http://www.cdc.gov/nchs/births.htm

— *Births to Teenagers in the United States, 1940—2000*, National Vital Statistics Report, Vol. 49, No. 10, 2001; Internet site http://www.cdc.gov/nchs/products/pubs/pubd/nvsr/49/49-13.htm

—*Deaths: Final Data for 2003*, National Vital Statistics Reports, Vol. 54, No. 13, 2006; Internet site http://www.cdc.gov/nchs/deaths.htm

—*Estimated Pregnancy Rates for the United States, 1990—2000: An Update*, National Vital Statistics Report, Vol. 52, No. 23, 2004; Internet site http://www.cdc.gov/nchs/births/htm

— *Fertility, Contraception, and Fatherhood: Data on Men and Women from Cycle 6 of the 2002 National Survey of Family Growth*, Vital and Health Statistics, Series 23, No. 26, 2006; Internet site http://www.cdc.gov/nchs/nsfg.htm

— *Fertility, Family Planning, and Reproductive Health of U.S. Women: Data from the 2002 National Survey of Family Growth*, Vital and Health Statistics, Series 23, No. 25, 2005; Internet site http://www.cdc.gov/nchs/nsfg.htm

—*Health United States 2005*; Internet site http://www.cdc.gov/nchs/hus.htm

— *HIV Testing in the United States, 2002*, Advance Data, No. 363, 2005; Internet site http://www.cdc.gov/nchs/products/pubs/pubd/ad/361-370/ad363.htm

—*Mean Age of Mother, 1970–2000*, National Vital Statistics Report, Vol. 51, No. 1, 2002; Internet site http://www.cdc.gov/nchs/births.htm

— *Sexual Behavior and Selected Health Measures: Men and Women 15–44 Years of Age, United States, 2002*, Advance Data, No. 362, 2005; Internet site http://www.cdc.gov/nchs/nsfg.htm

—*Teenagers in the United States: Sexual Activity, Contraceptive Use, and Childbearing, 2002*, Vital and Health Statistics, Series 23, No. 24, 2004; Internet site http://www.cdc.gov/nchs/nsfg.htm

—*Use of Contraception and Use of Family Planning Services in the United States: 1982—2002*, Advance Data, No. 350, 2004; Internet site http://www.cdc.gov/nchs/nsfg.htm

Glossary

age Respondent's age at the time of the survey interview, unless otherwise noted.

age at first sexual intercourse Respondent's age at first vaginal intercourse.

age of first sexual partner Age of respondent's partner at first vaginal intercourse.

baby boom Americans born between 1946 and 1964.

births expected The total number of births expected is defined as the sum of children already borne or fathered and additional births expected, including a current pregnancy if applicable. Respondents who were sterile or who were married to sterile partners were classified as expecting zero additional births.

breastfeeding duration The number of weeks that a singleton baby was breastfed. Babies born after 2000 are not included so that all babies could potentially have been breastfed for the longest category of duration shown, which is 12 or more months.

childcare arrangements Childcare arrangements were ascertained for working women who had at least one child, defined as a household member under age 13 who was the respondent's biological child, stepchild, adopted child, legal ward, foster child, or partner's child.

cohabitation Living with an opposite-sex partner, in a sexual relationship, outside of marriage.

couple agreement with respect to intendedness of pregnancy Couple agreement is based on the woman's report of her own attitude, and her report of the attitude of the father of the pregnancy, at the time of conception.

current contraceptive status Contraceptive status during the month of the survey interview.

Current Population Survey The CPS is a nationally representative survey of the civilian noninstitutional population aged 15 or older.

Taken monthly by the Census Bureau for the Bureau of Labor Statistics, it collects information from more than 50,000 households on employment and unemployment. In March of each year, the survey includes the Annual Social and Economic Supplement (formerly called the Annual Demographic Survey), which is the source of most national data on the characteristics of Americans, such as living arrangements. In June of every other year, the Census Bureau includes a special supplement in the CPS, which examines the fertility of American women.

fecundity status Fecundity status is determined by responses to questions asked in the survey interview, not by a medical examination. Fecundity status has three main categories: surgically sterile, impaired fecundity, and fecund. Women were classified as surgically sterile if they or their current husband or cohabiting partner had had an unreversed sterilizing operation (for example, a tubal ligation, hysterectomy, or vasectomy). Surgically sterile is further divided into contraceptive and noncontraceptive subcategories, based on the reasons for the sterilizing operation. Impaired fecundity includes women who reported that (a) it was physically impossible for them or their husbands or partners to have a baby for any reason other than a sterilizing operation (nonsurgically sterile); (b) it was physically difficult or dangerous to carry a baby to term (subfecund); or (c) they had been continuously married or cohabiting, had not used contraception, and had not had a pregnancy for three years or longer (long interval without conception). Fecund is a residual category and means that the woman or couple was not surgically sterile and did not have impaired fecundity. The percentage of currently married couples with impaired fecundity is higher than the infertile percentage because impaired fecundity includes problems of carrying babies to term in addition to problems of conceiving, whereas infertility includes only problems conceiving.

generation X Americans born between 1965 and 1976, also known as the baby-bust generation.

Hispanic origin and race In the National Survey of Family Growth, respondents were classified as Hispanic, non-Hispanic white, non-Hispanic black, or non-Hispanic other race, based on questions about Hispanic origin and race. The race choices were American Indian or Alaska Native; Asian; Native Hawaiian or Pacific Islander; black or African American; and white. Respondents could choose up to four groups. People who identified themselves as being of more than one race were asked to select one group that "best describes" them. Because of small sample sizes, Asians, Pacific Islanders, and American Indians and Alaska Natives are not shown separately. These groups are included in the totals of all tables, however.

HIV and AIDS surveillance During the 1980s, AIDS cases alone provided an adequate picture of HIV trends because the time between infection with HIV and progression to AIDS was predictable. This predictability, however, has diminished since 1996, when highly active anti-retroviral therapy (HAART) became available. Access, adherence, and response to HAART affect whether or when HIV progresses to AIDS. Thus, trends in AIDS cases alone no longer accurately reflect trends in HIV infection. AIDS trends do, however, continue to provide important information about where care and treatment resources are most needed. Before 1991, surveillance of HIV infection (not AIDS) was not standardized. Therefore, information on HIV infection (not AIDS) prior to 1991 is incomplete. Since then, the Centers for Disease Control and Prevention has assisted states in conducting active surveillance of HIV infections (not AIDS) with standardized report forms and software. Data on HIV infection (not AIDS) should be interpreted with caution. HIV surveillance reports may not be representative of all persons infected with HIV because not all infected persons have been tested. Over time, HIV infection may progress to AIDS and be reported to surveillance. Persons with HIV infection (not AIDS) who are later reported as having AIDS are deleted from the HIV infection (not AIDS) tables and added to the AIDS tables. All 50 states, the District of Columbia, and U.S. dependencies, possessions, and associated nations report AIDS cases to the Center for Disease Control and Prevention using a uniform surveillance case definition and case report form. The original definitions have been modified over the years to incorporate a broader range of AIDS-indicator diseases and conditions. Although completeness of reporting of AIDS cases to state and local health departments differs by geographic region and patient population, studies conducted by state and local health departments indicate that the reporting of AIDS cases in most areas of the United States is more than 85 percent complete. For persons reported as having AIDS, the reporting of deaths is estimated to be more than 90 percent complete.

infertility status Infertility is a measure used by physicians and others to identify couples who may need to be evaluated to see whether medical services could help them have a baby. In the National Survey of Family Growth, infertility is computed only for married and cohabiting couples. When neither the respondent nor her husband or cohabiting partner is surgically sterile, a couple is considered infertile if, during the previous 12 months or longer, they were continuously married or cohabiting, had not used contraception, and had not become pregnant.

intendedness (wantedness) status at conception The National Survey of Family Growth examined the wantedness status of pregnancies that ended in a live birth within five years prior to the interview date. These pregnancies were categorized as intended (wanted), mistimed, or unwanted based on the woman's responses to questions about wanting to have a baby, how soon she wanted to have a baby, and birth control use.

marital dissolution Dissolution of formal marriage includes death of the spouse and separation because of marital discord, divorce, or annulment.

menarche Menarche is defined as age at first menstrual period (in completed years).

metropolitan residence The respondent's address at the time of interview was classified into one of five categories according to year 2000 Census Bureau population counts and definitions of metropolitan statistical areas set forth by the Office of Management and Budget. The categories were (1) central city of one of the 12 largest metropolitan areas (listed below); (2) central city of any other metropolitan area; (3) in one of the 12 largest metropolitan areas, but not the central city; (4) in any other metropolitan area, but not the central city; (5) not in a metropolitan area. Categories 3 and 4 are sometimes referred to as suburbs of metropolitan areas. The 12 largest metropolitan areas in population size as of the 2000 census were

1. New York–Northern New Jersey–Long Island, NY–NJ–CT–PA
2. Los Angeles–Riverside–Orange County, CA
3. Chicago–Gary, IN–Kenosha, WI
4. Washington, DC–Baltimore, MD
5. San Francisco–Oakland–San Jose, CA
6. Philadelphia, PA–Wilmington, DE–Atlantic City, NJ
7. Boston–Worcester–Lawrence, MA
8. Detroit–Ann Arbor–Flint, MI
9. Dallas–Ft. Worth, TX
10. Houston–Galveston–Brazoria, TX
11. Atlanta, GA
12. Miami–Ft. Lauderdale, FL

The smallest of these areas, Miami–Ft. Lauderdale, was home to 3.9 million people in 2000. The total population of these 12 areas in the year 2000 was about 97 million, or about one-third of the population of the United States.

millennial generation Americans born between 1977 and 1994.

National Survey of Family Growth The NSFG, a survey of Americans' sexual and reproductive behavior, is taken every few years by the National Center for Health Statistics. It is based on interviews administered in person by trained interviewers in the respondent's home. Cycle 6 (2002) data are based on a nationally representative sample of the household population consisting of 7,643 females and 4,928 males aged 15 to 44. Interviews were carried out between March 2002 and March 2003. The NSFG data are collected through computer-assisted interviewing, with questionnaires programmed into laptop computers. Interviewers administered most of the questions, but some of the more sensitive questions were asked using audio computer assisted self-

interviewing. This mode of interviewing is a more private method of data collection because it allows the respondent to hear the questions and response choices over headphones or read them on the computer screen and enter a response into the computer without the interviewer knowing what the response is. The 2002 NSFG survey updates previous NSFG surveys taken in 1973, 1976, 1982, 1988, and 1995. In 1973 and 1976, the NSFG interviewed only ever-married women aged 15 to 44. In 1982 the survey expanded to include all women aged 15 to 44. Men aged 15 to 44 were included for the first time in the 2002 survey.

nonsurgically sterile Respondents were classified as nonsurgically sterile if it was physically impossible for them or their cohabiting partner to have a baby for any reason other than surgical sterilization. Nonsurgical reasons for sterility include menopause; sterility from accident, illness, or congenital causes; or unexplained inability to conceive.

nonvoluntary first sexual intercourse Two questions were used to ascertain the voluntariness or wantedness of first sexual intercourse among respondents aged 18 to 44. The first question asked how much first intercourse was wanted. The second question asked, "Would you say then that this first vaginal intercourse was voluntary or not voluntary, that is, did you choose to have sex of your own free will or not?"

number of husbands/wives or cohabiting partners Number of husbands/wives is the number of times a respondent has been legally married. Multiple marriages to the same husband/wife are individually counted. Respondents were also asked about the number of cohabiting partners they had ever had. Husbands/wives with whom a respondent also cohabited (outside of marriage) are counted only once, as husbands/wives.

number of sexual partners in lifetime/past 12 months Each respondent was asked to report the number or range of partners with whom they had vaginal intercourse. If a range of partners was reported, the number of partners was calculated as the average of the low and high numbers. In cases where the respondent reported zero partners for the low and one partner for the high number, the number of partners was set equal to one.

parity, or number of live births The number of live born children a woman has ever had. Multiple births (for example, twins or triplets) are counted as separate live births, although they represent a single delivery.

pelvic inflammatory disease A clinical syndrome resulting from the ascending spread of microorganisms from the vagina and endocervix to the endometrium, fallopian tubes, and/or contiguous structures.

percent change The change (either positive or negative) in a measure that is expressed as a proportion of the starting measure.

percentage point change The change (either positive or negative) in a value that is already expressed as a percentage.

postpartum A woman was classified as postpartum if she reported that she was not currently using a contraceptive method, was not trying to become pregnant, and her last pregnancy had ended six or fewer weeks before the time of interview.

pregnant or seeking pregnancy A woman was classified as seeking pregnancy if she reported that she was not using a contraceptive method at the time of interview because she or her partner wanted to become pregnant as soon as possible.

regions The four major regions and nine census divisions of the United States are the state groupings as shown below

Northeast
—New England: Connecticut, Maine, Massachusetts, New Hampshire, Rhode Island, and Vermont
—Middle Atlantic: New Jersey, New York, and Pennsylvania

Midwest
—East North Central: Illinois, Indiana, Michigan, Ohio, and Wisconsin
—West North Central: Iowa, Kansas, Minnesota, Missouri, Nebraska, North Dakota, and South Dakota

South
—South Atlantic: Delaware, District of Columbia, Florida, Georgia, Maryland, North Carolina, South Carolina, Virginia, and West Virginia
—East South Central: Alabama, Kentucky, Mississippi, and Tennessee
—West South Central: Arkansas, Louisiana, Oklahoma, and Texas

West
—Mountain: Arizona, Colorado, Idaho, Montana, Nevada, New Mexico, Utah, and Wyoming
—Pacific: Alaska, California, Hawaii, Oregon, and Washington

religion, current Respondents could choose from 28 religions or denominations. Responses were collapsed into five categories due to limitations of sample size: none or no religion; fundamentalist Protestant; other Protestant; Catholic; and other religion.

religion, importance of People reporting a current religion were asked how important religion was in their daily lives on a three-point scale of very important, somewhat important, and not important. Those who reported no current religion were coded as not important on this variable.

religion raised Respondents could choose from 28 religions or denominations to report the religion, if any, in which they were raised. Responses were collapsed into five categories due to limitations of sample size: none or no religion; fundamentalist Protestant; other Protestant; Catholic; and other religion. If the respondent was raised in more than one religion, he or she was asked to select the one with which he or she identified most.

rounding Percentages are rounded to the nearest tenth of a percent; therefore, the percentages in a distribution do not always add exactly to 100.0 percent. The totals, however, are always shown as 100.0. Moreover, individual figures are rounded to the nearest thousand without being adjusted to group totals, which are independently rounded; percentages are based on the unrounded numbers.

sexual intercourse In this book, the term sexual intercourse includes only vaginal intercourse between a male and a female. When other types of sexual activity are being referred to, they are labeled and described accordingly.

sexually transmitted diseases, notifiable There are four notifiable sexually transmitted diseases, meaning their incidence must be reported to health departments: Chancroid, genital infections with Chlamydia trachomatis, Gonorrhea, and Syphilis. HIV can be, but is not necessarily, a sexually transmitted disease and is nationally notifiable.

sexually transmitted infection (STI) other than HIV Respondents were asked about their experience with several sexually transmitted infections other than HIV. First they were asked whether they were tested or treated within the last 12 months for infections such as gonorrhea or Chlamydia. Then they were asked if they have ever been told they had genital herpes, genital warts, or syphilis. A "yes" response to any of these questions was considered a report of "any STI other than HIV."

sterilizing operation Sterilizing operations are tubal sterilization, hysterectomy, ovary removal, other female sterilizing operation, and vasectomy. In theory, respondents could report all five types of operations, but the most common combination of multiple operations was tubal sterilization first, with hysterectomy later.

surgically sterile (female, noncontraceptive) Surgically sterile means a woman is physically unable to have a baby due to an operation. Noncontraceptive reasons include medical reasons such as trouble with female reproductive organs or a high likelihood of miscarrying or having an unhealthy baby. Most of the women in this category had had a hysterectomy.

Index

relationship with sexual partner by, 11–12,
71–72
time between first sexual intercourse and
marriage by, 25–27
rhythm method. *See* Birth control.

same-sex experience:
as cause of AIDS transmission, 106,
108–109, 111–112, 114, 118, 120
as HIV risk behavior, 126–128
by age, 45–46, 66–70, 94–95, 98
by education, 96
by marital status, 69–70, 95
by metropolitan residence, 93, 97–98
by number of opposite–sex partners, 97
by race and Hispanic origin, 45–46,
67–70, 96
by sex, 45–46, 66–70, 87, 93–98
by sexual attraction, 87–88, 92
by sexual orientation, 87, 92
sexually transmitted infection by, 100–101
separation. *See* Marital status.
sex education, 28–29
sexual attraction
by age, 89
by marital status, 88, 90
by metropolitan residence, 91
by race and Hispanic origin, 91
by sex, 88–92
by sexual orientation, 87, 92
sexually transmitted infection by, 100–101
sexual intercourse: *See also* Anal sex; Oral sex;
and Same-sex experience.
age difference between respondent and
first partner, 4, 7–9
attitude toward condom use by experience
with, 227–229
attitude toward premarital, 50–51
average age at first, 4–6
experience, 34–37, 44–46, 54–58, 66–70,
76, 78
frequency of, 47–49
involuntary, 13, 17–19, 73–75
number of partners, 38–42, 59–65
reason for not having, 28, 30–31
relationship with partner, 10–12, 71–72
time between first and marriage, 25–27
wantedness of first, 13–16
sexual orientation. *See also* Sexual attraction.
attitude toward gay and lesbian adoption
by, 102–103

by age, 83
by marital status, 82–83
by metropolitan residence, 85
by number of opposite–sex partners, 86
by race and Hispanic origin, 84
by same-sex experience, 82, 87
by sex, 82–87
by sexual attraction, 87, 92
sexually transmitted infection by, 99–101
sexual partners:
anal sex experience by, 97
birth control use by number of, 216,
225–226
by sexual orientation, 86
HIV risk behavior by number of, 125–128
HIV testing by number of, 129, 135
in lifetime, 38–40, 59–62, 97
in past year, 38, 41–42, 63–65
oral sex experience by, 97
relationship with, 10–12, 71–72
sexually transmitted infection by number
of, 100–101, 145
sexually transmitted infection:
and HIV testing, 135
by HIV risk behavior, 127–128
by number of partners, 145
by sexual experience, 99–101
Chancroid, 137–138
Chlamydia, 136–138, 141
fear of, as reason for not having sexual
intercourse, 28, 30–31
genital herpes, 136–137
genital warts, 136–137
Gonnorhea, 136–138, 142
notifiable cases, 136–138, 141–143
pelvic inflammatory disease, 137, 145
prevention, as reason for using condom,
222, 226
syphilis 136–138, 143
treatment for, 136, 144–146
vaginal trichomoniasis, 137
smoking, during pregnancy, 271–274, 298
spouses, number of, 171, 174–175
states, AIDS cases by, 121–124
sterilization: *See also* Birth Control and
Condom use.
by age, 184–185, 219, 230–231, 233–236
by education, 186, 233–236
by marital status, 184, 219, 231, 233–236
by number of children, 185, 233–236